Casebook of Clinical Geropsychology

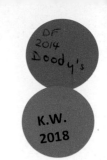

Casebook of Clinical Geropsychology
International Perspectives on Practice

Edited by

Nancy A. Pachana

Ken Laidlaw

Bob G. Knight

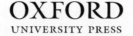

OXFORD
UNIVERSITY PRESS

OXFORD
UNIVERSITY PRESS

Great Clarendon Street, Oxford OX2 6DP

Oxford University Press is a department of the University of Oxford.
It furthers the University's objective of excellence in research, scholarship,
and education by publishing worldwide in

Oxford New York

Auckland Cape Town Dar es Salaam Hong Kong Karachi
Kuala Lumpur Madrid Melbourne Mexico City Nairobi
New Delhi Shanghai Taipei Toronto

With offices in

Argentina Austria Brazil Chile Czech Republic France Greece
Guatemala Hungary Italy Japan Poland Portugal Singapore
South Korea Switzerland Thailand Turkey Ukraine Vietnam

Oxford is a registered trade mark of Oxford University Press
in the UK and in certain other countries

Published in the United States
by Oxford University Press Inc., New York

British Library Cataloguing in Publication Data
Data available

Library of Congress Cataloging in Publication Data
Data available

Typeset in Minion by Glyph International, Bangalore, India
Printed in Great Britain
on acid-free paper by
Ashford Colour Press Ltd, Gosport, Hampshire

ISBN 978–0–19–958355–3

10 9 8 7 6 5 4 3 2 1

Whilst every effort has been made to ensure that the contents of this book are as complete, accurate and
up-to-date as possible at the date of writing, Oxford University Press is not able to give any guarantee
or assurance that such is the case. Readers are urged to take appropriately qualified medical advice
in all cases. The information in this book is intended to be useful to the general reader, but should not be
used as a means of self-diagnosis or for the prescription of medication.

Foreword

To my knowledge this is the first book of clinical cases in Geropsychology purposely designed to provide an international perspective on various aspects of clinical practice with older adults. Clinicians and clinical researchers from Australia, China, Netherlands, Norway, Spain, United Kingdom and United States have brought together case materials reflecting conceptual models and practices in their specialty area that are pertinent for addressing a wide range of age-related problems and issues encountered in clinical settings. The authors share many recent developments of clinical models in their specialty, along with illustrative cases to instruct the reader concerning the applicability of these clinical techniques within specific sociocultural settings. As such, this book offers the reader a broad spectrum of ideas and practices reflecting the "cutting edge" of clinical work in Geropsychology. The book is divided into three broad categories covering: a) various psychotherapeutic perspectives; b) issues of importance when completing assessments and formulating diagnoses; and c) approaches to specific groups within the older age range.

In the psychotherapy section, the editors have included six exceptional papers reflecting distinctly different psychotherapy modalities being employed with as many different types of patients residing in four countries with somewhat different sociocultural backgrounds. Beginning with the order in which they appear, Hinrichson deftly illustrates how an interpersonal therapy model for late-life depression can be an effective strategy when working with patients who have problems stemming from sexual orientation. Laidlaw and Wong sketch out a Cognitive Behavioral Therapy model (CBT) for the treatment of depression and anxiety, while highlighting adjustments to make this treatment modality maximally effective when working with older patients. This in itself is a laudatory effort, but they go on to awaken the reader to the challenge of formulating an expanded CBT model that would integrate relevant concepts and data from the literature on late-life development, such as "wisdom enhancement" and the "selection, optimization, and compensation" model. This is an exciting venture that is long overdue. Marquez-Gonzalez and her colleagues very aptly illustrate the application of Acceptance and Commitment approaches when working with informal caregivers of dementia patients who are experiencing distress. Garner and Evans outline the strengths of psychodynamic approaches and the influence of early developmental problems on older people's ability to deal with late-life stress. Halford, Chambers and Clutton present a brief treatment protocol that relies heavily on stress management and psychoeducational strategies to help couples cope with breast and prostate cancer. Gender differences in dealing with the accompanying stress are highlighted, with emphasis on how to minimize the impact of these on relationships, intimacy and sexuality in later life. Finally, Benbow and Goodwillie remind us of the importance of family systems as both a causal factor as well as a preventive or treatment component when working with older patients.

The last chapter in this section focuses on process issues in supervision. I applaud the editors for calling attention to this important topic in clinical work. What is arguably the most critical component of training in therapy, supervision is often conducted in a comparatively casual manner. However, the recent insistence on the use of evidence-based therapies is forcing the field to evaluate specific systems of supervisory training from this same perspective (cf. Rakovshik & McManus, 2010 for a review of this area). Yet old traditions fade slowly, and one can still find nearly as many different supervisory strategies as there are professionals doing supervision. This aspect of our clinical training must receive greater attention in the future. Though the accumulated data are not yet massive, it is now abundantly clear that students' therapy skills will not be developed properly, nor will the therapy skills of accomplished professionals, who are attempting to learn a new evidence-based therapy, be modified substantively without the experience of appropriate comprehensive and systematic supervision of their actual clinical work.

The second section will prove to be just as instructive for many readers. A predominant theme embodied in these six papers is the emphasis on how helpful accurate assessment can be in formulating an effective treatment and/or care plan. Nordhus and Hynninen discuss how CBT can be effective in treating patients with anxiety co-morbid with chronic medical disease or with cognitive impairment. A pivotal feature is their focus on how careful assessment of anxiety symptoms assists in the development of a treatment plan. James' focus on "challenging behaviors" evidenced by patients in residential care, which typically are reactions by the patient to some perceived toxic situation, truly highlights the importance of identifying potential antecedents, precipitating noxious unacceptable behaviors, which can then be incorporated into a treatment plan. Also with insomnia Simon convincingly illustrates the importance of comprehensive assessment of cognitive and behavioral processes prior and during the implementation of a treatment program. Roskowsky and Segal do a superb job in illustrating the significance of matching an appropriate treatment package with "A", "B" and "C" personality disorder clusters as outlined in DSM-IV-TR. Having specific information about a patient's enduring maladaptive traits clearly can lead to more effective treatment packages. Byrne's interesting paper on bereavement issues in later life shows us the importance of distinguishing between normal and "pathological" grieving, issues associated with grief in persons with dementia, and, importantly, offers comments on the draft DSM-V diagnostic criteria with respect to bereavement. Finally, Pachana, Squelch and Paton present an extremely useful and provocative paper on when and how to give neurocognitive feedback not only to referral sources but to patients as well. Their recommendations are sensible and clearly worthy of consideration in developing a feedback model that is consistent with local practice guidelines. Neuropsychologists will find useful material in this chapter to assist them in wrestling with the political, sociocultural and medical biases in communicating laboratory results, which may differ across cultures, governments and professions.

The third section of this work focuses on assessment and treatment issues in specific populations. Gallagher-Thompson and Thompson highlight problems encountered in working with outpatients above the age of 80 who were referred by physicians. Pot and Willemse use clinical examples to carefully outline possible roles for a Clinical Geropsychologist in a long-term care facility that emphasizes the multidisciplinary aspects of a person-centered care program. Using eight case examples in support of their arguments Chiu, Chan and Tsoh maintain that to reduce suicidal behaviors, timely and adequate assessment of risk factors and warning signs is a primary need, and service delivery for early intervention should be available at all levels of care. Finally, Hicken, Plowhead and Gibson have provided a thoughtful paper on the topic of capacity assessment, which is quickly becoming one of the most frequent problems in need of attention as the proportion of older-old persons increases. This informative work systematically covers the clinical and legal criteria for indexing capacity along with other relevant factors that arise in addressing this important legal/clinical issue. The authors also outline reasonable strategies to follow in order to minimize possible legal hassles and negative family reactions.

As a first in what may become a series, this book provides a wealth of information about models proving to be productive and case material showing how to apply the models in the clinic. Although the papers originate from different countries and reflect somewhat different sociocultural approaches in working with older persons, two important themes relevant to Geropsychology serve as a linkage among many of them. The first focuses on the uniqueness of each individual and his/her particular social system, irrespective of nationality, ethnicity or race. To achieve optimal effectiveness all clinical endeavors must identify these unique properties of each particular patient and modify assessments or treatments specifically to accommodate for them. The second is the recognition that because of broad age-related physiological, psychological and social changes, structural and procedural modifications are required in existing practices in order for them to be maximally effective. One set of authors (Nordhus & Hynninen, this volume) even re-labeled their treatment protocol as "Augmented" CBT.

On balance this is an excellent group of papers to introduce us to worldwide Clinical Geropsychology. As with most edited books some papers touch topics that are more timely. For example, if readers look at trends across time, it appears that what we've been doing over the last three decades or so is identifying existing treatment models that have been developed with a younger cohort in mind, and simply "tweaking" them to accommodate for age-related changes. In the process we have generally ignored some of the exciting models used to account for late-life developmental changes. These could conceivably assist us in developing more effective models and clinical practices as we move ahead in Geropsychology. Laidlaw and his group in Edinburgh have clearly laid down the challenge that this can and should be a major thrust of our conceptual and clinical efforts in the coming years. Another issue of major importance at the present time is the need to establish systematic guidelines for supervision when training professionals for clinical work. For too long supervision has been viewed as less important than other academic components in training programs. Although variations occur across major training programs, in general supervisors are paid less, seldom are given full academic credentials, and are led to believe that in the life of the student academic requirements have a much higher priority than supervision of clinical work. Only a few training programs around the US have encouraged careful systematic research in this area, and many supervisors assume they already know how to do supervision without formal training. Knight's chapter on supervision is a healthy reminder of its importance.

In a sense this publication stands as a testimony to the substantive advances throughout the world in Clinical Geropsychology over a relatively short time period. The first use of the term began to occur in the early to mid 70's. In 1974 Duke University sponsored a conference entitled, "Geropsychology: A model of Training and Clinical Service". The conference was subsequently published in 1977 by Ballenger Publishing Company, which may well have been the term's formal launch into professional use. At that time comparatively few mental health professionals were involved in any psychotherapeutic interventions with older adults, which as Garner and Evans point out in this book, was most likely due to Freud's insistence that psychoanalysis would not be beneficial for people over the age of 50. Although this specialty area has shown remarkable advances in this short time period, there is still much to be done. The questions for reflection at the conclusion of each chapter clearly provide broad brush strokes portraying what the future holds in store for Clinical Geropsychology around the world. With professionals like the contributors in this volume, there is little doubt that many new innovations and substantive advances will occur in the coming decade.

Larry W. Thompson, Ph.D.
Professor Emeritus, Department of Medicine
Professor Active Duty, Department of Psychiatry and Behavioral Sciences
Stanford University School of Medicine
Palo Alto, California, USA

Reference

Rakovshik, S.G., & McManus, F. (2010). Establishing evidence-based training in cognitive behavioral therapy: A review of empirical findings and theoretical guidance. *Clinical Psychology Review*, 30, 496–516.

Contents

Contributors

Susan M. Benbow
Visiting Professor of Mental Health
and Ageing
Centre for Ageing and Mental Health
Staffordshire University
Stafford, UK

Gerard J. Byrne
Head, Discipline of Psychiatry
School of Medicine
University of Queensland;
Director, Older Persons'
Mental Health Service
Royal Brisbane and Women's Hospital
Mental Health Centre
Herston, Australia

Suzanne Chambers
The Cancer Council of
Queensland and Griffith University
Queensland, Australia

Sandra Chan
Department of Psychiatry
Faculty of Medicine
The Chinese University of Hong Kong
Shatin, New Territories
Hong Kong

Helen Chiu
Department of Psychiatry
Faculty of Medicine
The Chinese University of Hong Kong
Shatin, New Territories
Hong Kong

Samantha Clutton
The Cancer Council of Queensland
Queensland, Australia

Sandra Evans
East London Foundation NHS Trust, City
and Hackney
The Wolfson Institute of Preventive Medicine
Queen Mary University of London
London, UK

Dolores Gallagher-Thompson
Professor of Research
Department of Psychiatry and
Behavioral Sciences
Stanford University School of Medicine
Stanford, USA

Jane Garner
Barnet, Enfield and Haringay
Mental Health NHS Trust
Chase Farm Hospital
The Ridgeway
Enfield, UK

William Gibson
Canandaigua VA Medical Center
Canandaigua, USA

Gillian Goodwillie
Consultant Family and Systemic
Psychotherapist
Head of Family Therapy
Wolverhampton CAMHS
Wolverhampton City, UK

W. Kim Halford
Professor of Clinical Psychology
Director of Clinical Psychology
Training Programs
School of Psychology
The University of Queensland
Brisbane, Australia

Bret L. Hicken
VA Rural Health Resource Center -
Western Region
VA Salt Lake City Health Care System
Salt Lake City, USA

Gregory A. Hinrichsen
Associate Clinical Professor of
Psychiatry and Behavioral Sciences
Albert Einstein College of Medicine
Bronx, USA

Minna J. Hynninen
Kavli Research Center for Aging and
Dementia
University of Bergen
Bergen, Norway

Ian A. James
Northumberland Tyne and Wear NHS Trust
Centre health of the Elderly
Newcastle General Hospital
Newcastle, UK

Bob G. Knight
Associate Dean,
Davis School of Gerontology,
The Merle H. Bensinger Professor
of Gernotology,
Professor of Psychology,
University of Southern California
Los Angeles, USA

Ken Laidlaw
Senior Lecturer in Clinical Psychology
University of Edinburgh
Clinical Psychology
School of Health in Social Science
Edinburgh, UK

Andrés Losada
Department of Psychology
Universidad Rey Juan Carlos
Madrid, Spain

María Márquez-González
Department of Biological and
Health Psychology
Universidad Autónoma de Madrid
Madrid, Spain

Inger H. Nordhus
Department of Clinical Psychology
Faculty of Psychology
University of Bergen
Norway;
Kavli Research Center for Aging
and Dementia
University of Bergen
Bergen, Norway

Nancy A. Pachana
School of Psychology
University of Queensland
Brisbane, Australia

Helen Paton
Older People's Health
Dunedin Hospital
Dunedin, New Zealand

Angela Plowhead
Portland VA Medical Center
Portland, USA

Anne Margriet Pot
Professor of Geropsychology
Department of Clinical Psychology
VU University Amsterdam;
Head Program on Aging
Netherlands Institute on Mental
Health and Addiction
Utrecht, The Netherlands

Rosa Romero-Moreno
Department of Psychology
Universidad Rey Juan Carlos
Madrid, Spain

Erlene Rosowsky
Massachusetts School of
Professional Psychology
Boston, USA

Daniel L. Segal
Department of Psychology
University of Colorado
Colorado Springs, USA

Simon S. Smith
Queensland Sleep Health group
Centre for Accident Research and
Road Safety
Queensland University of Technology
Kelvin Grove, Australia

Natasha S. Squelch
School of Psychology
University of Queensland
Brisbane, Australia

Larry W. Thompson
Professor of Research
Department of Psychiatry and
Behavioral Sciences
Stanford University School of Medicine
Stanford, USA

Joshua Tsoh
Department of Psychiatry
Faculty of Medicine
The Chinese University of Hong Kong
Shatin, New Territories
Hong Kong

Bernadette Willemse
Scientific Researcher
Program on Aging
Netherlands Institute on Mental
Health and Addiction
Utrecht;
Geropsychologist
Amaris Theodotion
Long-Term Care Facility
Laren, The Nertherlands

Introduction

Therapists listen carefully to their patients' stories; understanding is key to effective intervention. In time, experienced therapists can become adept at telling their patients' stories in order to guide the development and understanding of others.

The clinical case histories offered here cover significant problems and address contemporary issues in clinical work with older adults. The aim of this book is to provide the reader with insight into best practice in managing complex cases involving older adults from a geropsychology and/or geriatric psychiatry perspective. The book spans the international arena of practice, illustrating both universal themes in clinical work as well as regional practice issues that can inform health professionals more broadly. The cases encompass complex issues of diagnosis and formulation, assessment and intervention techniques, ethical and legal issues, and interdisciplinary perspectives that will appeal to a wide range of mental health professionals.

Each chapter is designed to inform the reader about the rich context in which clinical work occurs, including how the setting, the therapist's approach, and the nature of the problem interact to influence outcomes. Cases have been carefully chosen to reflect archetypal scenarios and provide practical, empirically informed guidance for assessment, formulation, and interventions. The cases are not clear-cut, and many will be open to multiple interpretations with respect to directions taken by the therapist. Although taken from the authors' actual clinical experience, all cases have been de-identified to preserve confidentiality.

The book does not endorse a single theoretical orientation, and indeed embraces emerging therapeutic techniques such as interpersonal psychotherapy, acceptance and commitment therapy and mindfulness, as well as incorporating more traditional approaches such as cognitive behavioral therapy and psychodynamic psychotherapies. Neuropsychological issues are touched on in several chapters, and psychiatric perspectives involving biologically based intervention strategies are included. Discussion points around the cases offer guidance for practitioners in managing emotional disorders in later life. References are selective and represent key readings in the area, with an emphasis on current issues and theoretical perspectives, rather than an exhaustive list of the extant literature in an area. As this is an edited volume, a range of expertise is provided in a single source, making this book an invaluable resource for anyone dealing with the mental health needs of older people.

Overall, this book provides a cogent picture of the unfolding of psychological issues in clinical practice with older adults, and affords a range of mental health professionals both empirical knowledge and tools as well as clinical insights into the successful treatment of a range of psychiatric disorders in later life. The text is designed to appeal to the clinicians wishing to update their practice with older adults, to educators looking for case material to enrich their didactic courses, and to students and fledgling practitioners looking for guidance in approaching casework. It fills a large niche in the clinical practice literature, and is written to provide both practitioners and educators with a useful guide from leading experts in the field.

Chapter 1

Sexual orientation issues in the context of interpersonal psychotherapy for late-life depression

Gregory A. Hinrichsen

Introduction

An important concept in gerontology is "age cohort" (Schaie, 1965, 1994). Persons born in different age cohorts have unique historical experiences that have enduring effects on world view, life expectation, intellectual abilities, and other characteristics. Another key gerontological concept is diversity among older adults (APA Working Group on the Older Adult, 1998; Fried & Mehrotra, 1998). In contrast to stereotypical notions of older adults as being much alike, researchers have found considerable variability among older people with respect to health, socioeconomic status, ethnic and racial heritage, political views, preference for social involvement, and an array of other factors. Although sharing common generational experiences with their own age cohort, subgroups of older adults also share unique life experiences. For example, the experience of being an African American raised during the 1930s was likely to be quite different than being a person of white Caucasian ancestry raised during the same time period. Cohort differences can also be a potential source of tension between older parents and their adult children who, despite sharing familial bonds, may hold differing norms and values that reflect the influence of their respective earlier-life cohort experiences.

Early on, sociologists recognized the power of social norms and values in guiding the behaviors of individuals throughout their lives (Rose, 1965; Rosow, 1974). They also speculated on the potential problems confronted by persons as they moved into later adulthood when their own norms and values could differ from younger generations—including their own children and grandchildren (Neugarten, Moore, & Lowe, 1965). Although a large body of research attests to the adaptability of most older adults in bridging gaps between self, larger society, and younger generations (Shanas, 1979), tensions do exist. The importance of understanding the cultural and historical experiences of people who receive health services is reflected in the emphasis on the development of multicultural competence among health professionals (APA, 2003; APA, Committee on Aging, 2009). One piece of multicultural competence that is sometimes forgotten is understanding that age—and the intersection of age and other factors such as race—are pieces of the diversity mosaic.

In mental health clinical practice with older adults, cohort differences in norms and values may come into play as part of the therapeutic picture. For example, some older adults have conflict with adult children because their views of family obligations differ, perspectives on childrearing are at odds, or commitment to religious values clash. A therapist's age and associated generational perspectives may not fit well with those of older clients and may erode the capacity of the therapist to engage the older adult, understand the complexity and nuances of difficulties which bring the older client into therapy, or offer therapeutic guidance to which the older client is receptive.

This chapter will discuss differences in generational expectations and experiences related to sexual orientation in the context of interpersonal psychotherapy (IPT) for late-life depression. Two cases will be reviewed in detail. In the first case, an older woman learns that her son is gay which leads to conflict between them and the onset of an episode of major depression. In the second case, retirement leads to depression in an older gay man who subsequently makes a suicide attempt. The cases are used as a vehicle for discussing sexual orientation issues in the context of geropsychological practice but also to illustrate the use of IPT in the treatment of late-life depression.

Sexual orientation and aging

Generational experiences of this cohort of now aged gay and lesbian individuals are quite different from those of young gay and lesbian persons. In earlier years, gays and lesbians faced job loss, imprisonment, forced psychiatric hospitalization, social ostracizing, and a host of other threats to social and emotional well-being (Kimmel, Rose, Orel, & Greene, 2006). Living the life of a gay person was dangerous and many lived lives cloaked in secrecy. Early political and academic focus on gays and lesbians barely discussed the presence of older sexual minorities. A common assumption was that being an older gay person was lonely and emotionally barren. Not unlike the larger society, older people experienced ageism within the lesbian and gay community. Gradually, there was acknowledgment of both bisexual and transgender individuals in the larger world of sexual minorities reflected in the inclusive and now commonly used terms LGBT (lesbian, gay, bisexual, and transgender). A literature has accumulated over the last 40 years which underscores the diversity and resilience of many older gay and lesbian people (Kimmel et al., 2006). However, studies suggest that the experience of older gays and lesbians in the health care system is not good. Many report negative reactions from health providers when identifying as sexual minorities and are therefore reluctant to disclose sexual orientation or even seek services. Further, there is a general lack of awareness of the complex social connections of older gay people in which long-standing partnerships are not recognized and the central role of friendships in providing vital social support is not understood (Brotman, Ryan, & Cormier, 2003). Congruent with contemporary models of psychotherapy with older adults (Knight & McCallum, 1998), psychotherapy with gay and lesbian older adults must be informed by a solid understanding of the larger cohort experiences of older adults and unique historical forces that shaped the lives of now aged gays and lesbians (David & Cernin, 2008). The interested reader is referred to *Lesbian, Gay, Bisexual, and Transgender Aging: Research and Clinical Perspectives* (Kimmel, Rose, & David, 2006), *Guidelines for Psychotherapy with Lesbian, Gay, and Bisexual Clients* (Division 44/Committee on Lesbian, Gay, and Bisexual Clients Joint Task Force, 2000), *Guidelines on Multicultural Competency in Geropsychology* (APA, Committee on Aging, 2009), *Guidelines for Psychological Practice with Older Adults* (APA, 2004), and the *Pikes Peak Model for Training in Professional Geropsychology* (Knight, Karel, Hinrichsen, Qualls, & Duffy, 2009).

A large literature attests to the critical role of "coming out" in the lives of gay and lesbian individuals. Coming out refers to disclosure of one's sexual identity to family, friends, work, and the larger community. The process can be complex both for gay and lesbian individuals as well as for family members who often grapple with new realities about the person (Ben-Ari, 1995; Strommen, 1989). To my knowledge, there is not a substantive literature on possibly unique issues faced by older adults (in contrast to young parents) whose children or grandchildren come out to them.

Interpersonal psychotherapy for depression

Interpersonal psychotherapy was originally developed as a time-limited, manualized treatment for depression. Theoretically, IPT was influenced by the interpersonal school of psychiatry best known by the work of Harry Stack Sullivan (1953) and attachment theory as articulated by John Bowlby (1969) and his associates. Empirically, IPT was undergirded by research that documented the adverse impact of stressful life events on mental health and the interpersonally damaging effects of depression on social role functioning. IPT was developed by Gerald Klerman, Myrna Weissman, and their associates (Klerman, Weissman, Rounsaville, & Chevron, 1984). The structure of IPT is outlined in a treatment manual first published in 1984 and subsequently updated and revised (Weissman, Markowitz, & Klerman, 2000).

IPT is delivered over 16 weeks in three phases of treatment: the initial sessions (weeks 1–3), intermediate sessions (weeks 4–13), and termination sessions (weeks 14–16). In the initial sessions, a diagnosis of depression is made, a depression severity rating scale often administered, and psychoeducation provided to the client about depression and its treatment. Depression is characterized as an illness that adversely impacts ability to function. A referral is made for antidepressant medication as needed. Recent life circumstances that appear tied to the onset of depression are explored with the client and the therapist administers the "interpersonal inventory" through which current and relevant past relationships are reviewed with the client. At the end of the initial sessions one or sometimes two problem areas are identified that will be the focus of treatment, and treatment goals and treatment structure are discussed.

The intermediate sessions focus on using therapeutic strategies to achieve goals that are established for each of IPT's four problem areas. The areas include: grief (complicated bereavement), interpersonal role disputes (conflict with a significant other), role transitions (major life change), and interpersonal deficits (problems with establishing and/or maintaining social relationships). The therapist also uses different techniques in conjunction with therapeutic strategies including, for example, exploration, encouragement of affect, communication analysis, and behavior change techniques. Throughout the intermediate sessions the therapist continues to evaluate the status of the client's depression, periodically administers a depression rating scale, and identifies the relationship between interpersonal stressors and change in depressive symptoms. Intermittently, the therapist also reminds the client of the number of sessions remaining in treatment.

In the termination stage, the therapist explores with the client feelings about the end of the therapy including feelings around loss of the therapeutic relationship. The therapist reviews treatment progress (and/or areas where progress may not have been made), provides encouragement and support for efforts made by the client during therapy, and makes an assessment of whether further treatment is needed after the planned end of therapy. For example, some clients may benefit by less frequent "maintenance" IPT sessions. In IPT, the therapist role is one characterized as patient advocate and is active (not passive). IPT primarily focuses on here-and-now issues. The therapeutic ethos is optimism, support, and encouragement.

IPT has been used in randomized, controlled clinical trials that have assessed its efficacy (alone or in combination with antidepressant medication) in the treatment of depression and other mental disorders. Among mixed aged groups of adults, IPT is effective in the treatment of acute major depression and in reducing the likelihood of recurrence of depression (among those initially treated successfully for depression). In clinical research trials, IPT has also been found useful in the treatment of depression in adolescents, different treatment formats (individual, group, couples, fewer treatment sessions), various clinical problems (medical problems, persons with HIV infection, marital difficulties), and in different cultures. Research studies have also demonstrated IPT's efficacy in the treatment of eating disorders. The reader is referred to

Comprehensive Guide to Interpersonal Psychotherapy (Weissman et al., 2000) for a review of IPT research studies as well as a review of IPT studies of depression (Mello, Mari, Bacaltchuk, Verdeli, & Neugebauer, 2005).

Interpersonal psychotherapy in the treatment of late-life depression

Three of IPT's four problem areas appear particularly well-suited to the life issues often seen among depressed older adults seeking treatment. The most common IPT problem area seen among older adults in IPT is role transitions including transition into the role of being a caregiver, assumption of the role as a person with health problems, residential move, and job change or loss. The second most common problem is interpersonal disputes including difficulties with spouse and adult children. When grief is an IPT problem focus it is typically related to loss of a spouse. Interpersonal deficit is a problem area that is rarely a focus of IPT treatment in older adults. IPT's collaborative, problem-focused, time-limited format is appealing to many adults and has been successfully used in clinical practice and taught to graduate students in psychology (Hinrichsen, 2008; Hinrichsen & Clougherty, 2006). The clinical treatment manual for IPT with older adults is *Interpersonal Psychotherapy for Depressed Older Adults* (Hinrichsen & Clougherty).

Although many IPT studies include "mixed age" adults (which include older adults), others have specifically examined the efficacy of IPT with older adults only. Two pilot studies provide evidence that IPT is useful in the acute reduction of depression in older adults (Rothblum, Sholomskas, Berry, & Prusoff, 1982; Sloane, Staples, & Schneider, 1985). Another study found that, compared with usual care, moderately to severely depressed older adults in primary care settings showed significant improvement after treatment with IPT (van Schaik et al., 2008). In a study of older adults who had been recently medically hospitalized, a brief form of IPT was associated with lower depressive symptoms 6 months after starting treatment compared with usual care (Mossey, Knott, Higgins, & Talerico, 1996).

The largest IPT studies with older adults are those conducted at the University of Pittsburgh. Two studies investigated the efficacy of "continuation/maintenance" treatment of major depression in older people. Study participants were initially treated with IPT and antidepressant medication. Those who improved were then treated further (continuation/maintenance) to investigate the utility of monthly IPT, medication, and the combination (compared with a control group) in reducing the likelihood of another episode of depression. In the first study, (monthly) IPT, medication, and the combination significantly reduced likelihood of relapse (Reynolds et al., 1999). In a similarly designed second study (in which the sample was 10 years older than participants in the first study), only medication reduced the likelihood of recurrence of depression and not monthly IPT (Reynolds et al., 2006). On the whole, evidence supports the efficacy of IPT in the treatment of late-life depression.

Clinical cases

Interpersonal role dispute

Case study 1: Sarah Goldstein: "It never dawned on me that my son was gay."

The initial sessions (weeks 1–3). Mrs. Goldstein was seen by the clinician for a diagnostic and assessment intake in an outpatient geriatric mental health clinic (name is fictitious and identifying information has been changed). This 69-year-old, white, widowed Jewish woman sought counseling at the clinic because of marked distress on recently learning that her son was gay. She described a long-standing warm and close relationship with her son characterized by frequent phone calls, visits, and shared activities. Mrs. Goldstein was shocked, dismayed, and disappointed that her son was gay. When she expressed discomfort to her son about his revelation he was hurt and angry. The frequency of phone calls decreased between them and when they saw each other both were uncomfortable. "It never dawned on me that my son was gay." Subsequently, Mrs. Goldstein began to feel depressed, less interested in taking part in her usual active regimen of social activities, ruminated about "what I did to make him gay," lost some weight, had problems sleeping, and associated symptoms of an episode of major depression. On the Hamilton Rating Scale for Depression (HRSD; Hamilton, 1960) she scored 26, indicating significant depression. She was in good physical health and had no history of prior episodes of depression or other mental disorders and was confused by why she "was no longer my upbeat self." She had an unmarried adult daughter who lived in her neighborhood. Her daughter had multiple sclerosis and Mrs. Goldstein provided ongoing practical, financial, and emotional support to her daughter with whom she had a conflicted relationship. The author told Mrs. Goldstein that he felt she would benefit from psychotherapy and that a referral to a therapist would be arranged. He also referred her to a clinic psychiatrist for medication evaluation.

Subsequently, Mrs. Goldstein was seen by a psychiatrist, prescribed an antidepressant, and advised that the clinician who conducted the intake would be the assigned therapist. Mrs. Goldstein expressed reservations to the psychiatrist about seeing the intake clinician for therapy and reluctantly shared that she wasn't sure she wanted him as her therapist because she perceived he was gay. The psychiatrist telephoned the clinician, advised of the situation, and said he had asked Mrs. Goldstein to meet with him at least once, convey concerns about his perceived sexual orientation, why this might be a problem for her, and make a decision about psychotherapy.

In the second meeting, the clinician thanked Mrs. Goldstein for being candid about her concerns about whether he was gay. She said she was embarrassed to have raised the issue but that she noticed that he wasn't wearing a wedding ring and that "you never know these days." "Yes, it's possible I'm gay. If I were, why would that be a problem for you?" She said that she felt that she needed to be candid about her son's situation and that she was afraid that if the therapist were gay and she expressed negative views of homosexuality that he would be offended. "Already you've been candid with me about your concerns and that's very important. Regardless of my sexual orientation, as a therapist I want you to be as honest as possible including any feelings of discomfort with homosexuality. That's why you're here, right?" The clinician told Mrs. Goldstein that if she was interested in seeing him for therapy, a time-limited psychotherapy for depression called "IPT" would be useful. He reminded Mrs. Goldstein that the symptoms she had discussed in the evaluation were part of a condition called major depression. "Major depression is an illness for which there are treatments including psychotherapy and medication. I'm very hopeful that at the end of psychotherapy—whether it is with me or someone else—you will be much improved." The therapist asked Mrs. Goldstein to think about whether she wanted to see the author as a therapist or for him to arrange for her to see another therapist. She said that she would think about it. A few days later, she left a message indicating that she would like to see him as a therapist.

In the third session, the therapist conducted IPT's "interpersonal inventory" through which additional information on significant current past relationships was gathered. Mrs. Goldstein's husband died of cancer when she was 57. She described a warm and loving relationship with her husband and experienced a deep loss at his passing. She had generally good relations with her siblings and a wide circle of friends and social engagements. She expressed concern and disappointment about her relationship with her 30-year-old daughter Rachel. Rachel was described as a promising lawyer who was diagnosed with multiple sclerosis in her twenties. She subsequently stopped working and currently lived on a disability income. Despite a previously good relationship, Mrs. Goldstein's ongoing efforts to be supportive to her daughter were met with frequent rebukes from Rachel. "She is not dealing with her health problems very well and she's very angry at everyone including me." Despite these ongoing difficulties, disputes with her daughter had not led to significant depressive symptoms for Mrs. Goldstein. "I can handle her. I can't handle this homosexual thing with my son Marc." "What would you like to change in your relationship with Marc?" asked the therapist. "I want him to get married like my friends' children are doing. That's what I want." "How likely do you think it is this will happen?" "Not very likely it seems," she remarked. The therapist finished up the session by providing his understanding of her problem and a proposed plan for therapy. "As I've said, you have what we call a major depression which is an illness that has been tied to your feeling depressed, thinking negatively, struggling to get through the day, and having sleep and appetite problems. The onset of depression appears tied to learning that your son is gay and the conflict with him that followed. Marc appears to want you to accept him which is not something you can do at this time. I'm proposing that we meet weekly for a total of 16 weeks in a psychotherapy called IPT. One goal of therapy is that your depression will be significantly improved. The other goal is that you will have a better handle on your relationship problems with Marc. Does this make sense to you?" asked the therapist. Mrs. Goldstein said that it did make sense but that she wasn't hopeful that things would improve. "I understand why you aren't hopeful—because hopelessness is often one of the symptoms of depression. I'm hopeful because this therapy alone or in combination with antidepressant medication has been found to be effective for most older adults who are treated with it. I want to emphasize that if there are issues or concerns you have about me or how the therapy is going, I'd appreciate knowing about them. Already you were candid about raising concerns about how my possible sexual orientation might affect therapy and I appreciate that."

The intermediate sessions (weeks 4–13). The therapist inquired about Mrs. Goldstein's depressive symptoms during the past week. She said she was feeling more upset and depressed since she and Marc had an unpleasant phone conversation. Marc asked her to come to his house to meet his boyfriend. She told Marc that she was not comfortable doing that and refused his dinner invitation. Marc said he was hurt and they abruptly ended their conversation. "Boyfriend? Is that what they call it? And now he wants me to go to dinner and meet this person like he's my son-in-law?" The therapist explored the differences in expectations between her and Marc. "Marc wants me to accept this situation and be positive and supportive. I'm still stunned on learning that my son is someone different than I thought he was." The therapist said he understood why Mrs. Goldstein would be uncomfortable meeting Marc's boyfriend when she had many issues to sort out with Marc first. The therapist also noted the connection between the recent phone call with Marc and increase in depressive symptoms. Different options were discussed for improving communication with Marc but it also appeared important for Mrs. Goldstein to have a clearer sense of why she was uncomfortable with Marc's homosexuality.

In the next couple of sessions the therapist encouraged the client to talk about her relationship with Marc. She described him as a smart, well-behaved, enthusiastic child. As a teenager he had many friends including girlfriends and did well in school. She was thrilled when he was accepted to an Ivy League school—something that was especially meaningful to Mrs. Goldstein since she was unable to attend college since her family could not afford the cost. Her own friends liked Marc and always inquired about him. "He's got everything Sarah—he's handsome, smart, and nice—you're a lucky mother." Indeed, she felt especially proud of her son. On graduation from college he obtained a prestigious and well-paying job. He called frequently, sometimes went on social outings with his mother, and introduced her to his friends. "I didn't hear much about girls but thought he was shy or just didn't want to tell me about who he was dating." When Mrs. Goldstein's daughter Rachel became ill, Marc was helpful to his mother and his sister despite angry outburst by his sister toward him. "With a sick daughter and a deceased husband, Marc was my rock."

In a subsequent session, the therapist asked Mrs. Goldstein to talk about her feelings about homosexuality. "I'm not a prejudiced person, Doctor. I have no religious problems with it. It's a topic that makes me uncomfortable. My generation was not raised talking about this. Girls weren't even supposed to talk about sex." She acknowledged that she didn't think she knew anyone who was gay and then began to wonder about people she had known in the past. "My friends Louise and May have lived together most of their lives—but I thought they were spinsters who shared an apartment together to save money." Beyond these observations Mrs. Goldstein was vague about her discomfort. He pressed her to talk more about concerns. "Well, I do wonder whether he could get AIDS." During the rest of the session she talked about her husband's long illness, the care she provided for him, and the hole that his loss left in her life. Tearfully she commented, "If Marc died of AIDS, it would be the end of my life too." "So it sounds like a big concern for you is that if Marc is gay, he might die from AIDS?" asked the therapist. "Yes. And how can a homosexual have a happy life?"

At the beginning of the next session, Mrs. Goldstein said that she and Marc had planned to go to a museum together the coming weekend and she said she was feeling less depressed. "Why do you think you might be less depressed?" "Because I'm going to see my son. But I'm also afraid that we'll have an argument." The therapist encouraged the client to make a plan for the outing with Marc. She said that she didn't want to talk about the "gay issue" but just wanted to have a good time with Marc. "What if Marc wants to talk about the issue?" asked the therapist. Mrs. Goldstein thought of different ways to respond to her son that would make it less likely they would have an argument. "What if I say to him: 'Marc, I know this has been a difficult time for both of us and I know you're disappointed that I can't be more accepting of the fact you're gay. I do want to talk more with you about this, but could you give me some time to sort this out?'" The therapist said he felt this was a thoughtful way to respond.

On the eighth session, the therapist administered the HRSD on which she had a score of 16. "You had a score of 26 when you first came to the clinic and now your score is considerably lower." She acknowledged that she was indeed feeling better and said that she and Marc had a good visit together the prior weekend. He told his mother that he understood that learning he was gay was a shock for her but that he loved her and now wanted to more fully include her in his life. They agreed they would talk more at a future time. It had been a difficult week for her daughter Rachel who was taken to the hospital but left against her doctor's recommendation because she didn't like the nursing staff. "How did that affect you?" "I was upset but this is not unexpected. She's home now. She won't take my calls but she'll call me in a few days, I know that." Did you notice a change of mood? "If you're asking me if I got more depressed because of Rachel the answer is no. I've told you, I can handle her."

In the next sessions, Mrs. Goldstein began to talk about her husband. She described a loving, warm relationship. "I was lucky enough to have a good marriage. That's something I wanted for Marc." "Do you think it's not possible for Marc to have a loving relationship with a man?" asked the therapist. I had never really thought much about that. "Do you wonder whether Marc has or has had a loving relationship?" "I wouldn't know. I've met some of his friends. They seemed like nice people—but I expected that since Marc was a nice person." "So it sounds like it's a possibility?" "Yes, I suppose." She returned to her fears about whether Marc might contract AIDS, her discomfort with news images of "men in dresses" at gay pride parades, and puzzlement over cultural changes during her lifetime.

In the next session, Mrs. Goldstein reported that her son had asked her to attend a meeting of a support group for families of gay people. "I told him I'd think about it but I know I'd be very uncomfortable going to such a meeting." Her son told her that a local chapter of Parents and Friends and Lesbians and Gays met in her area. Mrs. Goldstein said that she felt that going to such a meeting was premature. "After all, Marc and I haven't really talked much about this. Why should I go to a meeting of strangers and talk to them about it?" The therapist said that she made a good point and asked if she were ready to sit down and have a conversation with her son about the fact he was gay. "I'm nervous about this but I think it's time to talk." In this and the next session the therapist and Mrs. Goldstein discussed issues of concern that she would want to discuss with Marc. They reviewed ways in which the conversation might become heated and how to "cool" things down. There were three issues that were important for her to discuss with Marc. Did he have AIDS? Did he have a relationship? Why hadn't he told her earlier about the fact that he was gay. "I know it doesn't make sense why I want to know why he didn't tell me before. After all, I really wish I hadn't learned this. But I thought Marc and I had always been honest with each other. I felt a bit betrayed." The therapist said that it made sense to him why she would want to know why her son hadn't discussed his life more candidly.

In the next session, Mrs. Goldstein said she called her son and asked that they talk. "How did you say that to him?" asked the therapist. "I said Marc, I think I'm ready to talk with you about being gay. I'm still thinking about whether I want to go to that parents' support group." "That sounds like a good way to introduce the topic. How did Marc respond?" asked the therapist. "He said he really wanted to talk to me. And then it sounded like he was crying on the other end of the phone." "Why do you think he was crying?" "I'm not sure. This has been upsetting to both of us. Perhaps he was crying with relief that we could now talk." Mrs. Goldstein expressed apprehension that the conversation would lead to conflict and hurt feelings. In the remainder of the session, the therapist worked with Mrs. Goldstein to explore different ways to respond to her son so that the conversation would less likely lead to conflict as well as ways to manage her own strong feelings so that she was less likely to say something hurtful or provocative.

Mrs. Goldstein began the next session. "We had our talk." "How did it go?" "I think it went OK." She said that she and Marc met at his apartment. He made dinner for her and after dinner she said, "Ok, I guess it's time to talk." Mrs. Goldstein raised the issues of concern she had planned to discuss. "When he told me he didn't have AIDS I began to cry. I felt like a silly old woman thinking that everyone who was gay had AIDS but I needed to know." Marc shared with her that he had been in a 3-year relationship with Clark. "I remember meeting Clark at one of Marc's parties. He seemed like a very nice young man." Then Mrs. Goldstein laughed. "And Clark's a doctor. What Jewish mother wouldn't want her son to be married to a doctor? It's just that I never thought my son would be married to a doctor who was a man." Then Mrs. Goldstein said she raised the final issue of concern to her. That is, why didn't he tell her earlier he was gay. "Marc said he was afraid it would be too upsetting to me. He said that he himself had struggled with the issue and had seen a therapist about it when he was in college. He also wanted to be fairly certain that he and Clark would stay together before he introduced me."

Termination (weeks 14–16). Although periodically during the middle sessions the therapist reminded Mrs. Goldstein of the remaining number of sessions, he noted that they had only three remaining sessions and asked how she felt about this. She expressed surprise that the weeks had passed so quickly. "How do you feel about this?" "It's fine. You told me that this would only last 16 weeks." "But how do you *feel*?" pressed the therapist. "A little sad and nervous about ending." The therapist said this was a common response to ending therapy and that in the next couple of weeks they would talk more about it. Mrs. Goldstein said that she and Marc had had dinner together again. He asked if she would be comfortable having dinner with him and his partner Clark. She said she would but confided to the therapist that she was nervous about the meeting. "And what are you nervous about?" "Whether I'll like him and whether he'll like me." The therapist said that would be a perfectly expectable response on a parent's first meeting with a child's significant other. The remainder of the session focused on what would be the best circumstances for meeting Clark. She decided that she would invite both her son and Clark for dinner at her house.

In the next to final session the therapist again reminded Mrs. Goldstein of the planned end to therapy. He asked her to tell him more about how that felt for her. "Yes, of course, I'm sad about that. You have been very helpful. But I'm also guilty." "And what are you guilty about?" "About the way I behaved at the beginning."

"Wondering if you were gay and not wanting to see you. That was chutzpah." "I don't think it was chutzpah. It made perfect sense to me that you would wonder if it would make a difference in therapy if I were gay and you wanted to expressed negative feelings about learning that your son was gay. What struck me was that you were honest enough to raise the issue. I appreciated that."

In the final session, the therapist began by administering the HRSD on which Mrs. Goldstein scored 4. "This score indicates that you are not depressed. Further you don't have a major depression any longer." Mrs. Goldstein expressed relief on learning this and appreciation for the help provided by the therapist. "Well, I think you primarily have yourself to thank. After learning your son was gay you became depressed. You sought help—attended therapy, talked frankly about issues of concern, took action. You also took antidepressant medication. You were forthcoming and courageous." Mrs. Goldstein said that she had planned to have Marc and Clark over for dinner the following week and asked if she could call me and tell me how the dinner went. "Sure, I'd be happy to learn how that went." At the end of the session Mrs. Goldstein asked, "Would it be alright to hug you?" "Sure."

Mrs. Goldstein called 2 weeks later to say that her dinner with Clark and Marc had gone well. The reader may wish to reflect on these issues:

1. Consider the potential impact on the therapeutic relationship with the client for a therapist to reveal or not reveal his/her sexual orientation. What would be the therapeutic rationale for a therapist to reveal any personal information to the client?

2. Think about the advantages and disadvantages of assigning a therapist based on a client's preference for a therapist with a specific background. Would it depend on the type of request or the reason for a request? How might you respond to the following requests from prospective clients: "I want to see a female therapist because I was sexually traumatized by a man." "I don't want to see a foreign doctor because they aren't competent." "I want to see an African American therapist because he or she would better understand my problems than a white therapist." "Please don't assign me to a young therapist because they are inexperienced."

3. Reflect on whether the therapeutic relationship might have been deepened if the therapist had pursued in more detail Mrs. Goldstein's initial reluctance to see him as a therapist because of her concern that he might be gay.

4. Think about how you believe most clients perceive your sexual orientation. Are there aspects of your personal demeanor, dress, office environment, informal comments about your personal circumstances, or other factors that may lead clients to believe you are gay/lesbian or heterosexual?

5. Consider under what circumstances it makes good therapeutic sense to give clients information about self-help groups, brochures, or publications related to their concerns. Would it depend on the nature of their concerns (e.g. gay/lesbian issues, medical problem, substance abuse, alcoholism, or dementia)?

Interpersonal psychotherapy problem area: role transition

Case study 2: Bob Johnston: "I really don't want to talk about being gay, thank you."

Mr. Johnston was referred to the therapist from the inpatient psychiatric service. The written referral indicated that he was a 70-year-old, single, Catholic, white man who was hospitalized following a suicide attempt by taking an overdose of valium. He was diagnosed with major depressive disorder, severe, recurrent. Medical diagnoses included hypertension, elevated cholesterol, and arthritis for which he was taking three medications. He was referred for psychotherapy to help him address life issues that appeared to precipitate his suicide attempt. The prominent life issue that appeared tied to his depression and suicide attempt was retirement from his job as a high school teacher. He had a prior episode of depression about 20 years earlier following the death of a friend. Mr. Johnson had several brothers who visited him while in the inpatient service and who said they would be contacts for the therapist after his discharge from the inpatient unit. The therapist called the referring psychiatrist who said that during Mr. Johnson's inpatient hospitalization a brother said that Mr. Johnson was gay, a fact that Mr. Johnson had not disclosed to the inpatient staff. Prior to his discharge from the inpatient service, the therapist introduced himself to Mr. Johnston and established the date of the first appointment. During this visit, Mr. Johnston said that he was ashamed that he made the suicide attempt and "will not do it again."

The initial sessions (weeks 1–3). During the first session the therapist reviewed with Mr. Johnston what he had learned from the inpatient staff. Mr. Johnson confirmed that he became depressed following retirement as a teacher and had made a suicide attempt. He said that he did not currently have any suicidal thoughts and reiterated he would not make another attempt. The therapist asked questions to clarify the current likelihood of suicide and judged the risk was low. Mr. Johnston affirmed that he no longer had valium in his apartment and did not possess firearms. This was confirmed by his brothers to the inpatient staff who visited his apartment. Mr. Johnston had retired about 6 months earlier after many years as a high school teacher. After retirement, his days were poorly structured and he found himself with little to do other than watch television. He became increasingly depressed. Eventually, he had sleep and appetite problems, ruminated over the past with concurrent self-blame and reduction in self-esteem, had problems functioning (i.e. poor hygiene, unkempt apartment), evidenced marked anhedonia, and had thoughts of suicide. He refused invitations by his brothers to visit them and their families. He became convinced his life was not worth living, acquired valium from several area physicians by telling them he had muscle spasms, and then made a suicide attempt. He was found by one of his brothers in a semi-conscious state, medically hospitalized, and then psychiatrically hospitalized for 2 weeks during which he was treated with antidepressant medication and supportive group psychotherapy. On the HRSD Mr. Johnson scored 20 (significant depression) which was 8 points lower than on hospital admission. Mr. Johnston was especially polite during the session but appeared guarded and gave circumscribed answers to the therapist's questions. "So how do you feel about seeing a therapist?" "It's fine. I know that I am supposed to do this. No problem." "Why do you think you are *supposed* to do this?" "You know, the suicide attempt. I won't do that again." "The way you describe it, it sort of sounds like probation. But what had *you* hoped to get out of this?" Mr. Johnston said he wasn't sure. The therapist asked him to think about it for the next meeting.

In the next session, the therapist first inquired about depressive symptoms (unchanged from last session) and suicidal ideation (denied) and then conducted IPT's "interpersonal inventory" which reviews current and relevant past relationships. The therapist found Mr. Johnston's answers vague and it was difficult to get a good sense of his past and current social world. He evaded discussion of past or current romantic or close relationships. "Mr. Johnston, when I spoke with the inpatient psychiatrist she said one of your brothers said that you were gay. Is that accurate?" "I really don't want to talk about being gay, thank you." "I'm asking because I wanted to get a sense of you as a person. If being gay is part of your life, that's helpful for me to know." Mr. Johnston appeared annoyed. "I'm not here to talk about being gay, I told you that." "I agree," commented the therapist. "You're here not because you're gay but because your life changed, you became depressed, and you made a suicide attempt." With some reluctance Mrs. Johnston said that following the death of a friend in the 1980s he became depressed and went to see a therapist. Despite the fact that he saw the therapist to deal with his loss, Mr. Johnston said the therapist was most interested in helping him to change his sexual orientation. "So naturally you wonder if I'll do the same, right?" He nodded. "That's not the case. Remember when I asked you last session what *you* wanted to get out of therapy? I meant that. Would you think about that between now and the next time we meet?" He said he would.

At the beginning of the session the therapist inquired about depressive symptoms and suicidal thoughts. There had been little change in his depression and he avowed that he did not have suicidal thoughts. Mr. Johnston said that he had thought about the therapist's question about what he would like from therapy. He said that he knew that "life fell apart" after he left work. "I never really thought much about what I'd do after I retired." He felt that he could use some help figuring out how to spend his days. To the extent that he felt comfortable, the therapist asked him to tell him more about his past and current life. He had been a high school teacher throughout his life and loved his work. Although many of his colleagues retired in their late 50s and early 60s he remained teaching. He retired recently because financially it no longer made sense to work, found the commute to work increasingly taxing, and had more and more students with behavioral problems. He had good relationships with his brothers, their families, and several good friends with whom he socialized. In recent years however, his closest friends had moved or died and his network of social relationships had winnowed. "What you tell me makes good sense. For some people, a big change like retirement can be hard to manage and they become depressed. If you're interested in continuing to see me in therapy, I'm suggesting that we meet for a total of 16 weeks. One goal of the therapy is that at the end you will be significantly less depressed. The other goal is that you will find things to do in your new role as a retired person so that your life is more meaningful and that you have something to look forward to at the beginning of each day. I'm mindful of your wariness of mental health professionals. I'm not here to change your sexual orientation. Today, most mental health professionals don't see that as desirable or even possible since being gay or lesbian is not regarded as a problem. Nonetheless, I do believe that the more I know about your life, the better we can work together to achieve the goals. Does that make sense?" Mr. Johnston said that it did. "And please let me know if you have concerns about how the therapy is going or concerns about me."

The intermediate sessions (weeks 4–13). Mr. Johnston said he had been feeling more depressed in the past week. He had problems getting out of bed and had little structure to his days. He had fleeting suicidal thoughts but denied any intent. The therapist inquired about what he had previously done with his free time when he was working. He used to play cards with a group of friends on the weekends, visited with his two good friends Vick and Sid, saw his brothers and their families, and sometimes went to teacher union activities. Around the time he retired, however, Vick and Sid moved to Florida and the card game fell apart when several members began to have health problems. "So not only did your life change when you retired but it also changed because you lost two pillars of your social life—Vick and Sid and the card game. What about your brothers and their families?" He explained that now that his brothers' children were adults there were fewer family gatherings and the children now "had their own lives." "So it seems like the challenge now is to figure out how you can fill your life with other activities and people, yes?" The remainder of this session and next were devoted to thinking about different options for expanding his involvements.

Mr. Johnston began the next session by saying his friends Vick and Sid were coming to visit him from Florida. His affect was brighter than in prior sessions. "How has your mood been since learning they will visit?" He said he was feeling less depressed and looked forward to their visit. He reminisced about their long relationship and noted that Vick and Sid had been together as a couple for 40 years. "It must have been pretty tough for you to see them move away, yes?" He said he was very upset they left and considered moving to Florida too but didn't want to be that far from his brothers and their families. "But they are like family too." He said that he envied their long relationship and wished that he had been together with someone like they had. "Let me know if you're comfortable talking about this, but have you had a relationship with someone that lasted for a while?" He looked sad. "Yes, I did." He explained that he had had a 10-year relationship with Richard. There were problems and they eventually broke up. A few years after they broke up Richard was diagnosed with AIDS. Mr. Johnston provided care for him while he was dying. "Was that when you became depressed and saw a therapist?" He nodded. "So you went to see a therapist to talk about the loss of this very important person to you and the therapist wanted to help you change your sexual orientation. That must have been terrible for you," remarked the therapist. "He told me that my 'homosexual world was falling apart' because of AIDS and that there was still time to have a relationship with a woman. I don't really want to get into talking about this a lot. It's over. I've moved on." The therapist thanked Mr. Johnston for his candor and said that if he wanted to talk further about this part of his life, he should feel free to bring it up. The session closed on review of different options for re-establishing a social world for himself.

In the next session, the therapist encouraged him to talk about his life before retirement. Mr. Johnston said he had a great life as a teacher. He enjoyed teaching, felt he was good at it, and had a good rapport with the students. "I'm not bragging, but I got the 'best teacher' award more times than any other teacher in the school." He was active in after school activities and was the school debate coach for many years. He expressed sadness that this phase of his life had to come to an end. "Why did it end?" asked the therapist. "It was a long commute, many of my fellow teachers had retired, and there were more and more problems with the kids. I thought I was losing my edge with the kids and it wasn't so much fun anymore." He thought he'd spend more time with his friends but unexpectedly Vick and Sid decided to move and the card group fell apart. "I liked my old life. I wish I could get it back." "Well, I think you can have a new life but it will require some work," observed the therapist. "But I see why you feel sad. It's hard to say goodbye to a phase of your life that included meaningful work and good friends."

The visit with Vick and Sid went especially well and Mr. Johnston continued to show improvement in his mood. The therapist administered the HRSD on which he had a score of 12 which indicated "mild depression." "Of course I'm less depressed because my friends just visited me." "Excellent point Mr. Johnston! The more you're with friends and doing things you like, the less depressed you are." Mr. Johnston's brothers had a family barbeque to which Sid and Vick were invited. His brothers' children knew them well and called them "Uncle Sid and Uncle Vick." Sid and Vick expressed concern about his recent problems and also encouraged him to find new things to do. "They sounded like you," he remarked. He spoke with Sid and Vick about different options for enlargement of his social world: find a new card group, make efforts to contact former members of the card group, volunteer, and increase visits with his brothers and their families. Vick said that the local lesbian and gay community center had a card group. Mr. Johnston resisted the idea since he thought he'd be uncomfortable going to a gay organization. He explained that in prior years he had gone to a gay event and found the younger gay people unwelcoming. "In what way were they unwelcoming?" asked the therapist. "They couldn't believe how 'closeted' I was. I told them they didn't understand what it was like before Stonewall. Teachers could be fired for being gay. You could go to jail for being gay. You just didn't talk about it." Nonetheless, he agreed to check out the card group at the gay and lesbian center although he doubted he would go.

In the next session, he expressed sadness over Vick and Sid's return to Florida. Before they left they pressured him to make a call about the card group. To his surprise he learned the card group was for older gay men—and that, in fact, the gay and lesbian community center had activities just for older people. Vick and Sid had called former members of Mr. Johnston's card group and asked them to give him a call. Two of them did and invited him over for dinner. "They shouldn't have called our friends but I'm glad they did." He admitted that, in fact, these friends had telephoned him several times while he was depressed and that he did not return their calls. "That often happens when people are depressed—being with people feels like a burden so you avoid it. And people will stop calling," noted the therapist. Mr. Johnston said he appreciated "the kick in the butt" from Vick and Sid. The therapist asked Mr. Johnston to think more about what volunteer options might appeal to him. He said that his teacher's union had a volunteer program to tutor kids who had academic problems. He wasn't sure that he wanted to do that but he said he'd check it out.

Mr. Johnston began the next session by saying that Vick and Sid called him several times from Florida to see if he attended the card group. "I went just to get them off my back." Things went better than expected. He liked several of people he met at the card group and especially enjoyed the playful good humor of the group. He planned to return. "I'm so glad that things went well. Now let's talk about that volunteer job." He hadn't called the union but said he would. He'd been in more regular contact with his brothers and their families—and his niece called him and said how great it was to see him and Uncles Vick and Sid. "How's your mood been in the last week?" asked the therapist. "Better. And by the way, just so you don't have to ask. I haven't had any suicidal thoughts."

During the next several sessions the therapist worked with Mr. Johnston around ways to check out volunteer job options. He met with a union representative to talk about the tutoring program but didn't find it appealing since the program involved children with behavioral problems. Mr. Johnston thought it would be too stressful. He decided to volunteer answering phones and doing clerical work twice a week at the union hall. He continued to go to the card game through which he developed some new acquaintances who he thought he would see outside of the card group.

Termination (weeks 14–16). The therapist reminded Mr. Johnston that therapy would be coming to its planned end. Mr. Johnston expressed disappointment that therapy would end. "It's seems like we have just gotten to know each other." The therapist asked Mr. Johnston to talk about his feelings about ending. He said that he felt bad that initially he acted angrily toward the therapist when he brought up the issue of his sexual orientation. "I didn't know a straight guy could understand what it's like for an old gay guy." He wondered how he would do without therapy visits. "I relied on you more than I thought I would." The therapist underscored the many efforts that Mr. Johnston had made during therapy.

In the next session Mr. Johnston asked, "Is this therapy thing negotiable?" "What do you mean?" asked the therapist. "Could we continue?" Mr. Johnston acknowledged that he was doing better but could continue to use the therapist's continued support. The therapist underscored that Mr. Johnston had accomplished the goals they had set at the beginning of therapy: a significant reduction in depressive symptoms and transition to re-establishing a new life structure. "You've really made a lot of progress and it's a testament to your many efforts—you attended therapy sessions, you worked on issues during the week, and you continued to take antidepressant medication." They discussed different options for continuing. By the end of the session they agreed that after the end of planned therapy they would meet every other week, and then monthly until both therapist and client mutually agreed on an end to treatment.

In the final session, the therapist administered the HRSD on which Mr. Johnston had 7 which indicated some mild symptoms of depression. His major depressive episode appeared to be in remission. The therapist reviewed the course of therapy with him, congratulated him on his many efforts, noted that his work had resulted in significant improvement, and encouraged him to think about ways in which he could continue building on the therapeutic successes of the last 4 months.

The reader might wish to think about these issues:

1. In the context of this case, would the therapeutic relationship have been enhanced or complicated if the therapist revealed his sexual orientation if he were gay?

2. Consider ways in which a mental health setting may create an environment that is more or less welcoming to gay and lesbian older persons? How would you respond to mental health colleagues in the same setting who were reluctant to make a more "gay friendly" setting? What might be their objections?

3. Think about ways in which generational or "cohort" issues come into play in this case and with older clients you currently see in therapy. Which subsets of cohort issues are most relevant to conducting therapy with specific older clients you see?

4. Consider ways that mental health practice has changed during the lifetimes of older clients and how past practices/views of mental health may make them more or less amenable to receiving mental health care.

5. Think about how the dynamics of this case would have been different if the therapist were a young white, heterosexual woman and Mr. Johnston were a black, gay man?

6. Reflect on how what common countertransferential issues might be triggered for heterosexual therapists seeing an older gay or lesbian client. Depending on the therapist's gender, might these issues be different if the client were gay or were lesbian? For gay or lesbian therapists, how might countertransferential issues be similar or different from those of heterosexual therapists?

Conclusion

During many years of clinical work in a large, urban, outpatient geriatric clinic I found that very few clients identified themselves to me or other staff members as gay or lesbian and rarely did older clients talk about family members who were gay or lesbian. Therefore, the two cases presented here are not usual. Why would gay and lesbian issues rarely be evident in an urban setting? As in the case of Mr. Johnston, one suspects that some older gay and lesbian clients were reluctant to so identify for fear of how they would be received in the mental health system. Perhaps staff people didn't initially inquire about relationship status in a way that invited revelation of that information. (Instead of asking, "Are you or have you ever been married?" the clinician might ask, "Is there, or has there ever been, someone in your life with whom you've had a close, loving relationship?") Older clients might have been reluctant to talk about children or grandchildren who are gay and lesbian because of uncertainly about how the therapist would respond or because of embarrassment. This author once saw an older woman in therapy for an entire year before she revealed that early in her life she had romantic relationships with women. She called it "my lesbian phase." When I asked why she had never told me, she said that she needed to get to know me and trust that I would not judge her negatively about this part of her life. When asked how she came to that conclusion she replied, "When I talked about gay people in my earlier life, you seemed curious and accepting." For a generation during whose early lives mental health professionals classified homosexuality as pathological and some professionals avowed that sexual orientation could or should be changed, it makes perfect sense that being silent on the issue would be the prudent thing to do. It is therefore incumbent on the therapist not to assume that all clients are heterosexual and to convey this in a way that creates a feeling of trust and inclusion for those older clients who are gay or lesbian.

Seventy-five million members of the so-called baby boom generation will soon be turning 65 years of age. The generational experiences of this age group were different from those of their parents.

Social values and norms shifted in the 1960s and many gay and lesbian members of the baby boom generation came of age in the years that followed the historic Stonewall riots that marked the beginning of a slowly growing societal openness to gay and lesbian persons. Mental health professionals should therefore anticipate providing increasing services to older gay and lesbian baby boomers who will likely talk about their lives in ways that are more transparent than in the now exiting generation of older adults. In yet another cultural and generational shift, therapists should not necessarily assume that older gay and lesbian persons *aren't* married since some are now in states where it is permitted by law. Apropos to Division *Guidelines for Psychotherapy with Lesbian, Gay, and Bisexual Clients* (Division 44, 2000), therapists can conduct psychotherapy with aged gay and lesbian persons in ways that are sensitive, build rapport, and maximize therapeutic effectiveness.

I found that IPT was a useful modality for treating the issues that were presented in the two cases discussed in this chapter. Clinically, my colleagues and I believe that IPT is a well-thought-out, flexible, evidence-based treatment for working with depressed older clients who have a variety of life issues that nicely dovetail with IPT's problem areas (Hinrichsen, 2008; Hinrichsen & Clougherty, 2006). The collaborative, supportive ethos of IPT seems especially appropriate for working with clients of diverse backgrounds as evident in an IPT research study that included a sizable number of younger gay men who were successfully treated for depression (Markowitz, et al., 1999). Doing psychotherapy at the intersection of aging and sexual orientation issues is especially interesting and, by utilizing an effective therapy like IPT, this work holds the potential for improving lives and alleviating emotional suffering.

References

American Psychological Association (2003). Guidelines on multicultural education, training, research, practice, and organizational change for psychologists. *American Psychologist, 58,* 377–402.

American Psychological Association (2004). Guidelines for psychological practice with older adults. *American Psychologist, 59,* 236–260.

American Psychological Association, Committee on Aging (2009). *Guidelines on multicultural competency in geropsychology: A report of the APA Committee on Aging and its working group on muticultural competency in geropsychology.* Washington, DC: American Psychological Association.

APA Working Group on the Older Adult (1998). What practitioners should know about working with older adults. *Professional Psychology: Research and Practice, 29,* 413–427.

Ben-Ari, A. (1995). The discovery that an offspring is gay: Parents', gay men's, and lesbian's perspectives. *Journal of Homosexuality, 30,* 89–112.

Brotman, S., Ryan, B., & Cormier, R. (2003). The health and social service needs of gay and lesbian elders and their families in Canada. *The Gerontologist, 43,* 192–202.

Bowlby, J. (1969). *Attachment and loss, Volume 1: Attachment.* New York, NY: Basic Books.

David, S., & Cernin, P.A. (2008). Psychotherapy with lesbian, gay, bisexual, and transgender older adults. *Journal of Gay & Lesbian Social Services, 20,* 31–49.

Division 44/Committee on Lesbian, Gay, and Bisexual Clients Joint Task Force (2000). Guidelines for psychotherapy with lesbian, gay, and bisexual clients. *American Psychologist, 55,* 1440–1451.

Fried, S.B., & Mehrotra, C.M. (1998). *Aging and diversity: An active learning experience.* Washington, DC: Taylor & Francis.

Hamilton, M. (1960). A rating scale for depression. *Journal of Neurology and Neurosurgical Psychiatry, 23,* 56–62.

Hinrichsen, G.A. (2008). Interpersonal psychotherapy as a treatment for depression in late life. *Professional Psychology: Research and Practice, 39,* 306–312.

Hinrichsen, G.A., & Clougherty, K.F. (2006). *Interpersonal psychotherapy for depressed older adults.* Washington, DC: American Psychological Association.

Kimmel, D., Rose, T., & David, S. (2006). *Lesbian, gay, bisexual and transgender aging: Research and clinical perspectives*. New York, NY: Columbia University Press.

Kimmel, D., Rose, T., Orel, N., & Greene, B. (2006). Historical context for research on lesbian, gay, bisexual, and transgender aging. In D. Kimmel, R. Rose, & S. David (Eds.), *Lesbian, gay, bisexual, and transgender aging: Research and clinical perspectives* (pp. 2–19). New York, NY: Columbia University Press.

Klerman, G.L., Weissman, M.M., Rounsaville, B.J., & Chevron, E.S. (1984). *Interpersonal psychotherapy of depression*. Northvale, NJ: Jason Aronson.

Knight, B.G., Karel, M.J, Hinrichsen, G.A., Qualls, S.H., & Duffy, M. (2009). Pikes Peak model for training in professional geropsychology. *American Psychologist, 64*, 205–214.

Knight, B., & McCallum, T. (1998). Adapting psychotherapeutic practice for older clients: Implications of the contextual, cohort-based, maturity, specific challenge model. *Professional Psychology: Research and Practice, 29*, 15–22.

Markowitz, J.C., Kocsis, J.H., Fishman, B., Spielman, L.A., Jacobsberg, L.B., Frances, et al. (1999). Treatment of HIV-positive patients with depressive symptoms. *Archives of General Psychiatry, 55*, 452–457.

Mello, M.F., Mari, J.J., Bacaltchuk, J., Verdeli, H., & Neugebauer, R. (2005). A systematic review of research findings on the efficacy of interpersonal therapy for depressive disorders. *European Archives of Psychiatry and Clinical Neurosciences, 255*, 75–82.

Mossey, J.M., Knott, K.A., Higgins, M., & Talerico, K. (1996). Effectiveness of a psychosocial intervention, interpersonal counseling, for subdysthymic depression in medically ill elderly. *Journal of Gerontology: Medical Sciences, 51A*, M172–M178.

Neugarten, B.L., Moore, J.W., & Lowe, J.C. (1965). Age norms, age constraints, and adult socialization. *The American Journal of Sociology, 70*, 710–717.

Reynolds, C.F., III, Frank., E., Perel, J.M., Imber, S.D., Cornes, C., Miller, M.D., et al. (1999). Nortriptyline and interpersonal psychotherapy as maintenance therapies for recurrent major depression: A randomized controlled trial in patients older than 59 years. *Journal of the American Medical Association, 281*, 39–45.

Reynolds, C.F., III, Dew, M.A., Pollock, B.G., Mulsant, B.H., Frank, E., Miller, M.D., et al. (2006). Maintenance treatment of major depression in old age. *New England Journal of Medicine, 354*, 1130–1138.

Rose, A.M. (1965). The subculture of aging, a topic for sociological research. In A.M. Rose & W.A. Peterson (Eds.), *Older people and their social world*. Philadelphia, PA: David Company.

Rothblum, E.D., Sholomskas, A.J., Berry, C., & Prusoff, B.A. (1982). Issues in clinical trials with the depressed elderly. *Journal of the American Geriatrics Society, 30*, 694–699.

Rosow, I. (1974). *Socialization to old age*. Berkeley, CA: University of California Press.

Schaie, K.W. (1965). A general model for the study of developmental problems. *Psychological Bulletin, 64*, 91–107.

Schaie, K.W. (1994). The course of adult intellectual development. *American Psychologist, 49*, 304–313.

Shanas, E. (1979). Social myth as hypothesis: The case of the family relationship of old people. *The Gerontologist, 19*, 3–9.

Sloane, R.B., Staples, F.R., & Schneider, L.S. (1985). Interpersonal psychotherapy versus nortriptyline for depression in the elderly. In G. Burrows, T.R. Norman, & L. Dennerstein (Eds.), *Clinical and pharmacological studies in psychiatric disorders* (pp. 344–346). London: John Libbey.

Strommen, E.F. (1989). 'You're a what?': Family members reactions to the disclosure of homosexuality. *Journal of Homosexuality, 18*, 37–58.

Sullivan, H.S. (1953). *The interpersonal theory of psychiatry*. New York, NY: Norton.

van Schaik, A., van Marwijk, H., Ader, H., van Dyck, R., de Haan, M., Penninx, B., et al. (2008). Interpersonal psychotherapy for elderly patients in primary care. *American Journal of Geriatric Psychiatry, 14*, 777–786.

Weissman, M.M., Markowitz, J.C., & Klerman, G.L. (2000). *Comprehensive guide to interpersonal psychotherapy*. New York, NY: Basic Books.

Chapter 2

Enhancing cognitive behavior therapy with older people using gerontological theories as vehicles for change

Ken Laidlaw

Introduction

In this chapter, the basic elements of cognitive behavioral therapy (CBT) are sketched out for the reader and there is a very brief integrative review of the efficacy literature of CBT for late-life anxiety and depression. In most chapters, that would then leave room for a case example linking all the previous sections. In this chapter, it is my intention to do something *different*. New concepts and contexts are introduced for CBT with older people. Concepts such as attitudes to aging and wisdom enhancement, or profiting from "the wisdom of our years" are introduced and linked with some case examples to amplify their value as vehicles for change for CBT with older people. It is hoped that this chapter will enhance thinking about the application of CBT with older people as well as encourage developments in the creative maximization of standard techniques in CBT to enhance outcome for treatment for late-life depression and anxiety. This is an important endeavor as many more people are living longer and healthier (Laidlaw & Pachana, 2009), so there is a need for psychotherapists to become much more knowledgeable and more effective in working with older people to meet the needs of this new generation of older people (Knight, Karel, Hinrichsen, Qualls, & Duffy, 2009).

Cognitive behavioral therapy with older people

Cognitive behavioral therapy with older adults is a mainstream treatment approach for the alleviation of depression and anxiety in later life (Hendriks et al., 2008; Wilson, Mottram, & Vassilas, 2008). It is particularly appropriate as an intervention for older adults because it is skills enhancing, present-oriented, problem-focussed, straightforward to use, and effective (Laidlaw & Thompson, 2008). It is an active, directive, time-limited, and structured treatment approach whose primary aim is symptom reduction (Laidlaw, Thompson, Siskin-Dick, & Gallagher-Thompson, 2003).

Although cognitions are important for understanding the attributions people make about the meaning of their problems, or the challenges they face, behavior is equally important as actions can reinforce fears inadvertently. This is most commonly seen in anxiety disorders where people avoid situations because they are afraid of being overwhelmed and as a result develop attributions of personal inadequacy and weakness that in many cases cause more problems for them than was evident at the start of the development of an anxiety problem. Thus, avoidance may present an apparent short-term "solution" but this always results in bigger problems in the longer term. Thus, when using CBT with older people it is important that in-session dialogues are tied to out-of-session behavioral experiments because it is only through behavior change that symptom reduction can occur. CBT is therefore much more than a talking therapy; it is a *doing-therapy*.

The basic conceptual idea behind CBT is elegantly simple to grasp; that is, thoughts can often trigger mood-congruent affective responses which in turn can have an effect on behavior. So when someone thinks in a negative way this is associated with an elevation in negative moods such as sadness, and often as a result, there are behavioral changes, as people become more isolated and isolating. This is not a strictly linear process and therefore people may note that some behaviors they engage in can trigger thoughts. However, CBT is much more challenging to apply in reality and this often leads to a great deal of frustration on the part of practitioners. It requires applying the structure and the process of CBT consistently and effectively, while at the same time recognizing the idiosyncratic nature of a client's problems and individually tailoring treatment so that the client and therapist experience a unique therapeutic exchange. Additionally, the practitioner must adhere to agenda-setting, ask questions using a specific style (Socratic), and keep the focus in sessions on the changeable "here and now" orientation expected in CBT. This can be very daunting for therapists who may have many clients to prepare for in a day and so the discipline necessary to remain within mode of treatment with CBT can wane as the complexity of this apparently simple no-nonsense therapy sets in.

The application of CBT as a very challenging therapy can be an unpleasant surprise for many therapists. The myth that CBT is really a collection of techniques that can be picked up and applied in an unthinking fashion is one that has been inadvertently perpetuated by the ready availability of "cookbook" guides or manuals. Closer to the truth is that there are many excellent how to guides to CBT that may be useful as adjunctive reading when learning CBT in a properly supervised environment. Done poorly, CBT can be perceived as "mechanical and manipulative" (Beck, Rush, Shaw, & Emery, 1979) and will be uncomfortable and a poor fit for client and therapist.

Techniques do not make a therapy work, people do and it is in the sympathetic and skilled application of techniques allied to a good therapeutic treatment alliance that CBT becomes an effective and powerful treatment intervention for late-life depression and anxiety. CBT aims to be empowering of individuals and seeks to promote self-agency as it adopts a non-pathologizing stance to understanding how a client's problems may have developed (Zeiss & Steffen, 1996). As such, it can be a very attractive form of therapy for older people who often endorse strong cohort beliefs about personal independence and problem solving. To do CBT well requires great skill and ingenuity; one must be scientific as well as approachable and accessible. It is unhelpful if therapists are seen simply as experts; rather, a CBT therapist should be more comfortable with the role of coach than professor in working with clients. The goal ultimately is for clients to become their own therapists.

A treatment package of CBT can be considered to have three distinct phases: early, middle, and late, typically spread over 16–20 sessions (Laidlaw et al., 2003). In the early phase of treatment, taking place up to session 6 in some cases, clients are educated about the process of therapy and the nature of depression or anxiety itself (termed psychoeducation), socialized into a specific way of data gathering and self-monitoring and expected to become full partners in a collaborative process of discovery about the nature of the problems that has brought them into the therapist's office in the first instance. In this initial phase of treatment, a cognitive conceptualization is developed as a collaborative exercise. The conceptualization acts as a theory that explains the current difficulties and also predicts possible treatment obstacles and challenges. The conceptualization therefore links the overt levels of symptoms presentation to the covert level of presentation that often includes dysfunctional schemata (core beliefs) and underlying vulnerabilities endorsed by the client. Regardless of number of sessions, CBT is a brief form of psychotherapy with an expectation that treatment will terminate once symptom reduction has been achieved. It is often helpful and reassuring to the client if the therapist agrees to review therapy goals and progress periodically throughout treatment and initially after six sessions. Therefore, in order to maintain a client-focussed goal-oriented approach to treatment it is important to identify a problem list and set related goals for treatment outcome (Laidlaw, 2008). In the early phase of treatment however, setting up a working therapeutic relationship is essential as unless a trusting safe environment has been established it is unlikely that progress toward a successful resolution of goals will be fully realized.

During the middle phase of CBT treatment, the primary focus is on identifying and modifying negative automatic thoughts and developing related behavioral experiments that aid client self-discovery and hence symptom reduction. Often in CBT with older people, the client is not taught new skills but merely provided with a means of re-discovering old skills and competences that have been forgotten by the patient as they develop distress. In depression, the negative bias in cognitions results in the clients becoming excessively focused on negative attributes with the result that they are often self-blaming and rigidly punitive in their self-attributions. In anxiety, the clients often become so caught up on the "what ifs" of an impending disaster that they fail to realize that there are different ways to think about things. Often Socratic dialogue, a specific way of helping clients process information in subtle different ways, can help the client break through these unhelpful patterns of thinking. An example of this is Jean, a 78-year retired civil servant who was suffering from both anxiety and depression symptoms. She was expressing concern that she had experienced many headaches recently and although her general practitioner (GP) had carried out a range of assessments no cause had been identified and hence no cure was forthcoming. Jean had started to fret that her headaches indicated something was seriously wrong with her health. When the therapist asked Jean what she thought was the problem when symptoms were at their peaks, she replied, "I have a tumor in my head." The therapist did not seek to reassure the client that she did not have a tumor, but sought to help to process this further, by simply asking, "Jean, have you ever known anyone with a tumor?" Interestingly, Jean replied, "Yes, my mother." Once this fear was out in the open and being discussed, Jean was immediately able to de-escalate her own fears by herself. She stated that her symptoms were really quite distinct from those she witnessed in her mother and in the following week she did not experience any further problems with this fear. Here, the therapist did not seek to dissuade or reassure the client, but treated the idea with respect and the client with dignity. In the dialogue that ensued, the client did most of the reappraisal of her thoughts and fears were reduced to more manageable levels. This short dialogue shows the power of CBT, and the utility of the Socratic method. Socratic questioning does not involve following a roadmap, that is, taking a patient from "erroneous" attributions about situations to a "right" answer (from A to B). Instead Socratic questioning involves a joint process of discovery where the destination and elements of the journey may be and should be unknown at the outset, so that the journey is from A to wherever (Laidlaw, 2008).

In the middle phase of treatment, clients are taught self-monitoring skills to identify thoughts that are associated with negative mood and maladaptive behavioral response. Identifying and challenging negative automatic thoughts is termed cognitive restructuring and a common method of doing this is to use a dysfunctional thought record (DTR). The DTR is a form that has space for the patients to record their thoughts, feelings associated with their thoughts, and rational responses to these thoughts.

There are many versions of DTRs in CBT textbooks (see Greenberger & Padesky, 1995; Laidlaw et al., 2003). DTRs are generally poorly applied in practice and poorly complied with as homework tasks. Completing a DTR is a complex skill that therapists must master as well as clients. It is helpful to acknowledge with the client that identifying and challenging negative automatic thoughts may feel a little strange at first. After all, the therapist is asking the client to think about his/her thoughts and this can be a confusing and novel activity that will take time to become an intuitive skill (Laidlaw & McAlpine, 2008). Thus, in order to help the client master the process of examining and challenging his/her cognitions, it can be helpful to simplify the process as much as possible. Instead of presenting a client with a daunting blank five-column DTR, the process should be introduced in steps. First, if a weekly activity schedule (a simple schedule diary-grid form of a week's activities) has been used in early sessions, these can be useful for identifying negative thoughts. This is enhanced if the therapist has asked the client to rate his/her activities for enjoyment or pleasure. It is common that different activities at different times provide different enjoyment ratings and these can be examined for thoughts about these activities. The enjoyment ratings for activities can be used within session to infer and discuss what sorts of thoughts were associated with the activity and what was it about these activities that merited their ratings. It also introduces the notion that behavior and mood are linked. From this stage, the introduction of a simple three-column DTR can be used, with columns allowing description of situation, thought, and feeling. From these forms the therapist and client can in time agree to develop more complex forms of recording of thoughts and the skill of cognitive restructuring can be more easily mastered.

It is during the middle phase of treatment that homework becomes especially important as it is the test bed for implementing new understandings and new beliefs from within the sessions about the nature of the problems experienced by the client. Homework in CBT is an essential component of treatment and the vehicle by which the client develops the skills and competences to master his/her problematic situations. Homework can be poorly complied with in therapy, perhaps because homework is all too often vague in terms of task specifics, does not often follow after a discussion within therapy, and is therefore confusing for the client (Kazantzis, Pachana, & Secker, 2003). The therapist's main range of control in homework compliance is in the assignment of the task in the first place and therefore great care must be exercised in the negotiation and discussion of the planned homework (Tompkins, 2002). All too often, novice therapists are inclined to rush homework assignment by leaving it to the last few minutes of a treatment session, however, in reality homework can be set within a session at any time that it naturally arises as a topic to be tested out. If the therapist is curious about the outcome of homework and transmits this curiosity with an appropriate measure of enthusiasm and reinforcement then homework completion may be more likely (Tompkins), Finally, homework compliance can be improved if it is always the first item to be discussed in session as this transmits the importance of this task to the client.

In the final phase of therapy, two main tasks remain to be accomplished: (1) the agreement of an appropriate termination point for therapy and (2) the elaboration of a relapse prevention plan. It is important that the relapse prevention plan is at least role-played with the clients before they are discharged. Approaching the end of therapy can be an anxiety provoking time for the clients as they may develop fears about managing their problems on their own. Prior to ending treatment, it can be helpful to engage the clients in a review of what they have learned from therapy listing and what strategies might worked well for them and this can be usefully done as a homework task. At the end of treatment, intermittent or booster sessions can be agreed upon in advance of discharge. This can be useful in a number of ways. It allays the fears that the clients may have about dealing with problems alone and can break the simple habit of attending regularly for appointments. Booster sessions work in a number of ways as prior to termination clients become more confident in their own self-agency as their mood levels are maintained despite longer gaps between therapy sessions.

The efficacy of cognitive behavioral therapy for late-life depression and anxiety

A large number of systematic reviews and meta-analyses have concluded with a high degree of consistency that CBT is an efficacious treatment for late-life depression (Pinquart, Duberstein, & Lyness, 2006; Scogin, Welsh, Hanson, Stump, & Coates, 2005; Wilson et al., 2008).

Recent randomized controlled trials (RCT) in the United Kingdom also attest to the efficacy of CBT for late-life depression in primary care settings (Laidlaw et al., 2008; Serfaty et al., 2009). Although the evidence for CBT studies looking at depression co-morbid with physical illnesses is mixed, the suitability of CBT is less in doubt (Halford & Brown, 2009). It is arguable that outcome may be enhanced using augmented approaches to CBT that are more tailored to the circumstances of individuals adjusting to the onset of acute or chronic medical conditions.

Although CBT for late-life anxiety disorder has been criticized because the studies have tended to be conducted with a generally "young" older adult group of healthy, active volunteers and with studies conducted in university settings (Hendriks et al., 2008), a more recent RCT by Stanley et al. (2009) has answered many of these criticisms showing good outcome for CBT for late-life anxiety in primary care. Until recently CBT for anxiety in later life was difficult to quantify in clinical practice as there were limited measures for use with older people. The Geriatric Anxiety Inventory (Pachana et al., 2007) is recommended as it has been specifically developed for use with this population and differentiates between anxiety and depression and anxiety symptoms from physical symptoms associated with medical conditions.

Other recent developments in late-life anxiety include highly specialized CBT for people with executive dysfunction. This innovation in treatment provides a relatively new and exciting development for CBT of great promise. Mohlman and Gorman (2005) showed that outcome for CBT anxiety disorder was poor in older people with low levels of executive functioning abilities. Outcome was better for those individuals initially classified as having low levels of executive functioning when executive functioning was improved using attention-training and enhanced self-monitoring (see also Mohlman et al., 2008).

Thus overall, therapists and clients alike can be confident that CBT provides them with a powerful set of treatment interventions for anxiety and depression in later life.

Attitudes to aging and cognitive behavioral therapy

In many respects, CBT shares many more similarities than differences in applying interventions with older versus younger clients (Laidlaw et al., 2003). However, the main difference for therapists is likely to revolve around the context of an individual's experience of the aging process (Laidlaw & McAlpine, 2008). Although this may be most evident when dealing with physical co-morbidity and depression (Zeiss & Steffen, 1996), it is also evident when working with an individual's attitude to his/her own aging.

Consistent with the cognitive theory of cognitive therapy, it is hypothesized that mood-congruent negativity biases in depression may result in older people attributing their problems to aging rather than to depression (Laidlaw, in press). Thus, the problem confronting therapists is not a realistic appraisal of the experience of aging, but rather the issue is that depressed older people endorse negative attitudes to aging that are erroneous and are analogous to negative automatic thoughts in that they are plausible, distorted, and unhelpful. Examples of negative automatic cognitions in older people include, "Old age is a terrible time," or "All my problems are to do with my age," or "I'm too old to change my ways now" (Laidlaw & Pachana, 2009). Unless addressed by the therapist these cognitions may limit progress in therapy as problems are considered as being internal (an attribute of the individual, i.e. their age), global (all of their problems are because they are old), and stable (these problems as they are to do with aging are with them for the rest of their life). This can be daunting and challenging for therapists who are inexperienced and are unused to working with older people (for a fuller explanation see Laidlaw, in press).

Thus, consistent with cognitive theory of depression, older people may selectively attend to negative indicators of aging such as loss due to bereavement, or unwanted changes in physical health status such as the development of a chronic medical condition such as angina or some other long-standing limiting non-life-threatening condition that serves to activate the internalized negative age stereotype (the Diathesis). In the CBT model of psychopathology of Beck et al. (1979), the stress diathesis is an important explanatory concept. The diatheses are idiosyncratic vulnerablities that may predispose an individual to develop a depressive episode if there are certain stresses evident in the environment. "Cognitive vulnerability in the form of dysfunctional schemas and maladaptive personality are diatheses that remain latent in the non-depressed state until primed or activated by an eliciting event or stimulus" (Clark, Beck, & Alford, 1999, p. 292). In a stress-diathesis there is a person-experience interaction, where the development of depression may be explained by the activation of pre-existing vulnerabilities by experiences or circumstances that confront an individual. These diatheses or vulnerabilities are often deemed to be latent until activated by the stressors in the environment experienced by the individual. It is proposed that attitudes to aging may act as a diathesis for the later development of anxiety and/or depression in older people.

Encouraging consistent evidence for attitudes to aging acting as a stress-diathesis is found in the work of Levy and colleagues (Levy, 2003). Levy suggests that ageist societal attitudes are internalized from a very young age and can become negative age-stereotypes that are reinforced by an attentional bias to negative information about aging where eventually these beliefs become negative self-stereotypes. Negative age biases and stereotypes often operate outside the individual's conscious awareness much like latent maladaptive schemata mentioned previously. In interesting experiments reported by Levy presenting older people with subliminal positive or negative primes had an impact on function and outcome. Thus, individuals primed with negative words associated with aging performed more poorly on four memory tasks compared to those individuals primed with positive words. This same experimental paradigm generalized to handwriting and walking, including both gait and speed.

Thus, consistent with Levy (2003), it is proposed here that depression may act as a negative filter by which loss or change in age is perceived. Blending this idea with cognitive theory, consistent with the selective processing hypothesis (Clark et al., 1999) in depression, there is a negativity bias where individuals have a tendency to overlook positive information and selectively and preferentially attend to negative stimuli. "In depression, we find a mood-congruent bias for encoding negative material that is characterized by a heightened sensitivity for self-referent information involving themes of loss, failure, and deprivation" (Clark et al., p. 177).

In depression in later life, the negative self-referential bias often maintains a negative age focus. For example, Mrs. Rogers, aged 67 years has been referred by her GP because of her chronic depression, high levels of hopelessness and low level of suicidal ideation as she has stated an unwillingness to take antidepressant medication. Mrs. Rogers has stated in her sessions with her therapist that she thought her main problems were to do with her age and wondered about whether it was worth living as it (life) was only likely to get worse as she got older. She explained that aging was a terrible experience and warned the therapist that once age set in there was not a lot of joy in life. She stated she rarely smiled or laughed now and often felt on the verge of tears for no apparent reason. She also said "I forget a lot of things now. When I start talking I forget what I was going to say." As further evidence that her age was her main problem she said "I do a lot of sitting and not a lot of doing. I take a long time to get ready to go out now. When I do go out, I often can't be bothered and wish I were back home." She also noted that she avoids people because "If people talk to me, I cannot bear to answer them. I want to run away. I don't have the same interest [in people] as I had before. Sometimes I take the phone off the hook. I am more introverted now." Finally she said, "When I look in the mirror I just want to pack it in. I'm not happy compared with the way I looked before."

Therapists faced with such a coherent and eloquent list of the indignities of aging may be inclined to agree with their clients that their problems are indeed to do with age and then to commiserate with them, at the same time becoming passive in therapeutic orientation with a consequent lowering of expectations for outcome. This is fundamentally unhelpful to clients. It also ignores a large amount of evidence that in depression, thinking is overgeneralized, rigid, and biased (Kuyken, 2006). Looked at more closely, the therapist could see that each of the "negatives" linked by the client to aging are actually symptoms of depression, such as anhedonia, weepiness, sadness, hopelessness, apathy, etc. Although there is a great sense of despair described by the client, this despair is linked to depression, not aging *per se*. Working together, the therapist and client reframed the symptoms by reviewing the symptoms of depression in the DSM-IV (Diagnostic and Statistical Manual of Mental Disorders, fourth edition) (APA, 1994) section on depression. This was an open and collaborative approach to data gathering. The client was asked whether it was possible that depression was an alternative way to think of her problems. As she answered this was a possibility, standard cognitive restructuring techniques of asking what is the evidence for and against her belief that age was her main problem and then to compare this to seeing depression as her main problem were employed. Likewise Mrs. Rogers was asked what was the effect of thinking this way. Thus, a negative and nihilistic approach to thinking was challenged and modified using simple CBT techniques. In this intervention, the effectiveness of CBT techniques is enhanced as they are employed in an age-specific context.

From this example, it is hypothesized that the mood-congruent negativity bias resulted in Mrs. Rogers attributing her problems to aging rather than depression. The client has internalized negative societal values about aging and has developed an internalized negative self-stereotype of aging (see Levy, 2003). Thus, it is a pre-existing vulnerability that acts as a diathesis. The stressor that in effect activates this pre-existing vulnerability is her perception of negative personal changes associated with aging. In effect she is viewing her own aging through a lens distorted by depression. She selectively attends to negative indicators of aging such as unwanted changes in her physical appearance and losses of vitality that she attributes to age rather than depression that serve to activate her internalized negative age stereotype (the stress-diathesis). Thus, Mrs. Rogers' fears about aging equated to deterioration and dysfunction are apparently being realized. In this way, she develops a negative filter to identify other changes that are attributed to aging. In depression, loss of changes to appetite, poor sleep, and loss of hedonic pleasure (anhedonia) were attributed to age rather than depression. In this way she believes her problems to be due to an unchangeable aspect of herself, *that is, an outcome of her own aging consistent with stereotypical beliefs about the negativity associated with aging*. It was no surprise that Mrs. Rogers presented with a high level of hopelessness about the future and some suicidal ideation. The model of aging acting as stress-diathesis similar to the model of psychopathology first proposed by Beck et al. (1979) is illustrated in Fig. 2.1 developed by Laidlaw (in press).

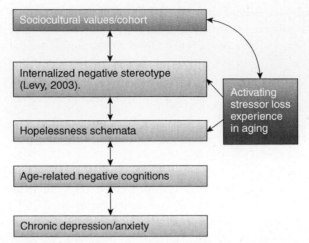

Fig. 2.1 A CBT stress-diathesis model of the negative internalized age stereotype.
Source: Adapted from Laidlaw, K. (2010). Are attitudes to aging and wisdom enhancement legitimate targets for CBT for late life depression? *Nordic Psychology, 62,* 27–42.

A final word about aging

The majority of older people live long and healthy lives and report high levels of satisfaction. Laidlaw, Power, & Schmidt (2007) developed a scale to examine the attitudes to aging in a large cohort of older people from a number of countries. Despite having a number of physical illnesses, many older people reported high levels of satisfaction with aging, indicating that negative attitudes to aging are not a universal experience amongst community dwelling older people. Chachamovich, Fleck, Laidlaw, & Power (2008) report that attitudes to aging are progressively and negatively influenced by increasing levels of depression. Attitudes to aging are therefore mood-state dependent, as individuals report more negative attitudes if they are depressed. Thus, depression is not an outcome of old age, it is an illness experienced in later life that may change an individual's attributions about his/her quality of life and attitudes toward it. It is a legitimate target for CBT therapists working with older people.

Levels of depression in later life are typically lower than for adults in middle age and in younger adulthood (Blazer, 2010). Moreover, in later life the aging paradox is in contrast to the notion that old age is a stage of life to be feared, as older people typically report high levels of life satisfaction at the stage of life most associated with cognitive and physical decline (Carstensen & Lockenhoff, 2003). Thus, when older people attribute their problems to age *per se*, this is inconsistent with the normative experience of aging. Blazer explains the paradox of low relative rates of depression in the presence of challenges associated with age in terms of three protective factors associated with aging such as, better emotional development, consistent with the work by Carstensen's theory of socioemotional selectivity theory (SST; Carstensen, Isaacowitz, & Charles, 1999), increased wisdom (Baltes & Smith, 2008), and resilience as older people cope better with stressful events as Blazer (2010) notes these are events that are experienced as being "on time" (p. 172), and thus are expected so that an older person may cope with these events better than is anticipated or expected.

Wisdom enhancement in late-life depression

Wisdom is a theoretically rich area in gerontology and provides a positive frame of reference when attempting to develop appropriate targets for work with depressed older people in psychotherapy

(Knight & Laidlaw, 2009). Wisdom also holds promise for augmenting CBT models for older people as it emphasizes "The acquisition of an expert system of wisdom ... requires concerted personal and societal investment of considerable time, effort, motivation, and structured experience" (Baltes & Smith, 2008). This description of the development of wisdom is not far from the experiences and expectations for a successful course of psychotherapy. Thus perhaps, wisdom is what CBT therapy provides people given that their beliefs about personally important and meaningful events are examined. The aim is to help clients to act on new ways of thinking in order to become more adept at managing ambiguous and complex scenarios with a presumed positive effect on outcome.

The concept of wisdom retains a high currency amongst many older people as it constitutes a commonly understood "folk theory" of aging and implies growth through adversity. It is not surprising that implicit theories of wisdom assume a positive correlation of wisdom with advancing age (Glück & Baltes, 2006), although age by itself is seldom sufficient to promote wisdom attainment. Wisdom enhancement may be about managing life's experiences and vicissitudes while dealing with ambiguity in the most pragmatic manner possible. Although there are many different perspectives on wisdom, the theoretical perspective adopted here is that of Baltes and Staudinger (2000). "Wisdom is expert knowledge about the fundamental pragmatics of human life." Additionally, Baltes and Staudinger discuss implicit and explicit theoretical perspectives on wisdom and define five criteria as the means of assessing wisdom behaviors. These are rich, factual, and procedural knowledge in the execution of decisions and activities. Lifespan contextualism covers the lifespan accruement of experiences across one's lifetime that informs an individual's development of self-identity. Another important criteria concern the relativism of values and priorities considered important for the individual. Therapy will only work if an individual is focussing on issues of high priority and can act within a value system that is meaningful to them. Baltes and Staudinger state that wisdom can be adjudged on how an individual deals with the recognition and management of uncertainty. This is also clearly of resonance for the work that is undertaken in psychotherapy. Often clients come into therapy because they have a challenging situation to deal with and there is uncertainty about how best to proceed. This can be seen in the transitions commonly experienced by dementia caregivers who can often experience great uncertainty in how they respond to challenging behaviors in loved ones where the caregiver is distressed at not knowing whether their responses to behaviors are calming or inflaming the situation.

The concept of wisdom as elaborated by Baltes and Staudinger (2000) is one that has good face validity for older adult therapists and their clients and corresponds nicely with the experience of older people participating in psychotherapy. When someone comes into treatment in CBT, his/her idiosyncratic way of seeing the world and understanding the problems is analogous to lifespan contextualism. In order for therapy to proceed, the therapist and client must agree on a shared sense of priorities and goals, and this is similar to the concept of relativism of values and priorities.

As CBT is skills enhancing there is an explicit recognition and respect for the richness of the factual and procedural knowledge clients bring with them into therapy. CBT explicitly acknowledges and values the client's skills and consistent with the goal of wisdom attainment, the pre-existing client competences can be promoted and supported by the therapist so that a different outcome may be achieved. In CBT with older people it is not always necessary to teach people new skills; sometimes the goal is simply to assist individuals to remember to use pre-existing skills and competences and direct these inwardly for better treatment outcomes. For example, Mr. Leckie is a keen cyclist. At the age of 77, he still regularly enjoys going for long cycle runs in the countryside with some friends. He has been diagnosed with generalized anxiety disorder and is very much concerned that he is not making quick enough progress in therapy. The therapist used Mr. Leckie's pre-existing skills and competences developed through cycling to help him decide whether he would wish to continue persevering with therapy. Mr. Leckie was asked how he would help a new member join his cycling team. He replied that the person would find it hard at first, but with practice, perseverance, and the support and encouragement of others he was pretty optimistic that anyone could become a competent cyclist. He added that it wouldn't happen overnight. The therapist asked Mr. Leckie to consider the wisdom of this advice before asking him what was the point of discussing this in therapy. Mr. Leckie was immediately able to see that this was the sort of advice he needed to follow in looking at his own progress in therapy, and that after a long struggle with anxiety and worry he couldn't expect progress to "happen overnight." Although this type of dialogue in CBT is neither new nor particularly innovative, cloaking it in the guise of wisdom enhancement is. It makes these ideas of growth through perseverance and challenge accessible. It allows the clients to see that therapy is an experience that is connected to many other experiences in their life and that the experience of learning new skills is not something that is beyond them.

Another interesting parallel between wisdom and psychotherapy is indicated in a research study by Baltes and Staudinger (2000) who noted that when individuals were asked to respond to dilemmas on their own, their answers were not considered high in terms of wisdom compared to responses generated in discussion with significant others or in groups, or when individuals were directed to consult an "inner voice." This is again analogous with the experience of therapy in that a "problem shared is a problem halved." Stated in this way, therapy sessions provide a nurturing environment for the growth of wisdom.

Wisdom enhancement strategy could potentially optimize already efficacious anxiety and depression treatments such as CBT. Drawing on experience, and becoming "wise" by reflecting upon and reframing narratives associated with past experiences may promote growth (Bauer & McAdam, 2004) and thus potentiate the effectiveness of CBT. Wisdom enhancement explicitly seeks to link people to their life experiences and thus contextualizes current episodes of depression within a lifespan perspective (lifespan contextualism). Often people construct personal narratives as a way of constructing meaning to their life and experiences (McAdam, 2001).

As depression in later life is often not the first episode of depression for many individuals this needs to be taken account of in CBT with older people. In these scenarios, individuals may construct personal narratives of failure or misfortune that increases hopelessness and compromises an individual's expectation for the possibility of change during a depressive episode. If left unassessed and unchallenged, such personal narratives reinforce a passive self-defeated perspective that may become an additional barrier to good treatment outcomes. A clinical example may illustrate this point. Elsie is a 71-year-old woman with a history of depression stretching back 50 years or more. She has experienced at least six separate episodes of major depressive disorder. She has been admitted to hospital for treatment of her depression and when the therapist meets Elsie in his outpatient clinic, it is evident that Elsie is very hopeless about her future prospects for recovery. She says, "I can't see me ever getting back to how I used to be," "I think I'll be in hospital for the rest of my life now." This can be very challenging to deal with in therapy. It is clear that no one knows what the future is and while it can be a useful intervention in its own right to point out to Elsie that she is making a "fortune-telling" error in her thinking, this may come off as unempathic. However, many other professionals meeting Elsie had sought to reassure her that she would recover and this is again a mistake as it is theoretically possible that she would not make a full recovery. To retain credibility as an open and honest co-worker with your client, it is crucial to avoid making promises that can't necessarily be delivered upon. Instead of providing reassurance the therapist sought to elicit hope for the potential of change by asking Elsie to make use of the "wisdom of your years." The therapist introduced the idea that by having previous episodes of depression she might be able to use those experiences to help her manage her current episode and recovery from it. The therapist asked Elsie, "When you were depressed before, did you ever think that you would not recover?" Elsie was able to see that she had thought this in every previous episode of depression. The therapist sought to help Elsie process this further by asking, "So, what does that tell you?" Elsie said, "well maybe I was wrong then and I'll be wrong this time." The therapist asked Elsie if she thought this might be possible whereupon Elsie said, "I have this image in my head. I can see myself sitting in the ward in 1973, here in this hospital, and I'm staring out the window." Elsie recounted that she clearly remembered thinking that she would be in the ward for the rest of her life. She recalled this as a vivid image. Elsie was able to use the vivid sense of having experienced a conviction that recovery was not possible for her to unseat some sense of her lack of recovery for her current episode. Thus, Elsie used the wisdom of her years to assist to her to better manage her current episode of depression. What made this image all the more powerful is that at that time, she did make a full recovery and she went on to marry and have a child. None of these experiences seemed at all possible to her at the time and this was powerful data for her to reflect on in managing her current sense of hopelessness and despair. Although again this is not necessarily straying too far from standard CBT techniques of cognitive restructuring, it is a novel use in therapy of lifetime experiences to help an individual better manage a current challenge. As CBT stresses the here and now orientation of problem solving, when working with older people with an extensive lifetime history, it can be confusing for therapists to know how to utilize this wealth of life experience. Wisdom attainment provides a convenient therapeutic vehicle in this regard. It is also very empowering for the clients to realize that they often have answers from using their own experiences.

Although aging offers numerous experiences of life and ample opportunity to develop wisdom, clearly not everyone learns from his/her experiences. Depression may block wisdom attainment because of the selective nature of recall on depression and the rigidly negative self-attributions that prevent individuals from looking at situations in a way that promotes learning through adversity (Joorman, Teachman, & Gotlib, 2009). Negative affect increases accessibility of mood-congruent material (Ingram et al., 1998). There may even be a false positive recall for negative information (Joorman et al.). In depression, people are more prone to ruminate rather than reflect on their experiences and hence become more self-critical and punitive as they review their actions (Watkins, 2008). In this way an individual may find it hard to identify positive memories and may be more likely to report many negative experiences over the course of a lifetime. This can provide therapists with a challenge when taking a history as a biased record may be provided. A useful technique for the therapist to employ when understanding an individual's personal narrative over the course of his/her lifetime without getting overwhelmed with negative recall is ask the client to construct a "timeline" within therapy.

The timeline can be located on a vertical line that connects the individual's birth date at the start of the timeline with the current date at the end of the timeline. The therapist can ask the client to put all notable events from life on this timeline. This is a task that can usefully be employed as a homework task in the first few sessions. By employing this simple technique the therapist gains an "edited" summary of the high and low points of an individual's life. It is in taking these elements from the timeline that wisdom enhancement comes into use. Wisdom depends on learning from experience but it is also evident in the execution of judgement where outcome depends on a decision and there is not an obviously correct solution. Thus wisdom comes into play in utilizing experience in making decisions. (Schwartz & Sharpe, 2005). Wisdom is evident when one learns from experience and elements that are registering on an individual's personal timeline will be important and personally meaningful. Bauer and McAdam (2004) note that themes arising in an individual's personal narrative are likely to reflect the things that are personally meaningful and relevant to them.

Perhaps wisdom can be enhanced by explicitly asking people to reflect on difficult life experiences in a structured way to see if they can identify anything good that may have come out of difficult experiences from the past and what they might use from this new learning to equip themselves better to deal with current difficulties. Similarly, McAdam (2006) talks of individuals developing "redemptive sequences" where a bad experience or event can be transformed into a growth experience by the individual. The emotional life of older people is more complex than has previously been recognized, Carstensen et al. (1999) introduced the concept of SST where the emotional life of older people can be better understood by considering the time-horizons shaping their experience. As people age, they are motivated by the perceived finite boundary to the time left to them in life to invest in more emotionally meaningful goals that promote changes to values toward the achievement of intimacy with a few valued others. This change in motivation and values promotes growth and change. There is also a literature on post-traumatic growth that resonates with the ideas presented here. "Post-traumatic growth seems closely connected to the development of general wisdom about life, and the development and modification of the individual's life narrative" (Tedeschi & Calhoun, 2004, p. 12).

Life crises are called crises for a reason and can result in significant and prolonged psychological distress (Tedeschi & Calhoun, 2004). Thus, one should never underestimate or minimize the impact of crises in an individual's experience. At the time when a person has experienced a life crisis he/she may have experienced a great deal of distress and this may have been a precursor to a depressive or anxiety episode. The affective component of the crisis and the subsequent change after the event is important in determining whether post-traumatic growth may take place (Tedeschi & Calhoun). Thus, looking back over difficult experiences should not be treated lightly and in the midst of depression needs to be considered carefully. If an individual is chronically and severely depressed, there may be more productive strategies that can be applied than having him/her review difficult past events; however, when cognitive restructuring work is proceeding in therapy this type of activity may promote additional opportunities to challenge the individual's self-attributions. In the aftermath of the crisis and looking back on how the individual coped, a more elaborated account may be possible that may be used to promote the sense of the individual having a resilience that he/she has failed to credit to himself/herself. For example, a more elaborated account of the struggles in the past with depression can be reframed as an example of resiliency. If the therapist is sensitive and careful in the way in which experiences are examined there may be a more elaborated experience of negative and positive connotations after difficult experiences where growth may be acknowledged. The key here is deliberate cognitive processing of prior experiences in a very supportive and structured way. By helping an individual to recognize his/her resilience in the face of difficult circumstance, this can be used to help the person deal with the "here and now" of the current difficult circumstances in dealing with anxiety or depression.

To promote wisdom enhancement the therapist may wish to ask the client to "Use the wisdom of your years …" as a way of promoting a more elaborated discussion of how to proceed in an ambiguous situation and to draw on previous experiences, good and bad, by asking "Using the wisdom of your years, what might be a wise thing to do" when discussing how to proceed with ambiguous and challenging circumstances. This is a Socratic discussion that is aimed at promoting increased sense of self-agency and the facilitation of focused problem-oriented thinking. In this way, this is similar to the approach adopted by Watkins, Baeyens, and Read (2009) who reduced depression symptoms and self-criticism by coaching dysphoric individuals to be more "concrete" and hence less overgeneralized in their thinking about events and experiences. This is consistent with the position adopted here in that when depressed an individual's appraisal of past situations can take on an overgeneralized negative character that can be difficult to challenge in any meaningful way. As CBT has a "here and now" orientation, the past can be assessed for what it may provide the individual in his/her attempts to deal with the current problems and this must proceed in a more concrete or focussed way if it is to benefit the individual. Data in the form of specific details about specific experiences provide the opportunity for learning from experience and through adversity. The dialogue should at all times be focussed and direct, and may enhance the wisdom of the individual as they attempt to manage their current challenging circumstance.

Questions for discussion

1. Although CBT has been shown to be efficacious with older people, is the evidence base the best we could have to prepare us to meet the needs of new and evolving cohorts of older people?

2. Is there a need to consider how to age-contextualize CBT for use with CBT?

3. How can the lifetime experiences of older people be usefully employed in therapy so as to reduce levels of hopelessness and passivity in depression and anxiety?

4. Can managing adversity be an opportunity to develop a positive framework for CBT with older people that challenges their beliefs about possibility for growth and change in any decade of life?

Summary

This chapter has sought to introduce a new set of targets for CBT therapists to consider when working with older people. The concepts of internalized negative stereotypes and wisdom attainment/enhancement are employed so as to afford better use of standardized CBT techniques in a more coherent age-appropriate context. However, it is important to emphasize that standard techniques in CBT are employed in this endeavor and all that has changed is the contextual framework for their use. This is important as the evidence suggests that CBT is an efficacious therapy and one does not wish to distance oneself from that strong body of evidence. In a sense this chapter attempts to encourage therapists to be more conceptually coherent in their thinking in how they individualize CBT for older people. This again is not new as Beck et al. (1979) emphasized that CBT is individualized to fit the client and approaches such as these outlined here help CBT to be a better fit for the needs of older people. As Laidlaw and McAlpine (2008) note most considerations of modifications to therapy with older people can be quite banal and procedural and this is minimally helpful for therapists and clients. It is hoped that gerontological theories can be examined and considered in terms of utility as vehicles for change in therapy.

References

American Psychiatric Association (1994). *The Diagnostic and Statistical Manual of Mental Disorders*, Fourth Edition. Washington, DC: APA.

Baltes, P.B., & Staudinger, U.M. (2000). Wisdom: A metaheuristic (pragmatic) to orhestrate mind and virtue toward excellence. *American Psychologist, 55,* 122–136.

Baltes, P.B., & Smith, J. (2008). The fascination of wisdom: Its nature, ontogeny, and function. *Perspectives on Psychological Science, 3,* 56–64.

Bauer, J., & McAdam, D. (2004). Personal growth in Adults' stories of life transitions. *Journal of Personality, 72,* 573–602.

Beck, A.T., Rush, A.J., Shaw, B.F., & Emery, G. (1979). *Cognitive therapy of depression.* New York, NY: Guildford Press.

Blazer, D.G. (2010). Protection from depression. *International Psychogeriatrics, 22,* 171–173.

Carstensen, L., & Lockenhoff, C.A. (2003). Aging, emotion, and evolution: The bigger picture. *Annals of the New York Academy of Science, 1000,* 152–179.

Carstensen, L., Isaacowitz, D., & Charles, S.T. (1999). Taking time seriously: A theory of socioemotional selectivity. *American Psychologist, 54*, 165–181.

Chachamovich, E., Fleck, M., Laidlaw, K., & Power, M.J. (2008). Impact of major depression and subsyndromal symptoms on quality of life and attitudes to aging. *The Gerontologist, 48*, 593–602.

Clark, D.A., Beck, A.T., & Alford, B.A. (1999). *Scientific foundations of cognitive theory and therapy of depression.* New York: Guilford Press.

Gluck, J., & Baltes, P.B. (2006). Using the concept of wisdom to enhance the expression of wisdom knowledge: Not the philosopher's dream but differential effects of developmental preparedness. *Psychology and Aging, 21*, 679–690.

Greenberger, D., & Padesky, C.A. (1995). *Mind over mood: Change how you feel by changing the way you think.* New York: Guilford Press.

Halford, J., & Brown, T. (2009). Cognitive-behaviour therapy as an adjunctive treatment in chronic physical illness. *Advances in Psychiatric Treatment, 15*, 306–317.

Hendriks, G., Oude, R., Voshaar, G., et al. (2008). Cognitive-behavioural therapy for late-life anxiety disorder: A systematic review and meta-analysis. *Acta Psychaitrica Scandinavica, 117*, 403–411.

Ingram, R.E., Miranda, J., & Segal, Z.V. (1998). *Cognitive vulnerability to depression.* New York: Guildford Press.

Joorman, J., Teachman, B.A., & Gotlib, I.H. (2009). Sadder and less accurate? False memory for negative material in depression. *Journal of Abnormal Psychology, 118*, 412–417.

Kazantzis, N., Pachana, N.A., & Secker, D.L. (2003). Cognitive behavioural therapy for older adults: Practical guidelines for the use of homework assignments. *Cognitive and Behavioral Practice, 10*, 324–332.

Knight, B.G., & Laidlaw, K. (2009). Translational theory: A wisdom-based model for psychological interventions to enhance well-being in later life. In V.L. Bengtson, M. Silverstein, N.M. Putney, & D. Gans (Eds.), *Handbook of theories of aging.* Second Edition. New York, NY: Springer.

Knight, B.G., Karel, M.J., Hinrichsen, G.A., Qualls, S.H., & Duffy, M. (2009). Pikes Peak model for training in professional geropsychology. *American Psychologist, 64*, 205–214.

Kuyken, W. (2006). Digging deep into depression. *The Psychologist, 19*, 278–281.

Laidlaw, K. (2008). Cognitive behaviour therapy. In R.T. Woods & L. Clare (Eds.), *Handbook of the clinical psychology of ageing.* Second Edition. Chichester, West Sussex, UK: John Wiley & Sons.

Laidlaw, K. (2010). Are attitudes to ageing and wisdom enhancement legitimate targets for CBT for late life depression? *Nordic Psychology, 62*, 27–42.

Laidlaw, K., & Thompson, L.W. (2008). Cognitive behaviour therapy with older people. In K. Laidlaw & B.G. Knight (Eds.), *Handbook of the assessment and treatment of emotional disorders in later life.* Oxford: Oxford University Press.

Laidlaw, K., & McAlpine, S. (2008). Cognitive-behaviour therapy: How is it different with older people? *Journal of Rational Emotive Cognitive Behaviour Therapy, 26*(4), 250–262.

Laidlaw, K., & Pachana, N. (2009). Aging, mental health and demographic change: Psychotherapist Challenges. *Professional Psychology: Research and Practice, 40*, 601–608.

Laidlaw, K., Thompson, L.W., Siskin-Dick, L., & Gallagher-Thompson, D. (2003). *Cognitive behavioural therapy with older people.* Chichester: John Wiley & Sons.

Laidlaw, K., Power, M.J., & Schmidt, S. (2007). The WHOQOL-Old Group. The Attitudes to Ageing Questionnaire (AAQ): Development and psychometric. *International Journal of Geriatric Psychiatry, 22*, 367–379.

Laidlaw, K, Davidson, K.M., Toner, H.L., Jackson, G., Clark, S., Law, J., et al. (2008). A randomised controlled trial of cognitive behaviour therapy versus treatment as usual in the treatment of mild to moderate late life depression. *International Journal of Geriatric Psychiatry, 23*, 843–850.

Levy, B.R. (2003). Mind matters: Cognitive and physical effects of aging stereotypes. *Journal of Gerontology; Psychological Sciences, 58B*, 203–211.

McAdam, D. (2001). The psychology of life stories. *Journal of General Psychology, 5*, 100–122.

McAdam, D. (2006). The redemptive self: Generativity and the stories that Americans live by. *Research in Human Development, 3,* 81–100.

Mohlman, J., & Gorman, J.M. (2005). The role of executive functioning in CBT: A pilot study with anxious older adults. *Behaviour Research & Therapy, 43,* 447–465.

Mohlman, J., Cedeno, L.A., Price, R.B., Hekler, E.B., Yan, G.W., & Frishman, D.B. (2008). Deconstructing demons: The case of Geoffrey. *Pragmatic Case Studies in Psychotherapy, 4,* 1–39.

Pachana, N.A., Byrne, G.J., Siddle, H., Koloski, N., Harley, E., & Arnold, E. (2007). Development and validation of the Geriatric Anxiety Inventory. *International Psychogeriatrics, 19,* 103–114.

Pinquart, M., Duberstein, P.R., & Lyness, J.M. (2006). Treatments for later-life depressive conditions: A meta-analytic comparison of pharmacotherapy and psychotherapy. *American Journal of Psychiatry, 163,* 1493–1501.

Schwartz, B., & Sharpe, K.E. (2005). Practical wisdom: Aristotle meets positive psychology. *Journal of Happiness Studies, 7,* 377–395.

Scogin, F., Welsh, D., Hanson, A., Stump, J., & Coates, A. (2005). Evidence-based psychotherapies for depression in older adults. *Psychology Science Practice, 12,* 222–237.

Serfaty, M., Haworth, D., Blanchard, M., Buszewicz, M., Murad, S., & King, M. (2009). Clinical effectiveness of individual cognitive behavioral therapy for depressed older people in primary care: A randomized controlled trial. *Archives of General Psychiatry, 66,* 1332–1340.

Stanley, M.A., Wilson, N.L., Novy, D.M., et al. (2009). Cognitive behavior therapy for generalized anxiety disorder among older adults in primary care. A randomized controlled trial. *JAMA, 301,* 1460–1467.

Tedeschi, R.G., & Calhoun, L.G. (2004). Posttraumatic growth: Conceptual foundations and empirical evidence. *Psychological Inquiry, 15,* 1–18.

Tompkins, M.A. (2002). Guidelines for enhancing homework compliance. *JCLP/In session: Psychotherapy in Practice, 58,* 565–576.

Watkins, E.R. (2008). Constructive and unconstructive repetitive thought. *Psychological Bulletin, 134,* 163–206.

Watkins, E.R., Baeyens, C.B., & Read, R. (2009). Concreteness training reduces dysphoria: Proof-of-principle for repeated cognitive bias modification in depression. *Journal of Abnormal Psychology, 118,* 55–64.

Wilson, K., Mottram, P.G., & Vassilas, C.A. (2008). Psychotherapeutic treatments for older depressed people. *Cochrane Database of Systematic Reviews,* Issue 1. Art. No.: CD004853. DOI: 10.1002/14651858. CD0044853.pub2.

Zeiss, A.M., & Steffen, A. (1996). Treatment issues with elderly clients. *Cognitive & Behavioral Practice, 3,* 371–389.

Chapter 3

Caregiving issues in a therapeutic context: new insights from the Acceptance and Commitment Therapy approach

María Márquez-González, Rosa Romero-Moreno, and Andrés Losada

Introduction

Caregiver 1: Carmen

Carmen is in her fifties, and is caring for both her father, who suffers from Parkinson's disease, and her mother, diagnosed with Alzheimer's disease. Carmen's parents are living with her, together with her husband and daughters. When you ask Carmen how is she feeling about her caregiving role, she smiles and says "It's a pleasure for me to devote my whole life to them. They cared for me all my life … now it's my turn to give them back all the love they gave me." She says she has no emotional distress, nor is she feeling at all depressed or stressed. She says that caring for a relative is a wonderful task to be involved in, and that one must fulfill that role with joy and happiness, with a "permanent smile on my face." In recent weeks, Carmen has been suffering from severe lumbago, which has forced her to stay in bed for several days.

Caregiver 2: Julia

Julia is a middle-aged woman, a primary school teacher who is caring for her mother who suffers from Alzheimer's disease. Julia comes to therapy because she wants to understand why, after all these years of care, she still feels anxious and sad when she interacts with her mother. She says "At this stage of the game I should be able to manage my negative feelings. It says very little of me as a caregiver that I still get caught up in anger and despair."

Caregiver 3: Ángela

Ángela is 70 years old and is caring for her husband, John, who has vascular dementia. Ángela's main complaints revolve around John's inability to understand her and his problematic behaviors—such as wandering and aggressiveness—which she thinks represent deliberate attempts to demand her attention, love, and affection. She is a highly protective caregiver, and almost never leaves her husband at home with other people because "My poor guy, he misses me a lot and reacts with anger and despair. I don't want him to suffer like that. So I don't want anyone else helping me in this. It's my responsibility."

Carmen, Julia, and Ángela share, at least, the following characteristics: (a) they are Spanish women; (b) they are devoted caregivers who place caregiving at the center of their lives; and (c) they find it hard to cope with one of the main challenges involved in dementia caregiving: acceptance. Carmen has trouble acknowledging that she is a human being and, consequently, has negative feelings and needs rest and nurturance. Julia is angry at herself for not being able to overcome uncomfortable feelings. Finally, Ángela is reluctant to admit that her husband has dementia and that he is no longer the intelligent and sensitive man he once was ... and keeps trying to reason and argue with him. Moreover, she will not accept any help from other people.

In this chapter, we present a brief overview of the sociocultural context of caregiving in Spain, placed within a broader Hispanic and Latin cultural context. We focus on the description of a framework for intervention with caregivers based on a contextual behavioral approach, specifically, Acceptance and Commitment Therapy (ACT). In order to help clinicians working with caregivers, we offer reflections and suggestions on the use of ACT with caregivers, as well as a guide for the assessment of the variables considered relevant within this approach, and a description of different therapeutic tools that can be used to achieve the objectives of this intervention model. The application of this approach is illustrated with examples of cases treated in our clinical practice. Finally, we briefly present preliminary data from an ACT-based group intervention and conclude with an integrative summary delineating the usefulness of an ACT approach for addressing complex psychosocial issues in family dementia caregivers.

Culture, gender, and caregiving in Spain

Various cultural and social aspects of Spanish society, such as the importance of the family and filial piety, are similar to those of other Latin or Hispanic cultures. In our country, however, historic events (e.g. the Spanish Civil War) and their correlates, both socioeconomic (lack of resources and difficulties in the access to formal education) and cultural (e.g. emphasis on traditionalism and conservatism, and strong influence of the Catholic Church), have contributed to the development of a profile in older adults, especially in women, characterized by a low educational level, conservative values, Catholicism, and the central role of family (Pérez, 2004; Sancho, Abellán, Pérez, & Miguel, 2002). In the Spanish cultural context, providing care for an older relative is highly valued as a moral obligation, as one of the purest manifestations of the values of familism and filial piety. *Good persons*, and specifically, *good women*, are expected to care for their relatives so as to allow them to stay in the community for as long as possible. Furthermore, cultural norms and the Catholic religion, so important for Spanish older adults, also dictate that the caregiving role should be fulfilled with patience, satisfaction, dignity, and even joy.

Although the study of the effects of religion and religiosity in the caregiving context remains scarce, and has yielded mixed results (Hebert, Weinstein, Martire, & Schulz, 2006), various studies carried out with non-caregivers have obtained data suggesting that Catholics, as opposed to those with other religious affiliations (e.g. Protestants), show higher distress reactions to stressors (Alferi, Culver, Carver, Arena, & Antoni, 1999; Park, Cohen, & Herb, 1990). Such results might be interpreted, albeit cautiously, in terms of the suppression of negative emotions (Danner, Snowdown, & Friesen, 2001). In this sense, it is interesting that a significant percentage (65.9%) of Spanish caregivers (predominantly Catholic) were found to report that none of 20 common behavioral problems (e.g. repeating questions, wandering, or agitation) of their relatives bothered them (IMSERSO, 2005), even when it is widely assumed in the caregiving literature that these behaviors are usually the most stressful factors for caregivers.

Reliance on the family is an issue that links different Hispanic and Latin cultural groups, and this characteristic has indeed been suggested as being positive for caregiving. However, research suggests that this issue is not clear. Losada et al. (2010) argue that familism is not necessarily positive for caregiving, finding significant associations between reports of family-oriented values and distress. This negative effect of familism on caregiving was interpreted in terms of a shift within Spanish culture in recent years, from a collectivistic tradition toward an individualistic way of thinking and behaving. This is similar to societal changes reported in other countries, where there has been a reduction in secondary caregivers' involvement (Wolff & Kasper, 2006). This may contribute to a phenomenon whereby having family-oriented values in an individualistic society that obstructs people from adhering to those values can lead to an increase in caregiver distress.

Although caregiving is gender-based throughout the world (women being the main providers of care), this is especially true in the Hispanic culture. And while recent decades in Spain have seen the guarantees for equal consideration of men and women increase (e.g. in the labor force), the reality is that caregiving continues to be a task done by females: 84% of caregivers of dependent older people are women (IMSERSO, 2005), compared to figures of around 67% in other countries (Wolff & Kasper, 2006). Indeed, the percentage of female caregivers in Spain has remained stable and even increased between 1995 and 2005 (IMSERSO, 2005).

In summary, the most likely profile of a Spanish caregiver is as follows: a woman in her fifties or sixties, caring for her mother or spouse, with low educational attainment, Catholic, and with strong familistic beliefs. She would very likely be the primary caregiver, since "it is her responsibility, and other relatives have their own life's struggles and obligations." At the same time as striving to be a good caregiver, this female caregiver would likely be trying to be a good mother, a good spouse and, in several cases, a good professional.

From change to acceptance: experiential avoidance and caregiving

Dementia caregiving is associated with high levels of depressive symptomatology and emotional distress, as well as with poor physical health indicators (Pinquart & Sörensen, 2003; Vitaliano, Zhang, & Scanlan, 2003). The majority of interventions with caregivers have been carried out within the stress and coping framework adapted to caregiving (Knight, Silverstein, McCallum, & Fox, 2000) and have mainly focused on reducing caregivers' level of perceived stress, burden, and depression by training them in effective coping strategies for dealing with stress (support-seeking, coping skills for managing behavioral problems, self-care, etc.). These psychoeducational and, especially, psychotherapeutic interventions can be considered as empirically validated, having shown success in reducing caregiver distress (Gallagher-Thompson & Coon, 2007). However, the effect sizes of these interventions are, at best, moderate (Pinquart & Sörensen, 2006), with the highest effect sizes corresponding to cognitive behavioral interventions.

Cognitive behavioral therapy (CBT) interventions with caregivers are aimed at challenging and modifying dysfunctional thoughts and beliefs that are considered to be at the root of caregiver distress (Gallagher-Thompson & Coon, 2007; Márquez-González, Losada, Izal, Pérez, & Montorio, 2007). Put another way, CBT encourages a **change** in maladaptive cognitions viewed as antecedents of caregiver depression and emotional distress. This change in cognitions leads to better coping with caregiving stressors, and thus helps caregivers adapt to their situation. Even though CBT-based interventions present the highest effect sizes among psychotherapeutic treatment, those effect sizes are no more than moderate, and their mechanisms of action have not been fully clarified by research to date (Pinquart & Sörensen, 2006).

Recently, some researchers and clinicians have begun to highlight the relevance of **acceptance** in the caregiving experience (McCurry, 2006; Spira et al., 2007). Caring for a loved relative involves high doses of unavoidable suffering, together with unchangeable losses and stressors. There appear to be two different areas of potential acceptance in caregivers: (a) acceptance of external situations and events that are associated with emotional distress (diagnosis of dementia, memory and attention deficits, some components of problematic behaviors, etc.) and (b) acceptance of internal events (physical sensations, emotions, thoughts, etc.). Caregivers' failure to accept these components of their experience has been found to lead to higher levels of distress. With regard to the first type of acceptance, avoidant coping styles (escape, denial, use of alcohol or drugs, and compulsive eating) have proven ineffective for dealing with caregiving stressors, and may even lead to heightened levels of distress (Knight et al., 2000). The other type of acceptance— the acceptance of internal events or an active tendency to allow the occurrence of aversive or painful sensations, emotions, and thoughts without making any attempt to modify either their content or their frequency (Hayes et al., 2004)—has been far less widely studied in caregivers. Experiential avoidance, that is, the tendency or desire to control and/or avoid the occurrence of uncomfortable emotions, sensations, and thoughts (Hayes, Wilson, Gifford, Follete, & Strosahl, 1996), can involve actively escaping from these unpleasant aspects through overt actions (distracting activities, substance abuse, compulsive actions, etc.) or covert ones (mental rituals or compulsions, thought or emotion suppression, denial etc.).

To our knowledge, there is only one recent study exploring the role of experiential avoidance in caregiving, namely, that of Spira et al. (2007). These authors found a significant positive correlation between this variable and caregivers' level of emotional distress, an association which remained significant even when the effects of problem-behavior frequency and caregivers' level of negative affect were statistically controlled.

Outside the caregiving field there is increasing evidence of the negative psychological implications of experiential avoidance (for a review, see Hayes et al., 1996). Attempts to avoid or suppress uncomfortable emotions and thoughts will not only be unsuccessful, but also exhausting, as they interfere with emotional processing, in such a way that the greater the level of avoidance, the more likely it is that these emotions and thoughts will return to the person, in a sort of "boomerang effect" (Campbell-Sills, Barlow, Brown, & Hofmann, 2006; Rachman, 1980). Another negative consequence of experiential avoidance is that people caught in this "trap of control" become involved in a pointless battle which can divert them from their values and their life goals (Hayes & Smith, 2005). This distance between individuals and their values eventually leads to increased emotional distress and depression (Orsillo, Roemer, & Barlow, 2003).

Returning to caregiving, the tendency of caregivers to avoid internal events (experiential avoidance) or unchangeable external situations can indeed result in greater depression and emotional distress in this population. Closely related to experiential avoidance are other relevant variables referring to caregivers' styles of experiencing and managing their emotions, such as limitations in emotional awareness, difficulties for processing, identifying, and being aware of feelings and emotions (*alexithymia*), or emotional suppression, which has been found to be significantly associated with experiential avoidance (Kashdan, Barrios, Forsyth, & Steger, 2006).

Identifying and targeting caregivers' patterns of experiential avoidance, limitations in emotional awareness and other difficulties of emotional processing and regulation would appear to be an important challenge for intervention in this area, and an approach that may help to improve our understanding of caregivers' distress and the effectiveness of interventions with this population.

Another important issue arising within caregiving research is the excessive focus by clinicians and researchers on the negative aspects of caregiving. Most interventions are focused almost exclusively on reducing levels of depression, perceived stress and burden, and usually ignore the positive aspects also inherent to the caregiving experience. It is not infrequent among caregivers to find positive subjective experiences, such as satisfaction, life meaning, a sense of purpose or coherence, self-actualization, growth or gratitude, which derive from the fulfillment of their values of love, sacrifice, familial obligation, filial piety, and reciprocity. These positive experiences are probably among the main factors explaining the fact that, in spite of primary and secondary caregiving stressors (problematic behaviors, emotional distress, depressive feelings, family conflicts, etc.), most caregivers remain in their role of caregiver for a long time—often until the death of the loved one. Hence, targeting values in psychotherapeutic interventions with caregivers, helping them to become more aware of them, to clarify and define them, and to develop actions that bring them closer to them, could be a promising pathway toward improving the effectiveness of such interventions.

A contextual behavioral approach to caregiving: acceptance and commitment therapy

There is considerable excitement in the fields of clinical and health psychology over the power of acceptance and commitment to help people reduce their emotional distress. Both the theoretical considerations reviewed above and the empirical evidence accumulated to date have crystallized in the form of a new therapeutic paradigm called ACT (Hayes, Stroshal, & Wilson, 1999). This approach emerges as a powerful therapeutic alternative for treating people with any type of psychopathology (mental disorders) or emotional distress involving some amount of experiential avoidance and the associated distance from life values. Evidence supporting the effectiveness of ACT has grown exponentially in recent years (Hayes, Luoma, Bond, Masuda, & Lillis, 2006).

Based on a philosophy of science known as functional contextualism, ACT is one of the "third wave" behavior therapies (Hayes, 2004). These therapies are considered to represent a "third wave" because, in contrast to the "second wave" behavior therapies (cognitive therapy), they are not focused on the elimination or change in the form, frequency, or content of internal events (thoughts and emotions), but rather target their functional associations with behavior, aiming to increase *psychological flexibility*, or the ability to behave in accordance with one's own values regardless of inner experiences.

ACT has proven especially useful for presentations or disorders that include unchangeable aspects, such as the emotional distress of parents of children with developmental disorders (Blackledge & Hayes, 2006) or people with chronic pain (McCracken & Eccleston, 2006). Dementia caregiving, as mentioned above, also involves many unchangeable aspects that caregivers should better learn to accept. In spite of this, however, and the promising results from empirical research on the effectiveness of ACT, the constructs considered to be central from this approach (experiential avoidance, value-driven actions, etc.) have not yet been sufficiently articulated in our models of intervention with caregivers.

Given this situation, we have adapted ACT for our clinical work with caregivers. In this chapter, we set out a rationale for intervention with this population, and describe some therapeutic tools for use in this context.

A working model for developing acceptance and commitment therapy interventions with caregivers

According to Hayes et al. (1999), ACT is not a set of new techniques to be applied "by the book," but rather a therapeutic *approach* based on a refined philosophy of the human condition (functional contextualism) and a rigorous psychological theory (relational frame theory and analysis of rule-governed behavior). In this section, we present an ACT-based model of intervention with caregivers, aimed at providing professionals with a framework within which they can design ACT-based tailored interventions for helping caregivers according to their specific and unique profile of vulnerabilities and difficulties, on the one hand, and strengths and resources, on the other. This framework focus on the two central modules of ACT, namely: (a) **acceptance** of uncomfortable internal events (emotions, thoughts, sensations) and the situations and stimuli involved in their emergence (e.g. dementia-related behaviors) and (b) **commitment** to personal values: clarifying and choosing valued directions in one's life and taking actions to move toward the chosen values. Within this framework, values and life directions are considered to be the *frame* of the intervention, as they represent powerful forces that guide human behavior. Helping caregivers to clarify and connect (or reconnect) to these forces may facilitate that they develop a sense of choice and freedom to value what they really want to value, and to follow the life directions they want to follow, instead of having the sense of coercion or "having to" value specific things and behave in specific ways. In this sense, they can learn to (re) connect with the personal values involved in caregiving and to remind themselves what they want their lives to stand for, in order to give back meaning to their everyday tasks and transform their daily caregiving experiences from an obligatory routine into a choice they make every day of their own free will.

This ACT-based working model for intervention does not pretend to be either exclusive or exhaustive, and it is compatible with and can be complemented by other therapeutic techniques of proven effectiveness in interventions with caregivers. In fact, in addition to these basic ACT components, we included other complementary therapeutic components that we have found very useful in our clinical practice with caregivers:

a. A starting module aimed at fostering *emotional awareness* and *understanding*

b. A module focused on helping caregivers to *"learn the dance between acceptance and change," that is,* to learn to adaptively analyze situations in order to opt for change, when it is reasonable and possible, or for acceptance, depending on the specific nature of the problem. We consider this ability to flexibly opt for acceptance or for change depending on the nature of the problem to be a central skill to be developed by caregivers, which is wonderfully described in the *Serenity Prayer,* "God grant me the serenity to accept the things I cannot change; the courage to change the things I can; and the wisdom to know the difference between them" (Reinhold Niebuhr).

Figure 3.1 shows the main components of our model of intervention.

The starting point: assessment of caregivers' profile of experiential avoidance and commitment to values

At the beginning of this chapter we described the cases of three female caregivers who had in common trouble for *accepting* different aspects of their caregiving experience. Carmen had difficulties accepting her negative feelings and her need for help in caregiving, nurturance, and rest. Julia did not accept the persistence of emotional pain and suffering in her daily caring for her beloved mother. Ángela had trouble accepting her husband's illness and his personality and cognitive changes. These different types of avoidance are not uncommon among caregivers. The cases of Carmen and Julia illustrate quite well the phenomenon called experiential avoidance, while the case of Julia involves the denial and non-acceptance of dementia-related changes and behaviors. The assessment of the caregiver's specific profile of avoidance is thus a first step in this approach to intervention.

As suggested in the section "Culture, gender, and caregiving in Spain," our cultural context may foster caregivers' experiential avoidance through the social rejection or punishment of moral and culturally "deviant" behaviors, such as the expression of some kind of negative feelings (anxiety, distress, anger) or thoughts (negative thoughts toward the care recipient, thinking it would be better if the person died, etc.) related to their caregiving role. It is not infrequent to find,

STARTING POINT: CONTACTING OUR EMOTIONS:
Fostering emotional awareness and understanding

LEARNING THE DANCE BETWEEN ACCEPTANCE AND CHANGE

God grant me the serenity to accept the things I cannot change;
the courage to change the things I can; and the wisdom to know the difference.
(The Serenity Prayer)

The Route Of Problem Analysis ⇨ | REALISTIC CHANGE

⇩

ACCEPTANCE

- Acceptance of internal aversive events (emotions, thoughts, sensations and needs) and of unchangeable dementia-related behaviours and situations (diagnosis, memory deficits, etc.)
  - Clean versus dirty discomfort
  - The paradox of "internal control"
  - Am I a Supercaregiver? Acknowledging my vulnerability and needs
  - Healthy Emotion Regulation

COMMITMENT TO VALUED LIFE DIRECTIONS
The centrality of Valued Life Directions (values)

Values involved in caregiving	Other valued life directions

• Clarifying and revisiting the values involved in caregiving: positive aspects of being a caregiver.
 	
• What does it mean to be a good caregiver?
    ○ Analysis of unrealistic expectations
    ○ Planning and involvement in committed actions.
	• Clarifying and revisiting caregivers' values in other life domains
	
	• Analysis of potential barriers to commitment
	
	• Take action: committed actions to get closer to personal values.

Fig. 3.1 Proposed model of ACT-based intervention with caregivers.

in our cultural context, caregivers who deny that they feel depressed about caregiving, while tears run down their cheeks. Likewise, many caregivers reject the word "burden" (in Spanish, *carga*) as a descriptor of their subjective experience and, in turn, highlight the positive aspects of caregiving as being more important for them.

Hayes et al. (2004) developed the Acceptance and Action Questionnaire (AAQ) to measure experiential avoidance. Although this instrument has appropriate psychometric properties and strong predictive validity, endorsing the role of experiential avoidance both as a correlate and as a predictor of emotional distress and psychopathology, in our opinion its items fail to address the specific types of experiential avoidance which are most prevalent in caregivers. In order to measure caregivers' level of experiential avoidance in the specific context of caregiving, we have developed the Experiential Avoidance in Caregiving Questionnaire (EACQ; see Table 3.1), that was based on the AAQ and on our clinical experience with caregivers. A 15-item measure, its responses are coded on a Likert-type scale that ranges from 1 ("totally disagree") to 7 ("totally agree"). Preliminary data obtained from a sample of 44 caregivers suggest that this questionnaire has adequate reliability (Cronbach's alpha of 0.72). However, this information should be taken cautiously, as a study with a larger sample is currently being developed, and more in-depth psychometric analyses on this will be performed.

Table 3.1 Experiential Avoidance in Caregiving Questionnaire

1.	A caregiver should not have bad thoughts about the person cared for.
2.	I always tend to excuse other relatives less involved in the caring, thinking things like "they're busier, they have their own lives...."
3.	I'm frightened at the emotions and thoughts I have in relation to my relative.
4.	I can't bear getting angry with my sick relative.
5.	You shouldn't feel rejection or other unpleasant emotions toward the person you're caring for.
6.	I can't bear having bad thoughts or feeling bad about having to care for my relative.
7.	Every time I get bad thoughts about my relative or my situation as a carer, I try to escape from them and amuse myself.
8.	It is normal for a carer to have negative thoughts and feelings about the person he/she is caring for (reverse-scored).
9.	It is normal to feel stress and depression when you are caring for a dependent relative (reverse-scored).
10.	When I feel bad about my situation, I try to amuse myself with some other activity so that the feeling quickly goes away.
11.	If a carer has negative thoughts toward his/her relative, the best thing for him/her is to do whatever possible to make them go away.
12.	I tend to "ignore" negative thoughts toward my relative that come into my mind.
13.	I try not to look into how I feel inside, because I believe that would make things worse.
14.	When you're caring for a sick person, it's better not to stop and think about what you're feeling or thinking.
15.	In difficult situations of the caring, in which I might need some type of support, I prefer not to talk to other relatives if it might cause conflict.

Other important variables to be assessed are emotional awareness and clarification of and commitment to values. Emotional awareness can be measured with the *Emotional Awareness* subscale from the *Trait Meta-Mood Scale* (Salovey et al., 1995) or with the *Toronto Alexithymia Scale (TAS-20*; Bagby, Parker, & Taylor, 1994). Values clarification and commitment can be measured with the Values Assessment Rating Form (Hayes et al., 1999).

Acceptance and Commitment Therapy-based intervention for caregivers: therapeutic tools

In this section, some of the components of the therapeutic approach outlined in Fig. 3.1 are described and illustrated through some exercises and metaphors we have found useful in our practice with caregivers. Examples of caregivers' experiences drawn from our clinical work with them are included to illustrate the applications of these therapeutic tools. Specifically, these examples are taken from the caregivers introduced at the beginning of this chapter. Comments about the use and the difficulties potentially involved in the application of these therapeutic tools are also included.

Starting point. Fostering emotional awareness and understanding

In line with emotion-focused therapeutic approaches (Greenberg & Paivio, 1997; Baker, 2001), we assume that emotions are powerful organizers of behavior and self-regulation, which act as *signals* that inform people about their transactions with the world, life situations, and people.

Emotions are essential experiences resulting from the fact that persons are *alive*, *in touch* with the world and other people, and affected by them in several ways. They can tell us important things about our position in the world, and about how we are affected by things that happen to us. Hence, emotions can be interpreted and used as *cues* for adaptive action, as they contain important information about the person (his/her relationship with the world and other persons, his/her response tendencies, etc.), which can help him/her cope successfully with life challenges and behave in more adaptive ways (Safran & Greenberg, 1988). This assumption is also consistent with Salovey and Mayer's (1990) model of Emotional Intelligence, whose components include the abilities of emotional clarity, emotional understanding, and effective utilization of emotions for guiding, thinking, and facilitating adaptive behavior.

Also, consistently with the construct of emotional processing, we assume that, even when they are painful or aversive, emotions have to enter awareness and accepted by the person in order to be fully processed, that is, "absorbed and declined to the extent that other experiences and behavior can proceed without disruption" (Rachman, 1980, p. 51).

In our clinical practice with caregivers, especially older ones, we commonly observe limitations in their ability to undertake psychological introspection and to be aware of and acknowledge their emotions, especially the more uncomfortable ones. Many caregivers also have difficulty labeling, understanding, and accepting their emotional experiences. Given this situation, we believe that a first step in intervention with caregivers may be to foster emotional awareness and understanding, necessary skills for building other abilities that constitute the focus of the other intervention modules. Specifically, the **objectives** of this module are to help caregivers:

a. to connect with their emotions and increase their emotional awareness;

b. to increase their ability for emotion labeling (naming their emotions) and discrimination (distinguishing between them);

c. to understand their emotions, acknowledging their intimate association with situations, experiences, thoughts, and bodily sensations, and the importance of emotions as fundamental cues for adaptive action; and

d. to increase caregivers' awareness of their reactions to their own painful emotions and to begin exploring their potential tendency to experiential avoidance.

Emotional awareness and understanding can be worked on with the caregiver through different exercises, such as the following one.

Exercise: "Contacting my painful emotions"

In this exercise, the therapist asks the caregiver to remember a recent situation in which she had felt a painful emotion (i.e. an uncomfortable or aversive emotional experience). The therapist tells the caregiver to try and recreate the scene and re-experience the emotion. It is sometimes helpful to ask her to close her eyes. A time is allowed for the caregiver to relive the experience. She is then asked the following questions, telling her that it is not necessary to answer them immediately, and that she can take her time to think about them:

- What emotions did you have?
- In which part of your body did you feel this emotion? What sensations did you have in your body while you were feeling that way?
- Did something happen in your life that could be related to these emotions?
- What were you thinking at that moment?
- How did you react to those feelings? What did you do then? Did you try to ignore, deny, avoid, or change them? How?

After reliving the experience, the therapist asks the caregiver these other questions:

- How difficult was it for you to recreate the experience?
- Are you usually in touch with your emotions?
- How do you usually react to your painful feelings? What do you usually do when you feel an aversive emotion?

The final step in this exercise is to ask caregivers to analyze their emotions at home, following the schema learnt in this exercise. To help them do so, they are given a self-record with the instruction to record and analyze some of their emotions: (What emotion am I feeling? Bodily sensations associated with this emotion; Situation associated with this emotion; Thoughts related to this emotion; and What did I do with my emotion? Did I do something to modify it?) and bring this material to the next session to work on it.

Example from a caregiver

When she refuses my help in dressing her, I usually feel a deep sadness … I felt it in my chest, like pressure … and in my throat … and then sadness changed to frustration, a sort of anger toward myself … I remember I thought 'every day the same story, once again … When will I overcome this feeling? When will I get used to this? Eight years caring for her and I still feel the same sadness … something is wrong with me'.

This exercise usually reveals the difficulty for caregivers to analyze their emotions and the factors associated with them. It seems especially difficult for them to be aware of the bodily sensations accompanying their emotions. This therapeutic tool is also helpful for exploring the presence of experiential avoidance, which can involve medication-related emotional numbness and secondary emotions related to the non-acceptance of the emotions felt (anger in the example). This exercise is also interesting for observing caregivers' repertoire of emotion regulation strategies, such as emotion suppression, and other potential barriers to the expression of emotions.

Acceptance of aversive internal events

Acceptance is one of the central modules of the intervention. As mentioned above, many caregivers have difficulty accepting aversive emotions. Many others have problems accepting negative thoughts about their relatives, or their situation, and still others have trouble accepting their vulnerabilities, needs, and weaknesses. It is also common to find caregivers who refuse to accept a dementia diagnosis or the dementia-related changes and behavior of their relatives. This module has the following **objectives**:

a. To help caregivers understand the concepts of "experiential avoidance" and clean versus dirty discomfort (Hayes et al., 1999), and analyze them in their own experience.

b. To help them understand the paradox of control, in other words, that excessive attempts at control of thoughts and emotions are the real problem, as well as the negative consequences of trying to avoid the unavoidable.

c. To train them in the appropriate alternative to avoidance: ACCEPTANCE of or openness to experiencing aversive emotions and thoughts (and the unchangeable situations associated with their occurrence) without trying to modify them, avoid them, or change them (WILLINGNESS).

d. To help them develop or enhance healthy emotion regulation strategies, which can in turn help them to accept their aversive internal experiences and accommodate to the difficult situations that generate them.

In our work with caregivers we have found the following exercises and metaphors to be very useful: "*the rule of private events*" (Hayes et al., 1999, pp. 120–122), "*don't think of pink elephants*," "*don't feel your tongue"* (asking them to notice their tongue, and then to try to suppress these sensations), "and "the *polygraph*"" (Hayes et al., 1999, p. 123). In this module, in order to keep track of caregivers' general degree of acceptance or openness to internal experiences (and its inverse, experiential avoidance), besides the self-recording task described in the exercise *"Contacting my painful emotions,"* we also use an adaptation of the *Daily Willingness Diary* (Hayes et al., 1999, p. 144) as caregiver homework. Our adaptation of this tool consists of a self-recorded task in which caregivers are asked to keep a daily record of the frequency (1—none to 10—extreme) of their main aversive experiential states (e.g. emotions such as anxiety, despair, or uncomfortable thoughts), and the degree of effort they have put into fighting against these states or remove them (*struggle*) (1—none to 10—extreme). We usually do not include the *workability* question of the original instrument, as we have found it to be rather complex for many caregivers to understand.

We have had difficulties, however, with the application of defusion techniques for building acceptance. In our experience, the successful application of deliteralization exercises aimed at defusing language and thought requires abilities for abstract thinking and metacognition on the part of the client. Beside the described tools for fostering acceptance, we have developed some new ones that are described below.

Exercise: "Isabel, the Supercaregiver"

In this exercise, the therapist reads to the caregiver the story of Isabel, "the Supercaregiver." This story is made up of two parts:

Part one:

Isabel cares for her mother, who has had Alzheimer's disease for 3 years. The illness has progressively taken away her mother's independence, and Isabel currently helps her mother with almost all her daily activities. Isabel has brothers and sisters, but they are not so close to her mother, and Isabel took on the caregiver role because she loves her mother and because she believes her mother deserves it, since she has been a really good mother. Since she began looking after her (giving up her job to do so), she has agreed to be the caregiver, and says she is HAPPY to have this opportunity to show her mother all her love. She treats her mother 'like a queen,' waits on her hand-and-foot, and says she is going to slow the illness and decline through her care. She also says that she has cared with energy and happiness since the first day, and is oblivious to any kind of depression because she does not allow herself to be influenced by circumstances. 'People who know me know that 'I'm made of iron,' and although nobody believes me when I say I've never had a negative thought or feeling, it's the truth, I'm really strong'. Her whole life revolves around her mother. Her aim in life is that her mother is well cared for and feels loved. The truth is that Isabel's mother usually behaves in an aggressive and rebellious manner, insults Isabel, and doesn't accept being looked after. Moreover, for a few weeks now, her mother has been showing some signs of not recognizing her daughter, asking 'Who are you?' at different times. In such circumstances, Isabel says that she always maintains a positive attitude, and never loses her smile: 'I'm not like other caregivers, who give up and put their relative in a home at the first sign of difficulties'. Isabel never has 'negative thoughts' about her mother; she always thinks in the positive, and never feels angry or resentful towards other relatives ... she understands them: 'Poor guys, they are busy with their lives and families'. Of course, she has never thought anything similar to: 'It would be better for her to die and not suffer'. She has complete control of her emotions and negative thoughts.

After reading the first part of the story, the therapist analyzes *several aspects of the story by performing the following questions to caregivers:*

> THERAPIST: What are your thoughts about Isabel? Do you know anybody who behaves like Isabel? Do you think it could be a real case? Do you consider yourself to be similar to Isabel in any respect? Would you like to be like her? Do you think it's possible for a caregiver to always feel strong and happy not to have a single moment of despair or weakness?

Is it possible for a caregiver to be free from suffering or any kind of negative emotion? Is it possible for any person, caregiver or not, to be always happy and strong?

Examples from caregivers
Example1

I strongly identify myself with Isabel, and I think she is a wonderful example to every caregiver. We all should be like her: positive. If we focus on the negative, it's much worse. I try to do my best and I think I'm pretty much like her most of the time.

Example 2

I think Isabel cannot be a real case, since it is impossible to be free from suffering. I think Isabel is trying to be the perfect caregiver, which is impossible, I think. But it's true that I find myself acting like her in many ways … this exercise has made me realize that I often set very high standards for myself.

After this first analysis, the second part of Isabel's story is told to the caregiver:

Part two:
But look what has happened to Isabel. For some weeks now she has not been sleeping well at night and has had pains in different parts of her body and a racing heart; she has also discovered that her blood pressure is really high … Furthermore, she has been suffering from severe headaches with no organic explanation according to medical examinations. Last week she lost her temper and shouted at her mother, and she does not know why. She spent all day feeling guilty for behaving so badly. Since that day there have been similar episodes. Isabel has begun to feel guilty and sad, and cannot understand what is happening to her or why she is unable to continue gently accepting whatever life deals her. She is angry with herself and frightened that she is no longer a good caregiver. Isabel does not like how she is feeling or some of the thoughts that are 'coming' into her head. That is why she does not want to spend a minute of her time thinking about how she feels. She does not stop doing things, always cleaning her house, and her mother is cared for 'better than a queen'. She has been to see her general practitioner (GP) about her sleep problems, and now takes medication at night and at times when she feels anxious. At home, her husband has noticed that she is nervous, and says that she loses her temper very easily. However, when asked 'How are you?' Isabel continues to give her best smile and say 'I'm always fine, thank God, with the same problems as always, but I never lose my smile, as you can see'.

After reading the second part of the story, the caregiver is asked the following questions:

THERAPIST: What are your thoughts about Isabel now? What do you think is happening to Isabel?

Through the discussion and analysis of the story, the following ideas are worked on with the caregiver. In caregiving situations:

- There are high doses of natural suffering and of objective and unavoidable pain and discomfort associated with the fact of watching a loved one's suffering and decline and coping with his/her problematic behaviors, memory problems, and dependence. This natural suffering is the ***clean discomfort.***
- It is normal for caregivers, as the human beings they are, to have negative thoughts (e.g. "I wish it would all end soon!") and negative feelings toward the care recipient (e.g. "Sometimes I feel like pushing him away").
- It is healthy for caregivers to acknowledge and ACCEPT these aversive internal experiences, and to allow themselves to have and express them.
- Many caregivers find it hard to acknowledge these internal events. Also, many caregivers feel guilty or angry at themselves for having these negative thoughts and emotions. This is the

dirty discomfort: feeling bad for having natural negative emotions and thoughts. People who experience dirty discomfort may be prone to avoiding the clean discomfort by engaging in **experiential avoidance**.

♦ Isabel, the "Supercaregiver" did not allow herself to have the natural aversive feelings and thoughts that can arise in caregiving situations (e.g. denial of negative emotions: "I have never had a moment of despair or weakness"). She avoided the clean discomfort (experiential avoidance) through several strategies, and eventually began experiencing dirty discomfort (guilt, anger at herself) and several health problems.

♦ The result of experiencing dirty discomfort and avoiding natural distress is an increase in suffering.

Once the caregiver has understood the concepts of clean and dirty discomfort and experiential avoidance, he/she is asked to identify examples of clean and dirty discomfort in his/her life.

Exercise: "My best friend ... and me"

This exercise is very helpful for bolstering caregivers' acceptance of their vulnerabilities and their need for rest, nurturance, support, and care. Also, it helps caregivers become aware of their "double moral standards," that is, the different consideration of other people's needs and rights and of their own needs and rights.

The therapist tells the caregivers the story of Encarna:

THERAPIST: I have known Encarna since childhood. I remember how they used to take us to play together in the park and we would spend hours there. We had some really good times together. She's one of my best friends. That's all a long time ago, but what's really special is that, even though nowadays we see a lot less of one another, she's someone I can rely on for anything. Whenever I've had a problem she's been the first to listen to me, support me. We know each other so well and there's so much trust between us that it gives me peace of mind to know that she's there for whatever I may need. A lot of things have happened to us in our lives, and right now Encarna is in a very painful situation. Her son has just died, aged 32, in a road accident. She has a granddaughter aged just 2, and the little girl's mother has to look after her alone without any income to support her. Encarna feels immense pain, has lost interest in everything, and constantly thinks' Why did it happen to me?' She cries a lot and feels angry and powerless, and doesn't understand why she has such feelings. Moreover, since all of this happened, Encarna's health has got considerably worse. She has muscular pain and headaches, and it takes a great effort for her to do anything at all.

Now, imagine that Encarna is your best friend. Think how you would behave toward her, if you would devote time to her, how you would advise her, if you would understand her situation. To help you reflect on this, answer the following questions: Is Encarna in a difficult situation? Does she need help? Would you help her? Would you listen to her? How would you help her?

Examples from caregivers

Example 1

She really needs help. I understand that she has feelings of sadness and pain because it's a very difficult situation. I'll try to help her realize that she needs to care for herself ... if she got angry or irritable I would understand that she is highly vulnerable, and I would forgive her.

Example 2

She needs to be nurtured .... I would give her treats, because she's weak and needs support ... I would look after her because she needs it.

The exercise continues with new questions for the caregiver:

THERAPIST: Now think about your own situation as a caregiver. Imagine to what extent you are Encarna? Which characteristics of Encarna could be applied to you? In order to reflect on this, answer the same questions that you answered for Encarna's situation, but as they apply to your situation as a caregiver, and think to what extent you behave in the same way towards yourself.

Are you in a difficult situation? Do you need any kind of help? Do you give yourself the help you need? How do you help yourself? Do you listen to your feelings?

The responses in this case are also discussed, and compared with those for the case of Encarna. Usually, it is easy to find some discrepancy between what caregivers would do for Encarna and what they would do for themselves. In our experience, this exercise is very useful with many caregivers, who realize that they apply a "double standard" for themselves and for other people. By asking them about why they make such a distinction between other people and themselves, we can help them to acknowledge their own needs of rest and nurturance and identify some barriers to fulfill these needs, which can be worked on in subsequent sessions.

Caregiving in the context of personal values: revisiting caregivers' life directions and commitment to them

We consider this module to be the most important, as it gives *meaning* and *direction* to the whole intervention. The analysis and clarification of and commitment to personal values should be the *frame* of the intervention or, in other words, the context within which the rest of the components are worked on.

In clinical practice with caregivers it is commonly found that, in the process of becoming caregivers, many of them have lost contact with their life projects; their lives have become *fused* with the values of sacrifice, moral/familial obligation, and love, which crystallize in the objective of *being good caregivers*. In many cases, this objective occupies their entire life. Even though the life values inherent in the objective of *being a good caregiver* may be excellent sources of self-actualization, personal meaning, and purpose in life, we find that many caregivers, in their every-day caregiving activities, are not consciously driven by them, but instead act in quite automatic and routine ways, as though they had lost contact with these values which are at the root of their caregiving role, as they led them to choose to be "good caregivers." In this module, the **objectives** of the intervention are:

a. To help caregivers recover their contact with the values that give meaning/purpose to their caregiving role and to enhance their awareness of those values.

b. To help them clarify other values and meaningful objectives in their lives.

c. To motivate them to increase their commitment to their values, in order to reconnect with their life projects.

d. To train them to live their lives in full awareness of their valued directions.

Several different exercises and therapeutic tools can be used with a view to attaining these goals. Some of them are described in the following lines.

We begin this module using an adaptation of the ACT metaphor called "*Gardening*" (Wilson & Luciano, 2002, p. 113). We have adapted this metaphor into an experiential exercise that consti-tutes one of the most important in the entire therapeutic program, as it sets the stage for working with caregivers' values. Caregivers imagine that their lives are a garden, and the plants in that garden are the things they care about, the valued areas in their lives, their values. They reflect on his/her life values and goals and their level of commitment to them.

Example from a caregiver

It has a central square with three plants: in the centre, my mother, and, at each side of her, my daughters and my husband. Wonderful trees surround this square, which represent work and personal growth, development, evolution … Around the square there are beautiful flowers representing other family members and my friends. There's a big area in the garden with flowers representing health … and the garden has a gorgeous door bearing the word 'THANK YOU'…Gratitude is very important to me.

Some caregivers have quite limited capacity for abstract thinking, and have difficulty understanding that plants represent important things in their lives. Others can imagine each plant in their garden as a person, but have problems thinking of plants as relevant areas in their lives.

Although this exercise is generally very well received by many caregivers, they may think that *"being a good caregiver is incompatible with other roles in life, because you have no time left for other members of your family, and even less time for yourself."* In fact, many caregivers, on doing the exercise, realize that they have focused excessively on caring for their relative and have left behind some other important persons and areas in their life. Hence, the "caregiving plant" is usually located in the center of caregivers' garden, and is the one which is cared for most carefully by them. Useful therapeutic work can be done with regard to this important plant of their garden, such as helping caregivers reconnect with the life values involved in caregiving and to understand the importance of living in full awareness of those values in their everyday caregiving activity. To help caregivers reflect upon these issues, some questions the therapist can ask them are the following.

- ◆ Why do you keep on being a caregiver?
- ◆ How did you become a caregiver?
- ◆ Did you decide it of your own free will?
- ◆ Why did you choose this role?
- ◆ If the "perfect professional caregiver" existed and offered to care for your relative, would you delegate the task to him or her?
- ◆ Would you stop being the primary caregiver?
- ◆ Does caring for your relative bring you positive emotions and experiences?
- ◆ What type of experiences?

After the questions, caregivers are asked to come up with a slogan or *motto* that summarizes the personal values involved in their caregiving activity. We suggest they write down this slogan and put it in a place where they can easily see it whenever they want, especially at times when they get *"lost in the jungle"* of caregiving (see next metaphor).

After discussing these questions with the caregivers in session, we try to help them become aware of the verbal rules governing their behavior, the *norms* they have with regard to being *good caregivers* (*What does it mean for you to be a good caregiver? Do you think your expectations are realistic, or that they might be somewhat idealistic?*). We try to guide caregivers to see how their "high standards" might be acting as barriers for getting closer to important values in their lives or for caring better for other "plants in their garden."

The final phase of this value-focused module deals with the drawing-up of caregivers' "personal constitutions." In this exercise, caregivers integrate and consolidate the insights and learning from the whole therapy, and especially the module focusing on values. We consider that this exercise provides an excellent closure to the intervention and functions as a motivating factor for caregivers to keep moving toward their personal values in their lives. An example of a caregiver's personal constitution is presented in Table 3.2.

Metaphor: "Lost in the jungle"

The therapist tells the caregiver the following story:

Imagine you are an explorer and you have organized an expedition to the Amazon rainforest to find a new route to the sea. Full of hope, you start out on your journey and plunge into the jungle, following a route you have mapped out from the beginning … You walk for several days, full

Table 3.2 My personal constitution

Julia's personal constitution

◆ My motto for caregiving (Exercise: My Caregiving Plant):

"I remain in my role as caregiver because … *I love my mother and this is my way of thanking her for all the love and protection she has given me all my life. This is my way of paying her back.*"

◆ Regarding the other precious plants in my garden:

"I commit to these values that are very important for me…"

◆ *My personal health*

◆ *My personal growth*

◆ *The love for my husband*

My duties	**My rights**
What specific actions do I commit to doing in order to get close to my values?	What do I have license for? What am I going to allow myself to do, to think, or to feel?
◆ *To do regular exercise: 1-hour walking every day.*	◆ *To feel sad for my mother, sometimes: it is normal to feel that way sometimes.*
◆ *Sleep and read more.*	◆ *To feel nervous and irritated with my mother, sometimes, without feeling guilty.*
◆ *Improve my diet (eat better than I do now).*	
◆ *Go to a movie with my husband once a week.*	◆ *To get angry with other people, without feeling guilty.*
◆ *Attend that course on Ancient Egypt at the Cultural Center.*	◆ *To delegate more to my daughters.*
◆ *Keep on caring for my mother the way I do.*	◆ *To ask for more help.*

On my way to my values, I know that my weaknesses or areas where I have to put in special effort to overcome barriers are …

◆ *Thoughts and emotions: I have to accept my painful emotions, it is natural to feel this way (acceptance of emotions and thoughts); I have to avoid trying to reason with my heart and being such a perfectionist. I have to escape from the formula "I am a Supercaregiver" and acknowledge that I also need nurturance.*

◆ *I am excessively focused on my mother and I am oversensitive to her emotional states; hence, I'm easily caught by the emotional blackmail she unconsciously uses….*

I commit to keep moving toward my values, performing my committed actions and trying to overcome my personal barriers.

Date: *7th April 2009*   **Signature**: *Julia*

---

of confidence, overcoming all the obstacles in your way, putting up with the terrible heat, and torrential rain … defending yourself against the wild animals you encounter … but full of hope. Suddenly you begin to feel tired … Although you have a compass, the map you are using as a guide is very general, and does not allow you to orient yourself well … One day you realize you might be lost … You've been walking for weeks, and you don't know where you are … Now you start to feel anxious … the wild animals you meet seem more savage, and start to scare you … you feel the oppressive heat is getting to you … and the torrential rain sweeps away with it the little strength you have left … Suddenly you see in the distance some higher ground, a high hill that stands out above the trees … and you decide to go toward it. When finally, your strength running out, you get to the top of the hill to have a look … from that height you have a view over the whole jungle. Far in the distance you can see the point you left from, and the whole way you have come so far … You've walked further than you thought … and you can make out, also far in the distance, the shining sea, your destination … All at once it is as though your strength had come back, and with it your hope and confidence, because you had lost sight of the meaning of your expedition … and you have just regained it …

After this, the therapist asks the following questions to caregivers:

- What does this story tell you?
- Do you see yourself as the explorer?
- In what sense does this story relate to your life?
- Do you feel you are lost in the jungle?
- What kind of jungle are you in?
- Have you found your hill from which to observe the whole path you have trod?
- Do you know where are you going?

The crucial message to be transmitted to caregivers concerns the importance of reconnecting with the values that make caregiving so important for them: sacrifice, love, filial responsibility, and so on. We consider that it is really helpful for caregivers to re-establish contact with and remind themselves of the life values that some time ago led them to accept becoming caregivers, the same life values they pursue every day when they keep choosing that role and trying to be "good caregivers." This attitude makes obstacles more like challenges than like problems.

At this point, the next step is to explain to caregivers that, in order to get closer to their values, they must set objectives that can be operationalized (translated) into highly specific **committed actions**. Caregivers commit to carrying out the specified actions during the week and to record their degree of success. They are also asked to describe the barriers or obstacles they encounter for performing their committed actions. Their success with regard to commitment to personal values and performance of the committed actions is reviewed each week and consultation with them. This exercise provides highly relevant information about potential *blockages* in caregivers' paths to their values. Such blockages may be related to different types of barriers, such as vulnerability to emotional blackmail, barriers to asking for or seeking help (dysfunctional verbal rules—"I am the only one who knows how to give him the care he needs"; fears—"we will have a fight if I ask for her help"; or lack of skills), and lack of time planning. All of these barriers should be identified and can be worked through in therapy, using the pertinent intervention techniques (skills training, exposure techniques, behavior experiments, etc.).

Preliminary data on acceptance and commitment therapy-based group intervention

With the aim of assessing the efficacy of an ACT intervention programme with dementia caregivers, 16 female dementia family caregivers took part in a pilot study in which we compared the effectiveness of an ACT-based group intervention in comparison to a control condition. Eight caregivers were in the ACT-based intervention condition (mean age = 61.88; SD = 8.66) and another eight were in the control condition (mean age = 58.75; SD = 7.92). Intervention and control groups showed similar sociodemographic characteristics, care recipients' age (78.00 and 78.25 years for the intervention and control groups, respectively), and functional status (Barthel index of 55.00 and 60.50 for the intervention and control groups, respectively).

The ACT-based intervention program consisted of eight weekly 2-hour sessions and its goals and contents were the ones described throughout this chapter (see Fig. 3.1). Experiential avoidance was assessed with the EACQ (see Table 3.1). Depression was assessed using the Center for

Epidemiological Studies-Depression Scale (CES-D; Radloff, 1977), an instrument widely used in caregiving research. Anxiety was measured by means of the Profile of Moods States (POMS; McNair, Lorr, & Droppleman, 1971) scale.

The results from this pilot intervention study revealed a significant decrease in caregiving experiential avoidance only in the ACT intervention group ($Z = -2.38$; $p < .05$). Pre- and post-intervention mean scores in experiential avoidance for the intervention group were, respectively, 60.63 (SD = 16.00) and 40.13 (SD = 10.18), and for the control group, mean score on experiential avoidance at pre-intervention was 60.00 (SD = 15.34) and at post-intervention 59.50 (SD = 17.55). Similar findings were obtained for depression and anxiety. Although, in this case, the post-intervention reduction in the intervention group was not significant, though a trend toward significance was found for both depression ($Z = -1.68$; $p = .09$) and anxiety ($Z = -1.78$; $p < .08$). Pre- and post-intervention scores for depression in the intervention group were 20.38 (SD = 14.06) and 13.50 (SD = 6.48), and for the control group 14.88 (SD = 9.55) and 17.50 (SD = 13.31). For anxiety, pre- and post-intervention scores in the intervention group were 14.25 (SD = 6.34) and 9.13 (SD = 4.58), and for the control group 15.50 (SD = 8.35) and 15.88 (SD = 8.73).

Summary

The model of intervention presented in this chapter sets out to offer a useful schema for developing psychological intervention with caregivers, in individual or group format, taking into account new insights from ACT. The proposed model highlights the importance of addressing relevant variables not usually considered in caregiving interventions, such as emotional awareness, experiential avoidance, acceptance of aversive internal events, and commitment to life values. Our proposal may be of particular interest for caregivers who have trouble accepting caregiving-related aversive emotions or experiences (high level of experiential avoidance), present low clarity regarding their life values and goals, or have a low level of commitment to those values. Also, the usefulness of an ACT-based approach seem to be especially high for caregivers with difficulties in emotional processing, that is, being aware of, acknowledging, and understanding their uncomfortable emotions.

Our proposal has been illustrated through real cases of caregivers who, to some degree, matched this emotional/motivational profile. The first caregiver, Carmen, presented a strong pattern of experiential avoidance that even involved the lack of awareness of her painful feelings. Medication, "compulsive caring," and emotion suppression were some of the avoidant strategies she usually displayed in her daily life. The Emotional Awareness and Understanding module was especially important for her, as she was able to acknowledge some painful emotions and understood the important connection between emotions and bodily sensations. The module focused on Acceptance was also essential for Carmen, as she discovered her tendency to avoid painful emotions and thoughts and her similarity with Isabel, the "supercaregiver." She also acknowledged her need to ask for help in caregiving in order to increase her commitment to her value of self-care. Consequently, she learnt to get more people involved in care. Julia, the second caregiver, had no trouble acknowledging her painful emotions, but she refused to accept some of them (e.g. frustration and sadness), and struggled to get rid of them, as she thought that, at that point in her life as a caregiver, she should be able to have them under control. Through the work on Emotional Understanding and Acceptance, she was able to assume that sadness and frustration are natural feelings in caregiving situations, and that it was not realistic to eliminate them or to try to "reason with her heart" (e.g. "I should be able to control my frustration"). She became progressively more able to avoid getting stuck in that fight, and to keep on living her life, despite the pain. The work on values and committed actions in order to approach them was also really helpful for Julia. Focusing on her needs and on the "other plants" in her garden (values non-related to caregiving), she improved her ability to tolerate caregiving-related painful emotions, and increased her satisfaction with her life. The exercises "My plant of caregiving" and the metaphor "Lost in the jungle" helped Julia to reconnect with the deep values involved in caring for her mother and with the positive experiences of purpose and meaning she obtained from her everyday caregiving experiences. Ángela had trouble accepting her husband's dementia and was completely focused on caring for him, ignoring her own emotions and needs. The work on Emotional Awareness and Acceptance helped Ángela to get closer to her emotions and needs for help and self-care. She learned to acknowledge her need for help from other persons in caregiving for her husband. In addition, working on her values through the exercises "My plant of caregiving" and "My personal constitution" helped very much Ángela, as she recovered the meaning and values involved in everyday care, which led her to have a better attitude to cope with her husbands' behavioral problems.

The objective of this chapter has been the presentation of an ACT-based model of intervention, which has been developed to offer some pathways to address some of the issues most frequently observed in clinical work with caregivers in our cultural context. Hence, this therapeutic model provides tools for addressing: (a) difficulties acknowledging, accepting, and/or expressing some negative or aversive thoughts and emotions; (b) difficulties to cope with dementia-related problematic situations which involve both modifiable and non-modifiable components; (c) lack of clarity, loss of meaning or connection with the personal values, and positive experiences involved in caregiving; (d) disconnection with one's own life goals; (e) low levels of commitment to personal values and/or lack of awareness of the barriers that hinder the committed actions to get closer to those values. In order to work on these issues with caregivers, we adapted different materials and exercises developed in the ACT framework, and developed new ones that we consider especially suited for working with caregivers. Also, we suggested some limitations and difficulties we observed in our clinical experience in the application of these therapeutic tools.

In this chapter, we have also presented the preliminary results from a pilot group intervention study analyzing the efficacy of an ACT-based intervention with caregivers.

These results suggest that ACT-based interventions may constitute a promising route to improve our ability to help caregivers to maintain their caregiving role in a way that allows them to remain involved in their life projects, consciously pursuing valued life directions. It is still early to draw definitive conclusions about this approach, but we hope and trust that more light will soon be shed on its effectiveness and prospects.

Final questions for reflection

1. Some caregivers find many difficulties in clarifying their valued life directions, as they have never thought about them. What strategies would you apply to help them discover their values?

2. In many cases, some barriers may exist for caregivers to approach some important value, as they face serious obstacles (e.g. limited time, limited financial resources, lack of social support, etc.) to reach the goals they have associated with that value. How would you manage these situations in therapy?

3. During the process of values clarification, some caregivers may discover that they did not choose to have "the plant of caregiving" in their garden, or that they do not really want to have it in their garden anymore. How would you deal with this situation in therapy?

4. What are, from your point of view, the main contributions of ACT for the intervention with caregivers?

Acknowledgment

The preparation of this article was partly supported by a grant from the Spanish Ministry of Science and Innovation (Grant PSI2009-08132/PSIC).

References

Alferi, S.F., Culver, J.L., Carver, C.S., Arena, P.L., & Antoni, M.H. (1999). Religiosity, religious coping, and distress: A prospective study of Catholic and Evangelical Hispanic women in treatment for early-stage breast cancer. *Journal of Health Psychology, 4*, 343–355.

Bagby, R.M., Parker, J.D., & Taylor, G.J. (1994). The twenty-item Toronto Alexithymia Scale-I. Item selection and cross-validation of the factor structure. *Journal of Psychosomatic Research, 38*, 23–32.

Baker, R. (2001). An emotional processing model for counselling and psychotherapy, a way forward? *Counselling in Practice 7*, 8–11.

Blackledge, J.T., & Hayes, S.C. (2006). Using acceptance and commitment training in the support of parents of children diagnosed with autism. *Child & Family Behavior Therapy, 28*(1), 1–18.

Campbell-Sills, L., Barlow, D.H., Brown, T.A., & Hofmann, S.G. (2006). Effects of suppression and acceptance on emotional responses on individuals with anxiety and mood disorders. *Behavior Research and Therapy, 44*, 1251–1263.

Danner, D.D., Snowdon, D.A., & Friesen, W.V. (2001). Positive emotions in early life and longevity: Findings from the nun study. *Journal of Personality and Social Psychology, 80*(5), 804–813.

Gallagher-Thompson, D., & Coon, D.W. (2007). Evidence-based psychological treatments for distress in family caregivers of older adults. *Psychology and Aging, 22*(1), 37–51.

Greenberg, L.S., & Paivio, S.C. (1997). *Working with emotions in psychotherapy*. New York, NY: Guilford Press.

Hayes, S.C. (2004). Acceptance and Commitment Therapy and the new behavior therapies: Mindfulness, acceptance and relationship. In S.C. Hayes, V.M. Follette, & M. Linehan (Eds.), *Mindfulness and acceptance: Expanding the cognitive behavioral tradition* (pp. 1–29). New York, NY: Guilford Press.

Hayes, S.C., & Smith, S. (2005). *Get out of your mind and into your life: The new Acceptance and Commitment Therapy*. Oakland, CA: New Harbinger.

Hayes, S.C., Wilson, K.W., Gifford, E.V., Follette, V.M., & Strosahl, K. (1996). Experiential avoidance and behavioral disorders: A functional dimensional approach to diagnosis and treatment. *Journal of Consulting and Clinical Psychology, 64*(6), 1152–1168.

Hayes, S.C., Strosahl, K., & Wilson, K.G. (1999). *Acceptance and Commitment Therapy: An experiential approach to behavior change*. New York, NY: Guilford Press.

Hayes, S.C., Strosahl, K., Wilson, K.G., Bissett, R.T., Pistorello, J., Toarmino, D., et al. (2004). Measuring experiential avoidance: A preliminary test of a working model. *Psychological Record, 54*(4), 553–578.

Hayes, S.C., Luoma, J., Bond, F., Masuda, A., & Lillis, J. (2006). Acceptance and Commitment Therapy: Model, processes, and outcomes. *Behaviour Research and Therapy, 44*(1), 1–25.

Hebert, R.S., Weinstein, E., Martire, L.M., & Schulz, R. (2006). Religion, spirituality and the well-being of informal caregivers: A review, critique, and research prospectus. *Aging and Mental Health, 10*(5), 497–520.

IMSERSO (2005). *Cuidados a las personas mayores en los hogares españoles*. Madrid: IMSERSO.

Kashdan, T.B., Barrios, V., Forsyth, J.P., & Steger, M.F. (2006). Experiential avoidance as a generalized psychological vulnerability: Comparisons with coping and emotion regulation strategies. *Behavior Research and Therapy, 44*(9), 1301–1320.

Knight, B.G., Silverstein, M., McCallum, T.J., & Fox, L.S. (2000). A sociocultural stress and coping model for mental health outcomes among African American caregivers in Southern California. *Journal of Gerontology: Psychological Sciences, 55*, 142–150.

Losada, A., Márquez-González, M., Knight, B.G., Yanguas, J., Sayegh, P., & Romero-Moreno, R. (2010). Psychosocial factors and caregivers' distress: Effects of familism and dysfunctional thoughts. *Aging & Mental Health, 14*, 193–202.

Márquez-González, M., Losada, A., Izal, M., Pérez-Rojo, G., & Montorio, I. (2007). Modification of dysfunctional thoughts about caregiving in dementia family caregivers: Description and outcomes of an Intervention Program. *Aging and Mental Health, 11*, 616–625.

McCracken, L.M., & Eccleston, C. (2006). A comparison of the relative utility of coping and acceptance-based measures in a sample of chronic pain sufferers. *European Journal of Pain, 10*(1), 23–29.

McCurry, S.M. (2006). *When a family member has dementia: Steps to becoming a resilient caregiver.* Westport, CT: Praeger Publishers/Greenwood Publishing Group.

McNair, D., Lorr, M., & Droppleman, L. (1971). *Profile of mood states.* Manual. San Diego, CA: Educational and Industrial Testing Service.

Orsillo, S.M., Roemer, L., & Barlow, D.H. (2003). Integrating acceptance and mindfulness into existing cognitive-behavioral treatment for GAD: A case study. *Cognitive and Behavioral Practice, 10*(3), 222–230.

Park, C., Cohen, L.H., & Herb, L. (1990). Intrinsic religiousness and religious coping as life stress moderators for Catholics versus Protestants. *Journal of Personality and Social Psychology, 59*(3), 562–574.

Pérez, L. (2004). *Envejecer en femenino: Algunas características de las mujeres mayores en España.* Madrid: IMSERSO.

Pinquart, M., & Sörensen, S. (2003). Differences between caregivers and noncaregivers in psychological health and physical health: A meta-analysis. *Psychology and Aging, 18*(2), 250–267.

Pinquart, M., & Sörensen, S. (2006). Helping caregivers of persons with dementia: Which interventions work and how large are their effects? *International Psychogeriatrics, 11*, 1–19.

Rachman, S. (1980). Emotional processing. *Behaviour Research & Therapy, 18*, 51–60.

Radloff, L.S. (1977). The CES-D scale: A self-report depression scale for research in the general population. *Applied Psychological Measurement, 1*, 385–401.

Safran, J., & Greenberg, L. (1988). Feeling, thinking and acting: A cognitive framework for Psychotherapy Integration. *Journal of Cognitive Psychotherapy: An International Quarterly, 2*(2), 109–131.

Sancho, M., Abellán, A., Pérez, L., & Miguel, J.A. (2002). *Envejecer en España.* Madrid: IMSERSO.

Salovey, P., & Mayer, J.D. (1990). Emotional intelligence. *Imagination, Cognition, and Personality, 9*, 185–211.

Salovey, P., Mayer, J.D., Goldman, S.L., Turvey, C., & Palfai, T.P. (1995). Emotional attention, clarity, and repair: Exploring emotional intelligence using the Trait Meta-Mood Scale. In J.W. Pennebaker (Ed.), *Emotion, Disclosure, & Health* (pp. 125–151). Washington, DC: American Psychological Association.

Spira, A.P., Beaudreau, S.A., Jimenez, D., Kierod, K., Cusing, M.M., Gray, H.L., et al. (2007). Experiential avoidance, acceptance, and depression in dementia family caregivers. *Clinical Gerontologist, 30*(4), 55–64.

Vitaliano, P.P., Zhang, J., & Scanlan, J.M. (2003). Is caregiving hazardous to one's physical health? A meta-analysis. *Psychological Bulletin, 129*(6), 946–972.

Wilson, K.G., & Luciano, C. (2002). *Terapia de Aceptación y Compromiso: Un Tratamiento conductual orientado a los valores* [Acceptance and Commitment Therapy: A behavioral therapy oriented to values]. Madrid: Pirámide.

Wolff, J.L., & Kasper, J.D. (2006). Caregivers of frail elders: Updating a national profile. *Gerontologist, 46*(3), 344–356.

Chapter 4

Psychodynamic approaches to the challenges of aging

Jane Garner and Sandra Evans

The unexamined life is not worth living
Socrates

The heart has its reason, which reason knows nothing of
Blaise Pascal

Introduction to the psychodynamic aspects of aging

As each of us ages and reaches a new phase in our development, we learn or become something new and we leave something behind. This is the challenge that continued existence poses. In relative youth, changes tend to be mostly rewarding—with some, but few drawbacks. The older we get after "a certain age" (which will not be described), this balance reverses somewhat and the gains become less obvious and losses more advertised: thus old age becomes something to be viewed with considerable ambivalence. Most of us would rather not die; at least, not now. Neither do we wish to become ill nor dependent. If we are to live to old age, illness may happen, and certainly the other—death is inevitable.

This chapter is presented from the perspective of two clinicians who are experienced in the psychiatry of late adult life. We are aware that the population we see for treatment tends to be skewed toward those experiencing difficulties, distress, and despair. Our older patients are often managing major mental illness—schizophrenia or bipolar disorder in the context of being older and consequently differently resourced to cope. Daily we witness some remarkably positive things—heart-warming and sobering—which give us a fillip to help us continue our work. We hope that these positive things will be evident in the clinical examples, but if not, and it all seems very gloomy, then we will have failed to convey the joys of working in this extraordinary specialty.

Psychodynamic therapy with the older person

Each person's experience of advancing years is different. The psychodynamic model of understanding the problem of aging is important in that it places particular emphasis on the uniqueness of people and their experience; and for those who need medical or social services it is also able to address the fears of staff working with this patient group. Increasing psychodynamic skills is a way of developing and enhancing communication with patients, regardless of their diagnosis or age, and is useful in settings other than psychiatric units—for example, hospices and medical wards (Terry, 2008). Not everyone is suitable for formal psychotherapy, nor would wish for it, but all clinical staff who work with older people could benefit from knowing psychodynamic principles and using reflective practice. This is particularly useful when working with patients experiencing extreme anguish (Davenhill, Balfour, Rustin, Blanchard, & Tress, 2003). Understanding psychosocial aspects of aging including our own fears and prejudices will not only increase the provision of therapies to older people, to whom they are currently rarely offered, but would also augment our usual psychiatric interventions and management (Kitwood, 1988; Evans, 1998).

When Freud wrote of the ineducability of people over 50 indicating that too much material would be presented by older patients to be analyzable, it is doubtful that he could have imagined how these words might have impeded the progress of psychological therapies in this age group. This has only changed relatively recently. At present, our U.K. health service is planning to offer talking remedies as standard for most patients; including older people (improving access to psychological therapies, IAPT, 2009—part of a U.K. Government drive to reduce the impact of mental illness on the Nation's wealth).

Psychoanalytic theory is a theory of development. Nowadays analysts see development continuing throughout life. Those lending themselves more to this lifespan approach were Erikson, Kohut, and Bowlby. Group theory also adds the social dimension and the real external environment to the psychological framework. This perspective is extremely useful in studying older people, and allows us to reflect on the changes that aging has on interpersonal relating (Evans, Chisholme, & Walsh, 2001; Evans, 2004a and b).

The underlying assumptions in psychodynamic work are that there is an area of mental life of which we are usually unaware—the Unconscious; an area of our existence peopled by figures (objects) from our past, which nevertheless interact with our current experiences and influence our behavior and emotional state. These internalized people, unconsciously remembered positive and negative, become our "internal objects." As our developmental pathway unfolds, each stage of our development remains with us and may be reactivated throughout life by personally potent environmental or relationship factors. Our symptoms and personality difficulties often have meaning which may be hidden from our conscious minds, but may infect relationships with family or friends or hospital staff, etc. These difficulties are much more likely to become active at times of emotional upheaval and crisis such as illness or loss. A relationship with a professional or therapist, sensible of these ideas may be therapeutic as well as diagnostic. If these assumptions are accepted, there is no good reason why they will not also be applicable to older people. There is no evidence that older people who are able to access therapy do less well than younger ones, but plenty of evidence that therapy is not offered because of agism and ignorance. Using psychodynamic ideas for the treating team is very useful, even when the patient is not directly receiving therapy (Stern & Lovestone, 2000).

Clinical illustration: Mrs. R

Mrs. R's case illustrates this well. She was in her eighties when she began to suffer from the effects of a number of physical illnesses—mostly cardiovascular—which plunged her into a state of mild confusion.

Mrs. R had been one of life's eccentrics as far as anyone knew. She was "known" by services for many years after her husband's death because she complained endlessly to the council and the police about her neighbors. There was never any substance to her complaints, neither was she actually psychotic, but she was provocative and capable of minor acts of vandalism. At those earlier times her family doctor had tried to have her assessed but she always declined a psychiatric appointment. She was thought to be exhibiting features of a paranoid personality structure. After her eventual diagnosis and treatment, it was considered that her husband's death had unmasked a previously undetected problematic personality trait (Reich, Nduaguba, & Yates, 1988).

She could have been seen in lay terms as a "cup half empty" sort of person. She did not see the benefits of having her own comfortable house, and she always seemed to feel that others were better off than her. She supposed that people were hostile toward her, rather than the opposite which was that she was not community spirited. She would describe herself as a "private person," and indeed it seemed that after her husband's death no one was able to say much about her at all. As the years progressed she became more frail and dependent on formal carers employed by the local authority. She did not treat them well, finding fault with all their completed tasks. Her admonishments were peppered with racist insults, often leaving the carer with difficult feelings toward her. She was Jewish but her own personal history and experiences of the time of the Holocaust was not known, and could only be speculated upon. She was singularly unforthcoming about her life.

Mrs. R's confusional state seemed to have been precipitated following her dismissal of the most recent carer at home—she did not take tablets or food regularly. She became increasingly ill as a result, and yet refused offers of help, perceiving increasingly their concerns and insistence as a threat to her liberty. She began to behave as though she were under siege. When she was at risk of grave decline from her untreated illness and was taken to hospital under the mental health act, she accused her rescuers of being "Nazis."

On the ward she recovered considerably once her physical equilibrium was restored, but was clearly in an early stage of dementia. She oscillated between being sweet and emollient, and being accusatory. It became apparent that the ward staff were "split" into those who would do anything for her, and those who although behaved professionally, did not warm to her. They would be accused of all kinds of abusive acts—patently untrue (although she had been deprived of her freedom; albeit in her best interests). Some allegations were so serious that it was required that the police were called; and staff only attended to her personal care in pairs. Clinical case discussion with all staff revealed that many felt intensely guilty when interacting with her—although on close reflection, there was no logical reason to do so.

Case reflections on Mrs. R

Mrs. R, like many older patients in a state of confusion, arrive without care staff knowing the sort of facts about her own history that give clinicians some guidance and confidence; like a roadmap in an alien country. The crisis which precipitated her institutionalization, generated powerful, undigested feelings which were projected actively into her carers, and which resonated with them. Bringing these thoughts and feelings together during case management meetings, was a bit like bringing the split parts of her mind together. This enabled staff to act as a united team to help her in the most kind, professional, and humane way possible, despite all the threats and accusations (Main, 1957). They were able to conjecture a bit on what might have befallen Mrs. R in her earlier life for her to perceive the world about her in such a way as to add to her distress and feelings of persecution. These "projective identifications" were a clue to her internal world, and could only really be accessed and discussed in an environment where the staff were able to talk freely and without fear about her, and how they had been made to feel. Tolerating her projections and behaving with kindness seemed to moderate her behavior and as time went on it became less extreme.

Stigma, prejudice, and agism

Sadly we still live in an ageist society. The old are considered not to have gained experience but to have lost youth. They are considered a burden on the young, and on the tax payer. To grow old in our kind of Western society is to risk feeling alienated from youth, and to worry about the impact of increased frailty on our day-to-day lives. We carry with us negative and stereotyped images of old age in our conscious and unconscious minds, and use the images as a repository for all the things that we feel anxious about—hearing loss, dementia, and ridicule. The concept of introjected negative images links well with a more cognitive model researched by Levy (2003). Old age becomes a place we don't wish to visit, like the stereotyped care homes where people sit and wait. Staff who work with older people need to carefully examine their own attitudes and feelings; idealization, envy, or pity are as unhelpful as more overtly negative thoughts. For example, why do we congratulate people for seeming younger than their years?

Older people over many decades have introjected the prevailing attitudes. Bill thought of himself as a dirty old man as he continued to have a potent sex drive in his late 80s. Jean who was offered therapy for her depression felt that it should be given to a younger person, "I've had my innings, dear."

The consequences of agism can be serious and dramatic, not only poor taste birthday cards or jokes. The richness of interaction with others in a meaningful and sustained way (even or perhaps especially during supportive care in their own homes) is often absent and adds to any existing feelings of loneliness. Individualized care packages may be helpful, but may reduce the offers of a community for older people to be with others and to associate with their peers. The common complaint of not wanting to join any activity targeted at pensioners because it is "full of old people" is an aspect of a malignant projection of all that is decrepit, disgusting, and abhorrent into the group of elderly people (Evans, 1998). It is similar to a common complaint of group therapy patients (younger as well as older) that the group they have joined is full of "saddos and losers." The hatred of what is inside the self—dependence and fear or frailty and depletion, is projected onto the group which becomes the embodiment of all that is hated and feared. The danger occurs if this group or community is avoided totally. If avoidance wins out, then the opportunity to take back projections is also lost, that is, to see that the other person contains aspects similar to oneself, and that these are not so terrible.

Good aspects and strengths may be discovered or rediscovered too. Therapy space for older service users is important and people should have the opportunity to have their therapy in groups—not merely because it is also cost-effective and an efficient way of working, but more importantly because there is a positive therapeutic benefit from having therapy together (Hearst, 1988; Evans et al., 2001; Evans, 2004). This applies equally to the creative therapies such as art, music, and dance therapies which can be so helpful to people who might be losing their capacity to speak due to stroke or dementia (Darnley-Smith, 2004; Violets-Gibson, 2004).

Addressing the issue of older people accessing services available to other groups of people is so important because older adults are still not being offered the same services as younger patients (Age Concern, 2007; Healthcare Commission, 2008). For example, a referral for therapy simply may not be considered by the treating doctor. Even when no barrier exists in theory, in practice there is a huge gulf between what older people actually get and what they are supposed to receive; including psychotherapy. Governmental initiatives to eliminate discrimination are welcome, but need to be more sophisticated if access problems continue to prevent real equity of provision. Access may be difficult because of the physical environment, because the wait for treatment is too long and unrealistic for the person's age, or the clinicians offering the therapy have little "cultural competence" for working with older people. People should not be treated in the *same* way, that is, identically but with *equality*, that is, fairly, equitably, and impartially.

Themes in psychological work with older people show some differences from work with younger adults and some modifications to the therapeutic process may be necessary (see Table 4.1).

Table 4.1 Themes and modifications: special considerations when working psychotherapeutically with frail old people

---

◆ More emphasis on rationale of treatment at the beginning
◆ Refocus ideas of change
  • Realistic goals
◆ Loss
  • Actual
  • Potential
  • Specific
◆ Mourning—liberation
◆ Adaptation to biological reality
◆ Adaptation to social reality
◆ Dependency
◆ Incorporating life review
  • Developmental tasks in later life
◆ Time
◆ Dementia
◆ Death
◆ Families and shifting family dynamics
◆ Confidentiality
◆ Transference/countertransference
◆ Need to respond to the strengths of older people

Time may need to be spent at the beginning of treatment looking at the patient's reluctance to engage because of his/her age and therefore feeling undeserving of therapy.

Practical modifications may need to be made, for example, seeing the patient in a ground floor room if there is an unreliable lift, giving a helping hand out of the chair if that seems necessary—this needs then to be spoken of, perhaps it is a despised or pleasurable aspect of increasing physical dependency. Whatever the setting, there needs to be a neutral space without external distractions, possible to contain the unfolding relationship between patient and therapist.

In psychotherapeutic work with the older client, there is a requirement to refocus ideas of change. The options of taking new routes through life, in terms of life style or behavior, which may be open to younger patients, is rarely available to the older, because of the constraints of their external world. The aim of treatment is neither youth nor happiness but coming to an acceptance of what is or changing what may be changed internally; perhaps an altered relationship with internal objects, in order that the highest quality of life may be achieved in whatever circumstances the patient finds himself/herself. A focus for work could be chosen, a complete reconstruction of a lifetime of history may not be needed.

Loss is inevitably the most common theme. Over the years, we may lose many things; parents and siblings, spouse, friends, employment, financial status, physical strength and health, independence, home, etc. The ability to face loss is founded in very early capacities to bear psychic reality. In working with older patients, the therapist needs to be open to recognizing what is being experienced in relation to later life and what has been revived from earlier times. An ostensibly small loss may precipitate intense grief, touching previous losses inadequately mourned.

Clinical illustration: Mr. A

It was the death of a caged bird, a 15-year-old cockatiel, which brought Mr. A, a 71-year-old retired business manager, to services. He was referred by his general practitioner (GP) for depression. He lived alone, had never married. At work he had had a friend, Beverly, whom he often joined in the staff canteen. He had a fantasy of a longer-term and more intimate relationship but he had never approached the subject with her. His previous rare sexual encounters, he had thought of as necessary but squalid, with strangers. When he retired he did not contact anyone from work, not even Beverly. He had cordoned that off in his mind as an episode that was over. Now with the loss of the pet and sensitive understanding from the junior doctor who had taken Alan on as a training case, feelings of loss felt as if they were overwhelming him. He had actually lost his friend by not contacting her. He had also lost the potential of a more intimate relationship. He identified himself with the bird in the cage and had suicidal thoughts. His cage was a rather inflexible father and childhood experiences, which left him very capable of "behaving properly" but less skilled at expressing emotions. The most difficult times in therapy were when the doctor was about to go on study leave or annual which he experienced as further loss.

Over 18 months Mr. A gradually learnt to appreciate what his parents had been able to give him and acknowledged what their own personalities and upbringing caused them to be unable to give. Having lived a rather isolated life he now joined a couple of adult education classes, while acknowledging that would probably give acquaintanceship. He also felt he could keep himself open to more intimate possibilities.

Case reflections on Mr. A

Actual losses occur alongside the fear of anticipated future losses and the loss of possibilities—all those things that in younger life one might do or be in the future, which will now never happen. Each loss is specific and particular. Murphy (1982) noted that the "social origins of depression in old age" were often life events that are not ordinarily considered as severe or problematic to younger people; for example, the death of a neighbor's cat who spent some of its day with the nearby older person.

Loss, a common theme in therapy with older people, needs to be acknowledged and given time to work through psychologically.

Pollack (1982), an American training analyst, wrote of mourning—liberation being the focus of work in later life. Aging well depends on the ability to mourn for the self, those aspects of life which are lost. The ability to mourn opens up possibilities and freedoms in the years that are to come. For those with sufficient internal resources, aging itself with the inevitable losses and traumata, may be a spur to positive development. Some analysts have written of the exigencies of age, inducing courage, and strengthening the personality. Any successful psychotherapy involves loss—the giving up of maladaptive, infantile ways of being. In order to move on through life things need to be given up also through adulthood. All that is lost leaves its mark and adds to the molding and the richness of the personality.

Physical health problems and handicaps are common; they may accumulate and be chronic with advancing years. One of the skills in working with older patients is in understanding and acknowledging this biological reality while incorporating it into the therapy along with its symbolism and meaning, the transference, and the intrapsychic world. Much psychotherapy in the health service, as more is learned about the complex inter-relationships of etiological factors, is about coming to acceptance of biological reality—genetics, alterations in neurotransmitters, structural and functional neuroimaging changes, etc. The body-mind relationship is emphasized in child development and therapy but it tends to be ignored in work with adults. Nevertheless, as one does not become old suddenly, adults of many ages are preoccupied by bodily changes. One only has to switch on the television to see how deeply our bodies' appearance and function affect our lives. The patient may avoid introducing this into the session for fear of activating the painful feelings that the narcissistic injury of aging may bring. Therapists may have similar fears for themselves and their own bodily decline. This should not be an excuse for them not to approach the topic. Psychological mindedness is an important mitigating factor in dealing with adverse experiences.

Social reality may also be grim; mobility problems may exacerbate isolation and there are financial constraints. Managing on a pension is usually possible, but over time may feel oppressive. Moving away may have helped offspring find employment but leaves parents and grandparents with a diminished practical role in the family. The anonymity of people in some housing blocks, roads, and areas may be appealing at some stages in life but when older, may feel like alienation. If the only person seen is the one delivering Meals on Wheels, then this needs to be acknowledged along with other social realities, in the therapy.

Old age is likely to be associated with increasing dependency or fear of anticipating dependency. The way in which early experiences of physical and emotional dependency are remembered consciously and unconsciously, greatly determines the capacity to face this time of life (Martindale, 1989). Being dependent on family or staff brings once more to the fore the capacity for trust, first negotiated by the baby. Perhaps fears that the caregiver will not have sufficient goodwill in order not to hate or be disgusted by the frailty and dependency presented. A referral may be made for anxiety or depression if the patient is not consciously aware of the dependency fear. Some react with pseudo-independence, turning down all attempts to help despite major difficulties. Some become overly dependent, able to do much more for themselves but instead appearing "needy" and possibly demanding. Complaining and denigrating others' attempts to help may be understood as an ego-defense mechanism—installed to prevent the pain of the narcissistic wound—the perceived damage to the sense of self that frailty can bring (Hess, 2004). Good enough experiences in early life can be transferred onto carers in late life. Being able to appropriately accept help is a strength.

Timing of sessions and of therapy needs to be related to the individual. Some older patients work well and quickly to make changes, recognizing they do not have decades to spend "on the couch":

> Depend upon it Sir, when a man knows he is to be hanged in a fortnight, it concentrates his mind wonderfully.

> (Boswell, life of Johnson, 1777)

Other patients may fear discharge, perhaps linking it with death, they may need to know that the therapist or that the institution where they work will be available to them until their death (Martindale, 1989; King, 1980). It may be sufficient to say they may return—having that possibility may mean they do not actually need to come back. It may be better to terminate work gradually.

For patients whose cognition has slowed, interpretations may be better taken more widely spaced and sessions held regularly but less frequently so that there is time for material to be assimilated. The time represented by sessions with a beginning and an end, and the endings involved when the therapist takes a holiday can be linked to the patient's concern about the passage of time. The loss involved in the ending of therapy will have been anticipated from the beginning and linked with previous and potential future losses.

Dementia is not inevitable in old age, 25% of over 80s have a dementing illness (see later paragraphs), therefore 75% do not. However, it holds a fear for patients and perhaps also for therapists, so may be another reason for the reluctance to take on older patients. Dementia is not a contraindication to psychodynamic understanding (Garner, 2004a; Evans, 2008) and therapy.

There are different psychological views of death, reflecting differences between clinicians and between patients. For some (Knight, 1996), the task of negotiating death is one of middle life so that older people have often come to terms with their own mortality. For others, death remains a persecutory or depressive anxiety (Carvarlho, 2008). Some conceive of the unconscious as time-less with an eternity for itself, so death is not a possibility, there is no "not being" but numerous worries about the time leading up to the physical death—increasing dependency, pain, and physical disintegration. It may be of clinical significance to examine the patient's anticipated "life after death." In western culture we construct individual destinies, a Christian investment in the body, which is tormented, killed, and finally reborn. Other cultural and religious traditions invest less in the body and death; current experience is considered more transitory. Clinical views need to be linked to cultural concepts in this and other respects.

Families, if they are involved, may be helpful in bringing the patient to appointments for therapy, but it needs to be considered whether that is a useful idea or whether hospital or public transport will give the patient more psychological space. Families may be resistant, or may be resentful of the therapist's relationship with the mother/father. They often have the capacity to sabotage appointments and may act on unconscious feelings of fear or envy, or they may be a positive facilitatory influence on the process. Along with the infantilization which may accompany agism, is also the frequently expressed notion that families have a right to know what is being discussed: the rules of confidentiality apply whatever the age of the patient. With aging of the older generation, power relationships may change. The once powerful dictator may fall and family dynamics shift as Shakespeare described so eloquently in King Lear (Shakespeare, 1971; Hess, 1987).

Therapeutic alliance and transference

Concepts such as therapeutic alliance, staff/patient collaboration, transference, and countertransference apply in all our interactions with patients. In psychodynamic work, understanding the concepts and the manifestation of the transference/countertransference relationship is the therapist's guide to the unconscious. The patient's history is not only a collection of facts from the past but can also be experienced by the therapist in the relationship with the patient in the present. The countertransference allows some understanding and reconstruction of the patients' relationship with their internal objects. The therapist needs to understand their own relationship with their own internal objects so it is clear which feelings belong to the therapist and which to the patient. This is the reason for personal therapy to be part of training and the necessity for good supervision. Within the health service the therapist may feel they are being driven by the patient to act as a social worker, nurse, or doctor, as well as son/daughter, etc. That needs to be understood along with an ability to maintain the containing therapist role and not to feel compelled to act and to do rather than to be.

Although in part the patient may envy the therapist his youth, health, sexuality, holidays, within the relationship the therapist may also be seen as spanning generations; child, sibling, parent, grandparent. Not only the early years but also the adult past is a source of (positive, negative, sexual, etc.) transference; representing employer, employee, partner, friend, etc.

Understanding these ideas and using them in work discussion groups and supervision will aid psychiatric work generally, indeed any work involving the care of patients. It may be helpful to discharge someone quickly but only if that fits into a thoughtful clinical plan, not because their dependency or habits irritated or disgusted staff, or conversely, as illustrated in the following vignette:

> Lucy, a student nurse, seemed very involved with Mr. Thomas, an 85 year old retired headmaster, a widower, admitted with depression from his residential home where he was living due to mobility problems. She did not want him discharged back, being adamant that he receives better care in hospital—she seemed to be saying he received better care from her. Sensitive discussion with Lucy helped her understand that Mr. Thomas was the wise, polite, charming, idealised grandfather she had never had. Her own grandfather had spent time in prison for house breaking and when out she had thought him vulgarly over familiar and uncouth with her and her friends. The situation had some resolution with Lucy being involved in preparing Mr. Thomas for discharge and in writing the care plan which was being suggested to the residential home.

Particular and powerful feelings may be evoked by working with patients who are older, perhaps much older than the therapist, maybe with physical problems or a dementing illness. Treating life in decline has been described as a blow to medical narcissism. Personal feelings of inferiority may be stimulated in identification with the patient. The relationship being ostensibly unequal and the therapist seeing himself/herself in the more powerful position may have evoked unhelpful feelings of pity or sadism. The patient idealized or denigrated may be seen as grandparent, parent, or the therapist's imagined self in old age. Feelings of anger, hatred, or fear that have not been worked through can be dangerous. Winnicott (1947) introduced the idea of the "good enough" mother, extended this thoughtfulness to those seeing patients. His seminal paper "Hate in the countertransference" gives permission to face unacceptable negative feelings about patients rather than using the defenses of denial and projection. The capacity to tolerate hate without doing anything about it depends on being completely aware of the hate. Winnicott comments that the circumscribed time of the therapy is not only containing for the patient but also permits the therapist to bear the difficulty of the work and the negative feelings which can be aroused.

Dementia

Although dementia is not inevitable in old age, it is a significant cause of illness and disability in people as we all age. Therefore, the awareness of it, the anticipation, and the experience of it in self or others—particularly peers—is a very particular challenge that aging poses. Only now in the early part of the twenty-first century it is being dealt with as an illness process by the U.K. Department of Health, and not as a normal part of getting old. As a consequence, it had not previously been treated or researched in the same way as cancer or heart disease has been for years. The National Dementia Strategy (Department of Health, 2008) exhorts us to diagnose dementia at an early stage, so that treatment and management plans can be instituted early. It is anticipated that this strategy will reduce the distress associated with ignorance and despair.

This laudable goal demands that we think of the sufferers' experience as well as that of the carers. This will need to be addressed in accordance with the degree to which the illness has progressed, and the emotional needs of the patient and their family. It will inevitably require support for those who react adversely to the bad news of a terminal and horrible illness. In an essay looking at psychoanalytic aspects of dementia, the author (Evans, 2008) divided dementia into three arbitrary stages, mild, moderate, and severe, to describe the gradual progression of the person from mildly confused to a state of utter dependence, through the neurodegenerative process. The purpose was to demonstrate that at each stage there are changes occurring that give rise to new challenges. These challenges are to the sufferers and their family and carers, to cope with loss, but also to maintain communication. Psychoanalytic understanding, with its emphasis on the unconscious, and on non-verbal communications, is a particularly useful paradigm with which to address the difficulties of people whose unconscious is becoming less protected by their conscious minds, and whose verbal skills and conscious memories are diminishing. In dementia care, it is helpful if the carer/clinician is able to tune in to the patient through examination of his/her own affects and mental states. This is over and above simple empathy and may require specialist supervision to help understand what is being communicated.

In early dementia, there is often a great deal of anxiety felt by the sufferer who may be fully aware or only aware at some level of consciousness, that something is amiss. Personal resources are dwindling. This experience of loss may be so painful that the sufferer blocks it from their mind completely, using denial as an ego-defense mechanism. Considerable psychological work may be required to help that individual come to terms with his/her loss (Sinason, 1992). One needs to be fully aware that the lack of insight into the dementia may also be part of the destructive neurological processes on cognitive function—particularly if the frontal lobes are involved (Morris, 2009). If the knowledge is somewhat less painfully experienced, simple counseling may help them through it. In some situations, the loss may resonate with earlier, as yet unresolved losses and threaten a more depressive breakdown (Waddell, 2000). For example, in the previous clinical illustration of Mrs. R, part of the presenting problem was that she was beginning to lose her mind. The fear of being out of her own control was projected onto her carers whom she perceived as "Nazis." In an odd way, it may have been less painful for her to deny the reality that she was losing control, and believe that others were controlling her, rather than admit to her dementia. It is not hard to see how an earlier real threat, experienced when the patient was young, can become superimposed on another real-lived experience; with the potential for re-traumatizing and causing greater anxiety. Not to take that history into account risks losing the opportunity for understanding the patient and her fears, but also robs the staff from a chance to understand why they may be experienced as persecutors, and feel guilt. If the patient has sufficient cognitive function to hold on to the information, they may be helped psychodynamically. In this example by suggesting to Mrs. R that she has experienced us *as though* we were Nazis persecuting her, but that the *reality* is that she is unwell and in need of our help. Although it is difficult for her to trust us, part of her wants to trust—and to feel safe.

This early stage of dementia may be an opportunity for people to receive a dynamic psychotherapy previously not undertaken, in order to vent, even to resolve conflicts. The loosening hold of the conscious mind makes unconscious processes more overt and less inhibited, and therefore more available for and less resistant to change (Sinason, 1992; Evans, 2008). Even dreams can become more accessible.

As the dementia advances, verbal skills may be lost, and therefore opportunities for therapy in media other than words should be made available. Art therapy can assist a person to access in order to express, feelings about loss and grief. One patient who did not understand what was happening to her consciously, painted a series of tulips that gradually diminished in color and complexity (Iyemere—personal communication). It was possible to work with her through mirroring her work in words, to help her to understand that she was experiencing herself as losing color and complexity. This work helped her to be less anxious, as though the experience of sharing this understanding was powerful enough to reduce her sense of isolation and fear. Byers (1995) describes in greater detail how this works in Art Therapy, and Darnley-Smith (2004) and Violets-Gibson (2004) use the medium of music to aid communication and to evoke emotions with which one may access important memories.

In the more advanced severe dementias, people's dependency is absolute. Communication through the process of projection and projective identification is extremely important, and it is no surprise that many excellent carers in residential and nursing homes are largely "unskilled" women who have raised children from infancy, and thereby understand the need for tuning in to the dependent patient in order to understand their needs. Equally of critical importance is the need for sophisticated clinical supervision for these workers. The exposure to painful states of mind is a daily occupational hazard in some care homes (Davenhill et al., 2003). The staff too need containing, and a sensitive management structure in place to provide these skills. They also need support and the acknowledgment that the work they are doing is difficult but essential.

Abuse

The etiology of individual and institutional abuse, which is so common in supposed "care" services, is complex and involves a combination of factors always including agism.

Abuse can and does sometimes come from the patient too. Occasionally, genuine changes to the brain such as a frontal-lobe dementia may present with gross personality changes, causing previously fastidious people to swear or use acts of aggression and hostility. However, it is still the case that the more aggressive and less likeable residents in a care home are those who are more at risk of being abused themselves.

Far less extreme examples than the thankfully rare brutalizing of older vulnerable people occurs on a daily basis in the most well-meaning of settings. Older people are often denied an acknowledged emotional life even when in residential homes and hospitals where they receive a reasonable level of biological and social care. Failure to place life partners together in care homes, or thoughtless separation of people who have struck an important friendship is a regular event within many institutions. Recognition of this practice may help us to acknowledge and begin to address some of the darker forces within our own psyche which can allow us to accept substandard practices, or consider them expedient or pragmatic.

Clinical illustration: Mr. H

Mr. H was referred to an old age psychiatry service. He suffered from a long-term bipolar disorder—probably genetically inherited and was managed by services for younger adults until he reached 65 years. Of significance was the aggressive manner which he displayed whenever he needed help. It was a life-long trait and would worsen the more desperate he became. He had served time in prison as a much younger man for assault and criminal damage, but latterly was more inclined to destroy property rather than hurt others. Inevitably, this behavior became more prominent when he became anxious and as his physical health began to deteriorate. As he got older this behavior had started to re-emerge. Recently, he had been thrown out of several accident and emergency departments for abusive and threatening behavior when he had had real concerns about his health. Because he was an older patient he "graduated" to a psychiatric service specifically for his age group. The new team seized the opportunity to take a full history—including his early childhood experiences. His mother had been severely mentally ill and had in her wretchedness, been unable to attend to his needs. It is likely that it was this dynamic which set him on his course of aggression. His spell in a reform school and later in prison seemed to have been containing—by relieving some of these feelings, and he had made a strong and positive attachment to institutions (Adshead, 1998).

This positive feeling toward hospitals allowed the possibility of making a good therapeutic relationship, if only he could keep the aggression under control. Some of his internal objects were persecutory, and these were the predominant transferences he would make when he was frightened; consequently bringing out all his anger and aggression. The fear experienced by the clinical staff when confronted with his aggression would have no doubt mirrored his own; that he would be denied the medical treatment he needed, and that he would be abandoned to a miserable fate—possibly even his own death. This fear could be understood as a communication of the state of his internal world, projected into them—in addition to their own understandable and genuine alarm at his abusiveness.

Case reflections on Mr. H

Clearly one can only begin to understand the connection between the past experiences and current illnesses and behavior, if the patient's own personal history is taken in a sensitive, searching, and systematic way. This kind of psychodynamic history taking allows a number of therapeutic changes to occur, and presents the opportunity for further work, by providing a focus on which to concentrate precious resources (Wesby, 2004).

An interested and sensitive clinician asking about and listening to their life story can be an important first in someone's life. It cannot be underestimated how profoundly positive a good history taking can be for the patient—at any age—and how it binds the clinician and patient together in an important endeavor—described as the Therapeutic Alliance.

For the patient, the opportunity to construct a narrative from his/her own experiences, can provide not only an important step toward understanding and taking control of the predicament, but also paradoxically, a step away from the overwhelming experience. Putting a feeling into words can help move it away from being merely an emotional mire, into thoughts. Bion (1962) described this as being a maternal task, helping a developing infant by applying her mind to her infant's experiences; in order to help the child cope with and have his feelings "contained," that is, to be held in a well-functioning mind that can know that howsoever overwhelming the feelings are for the infant, it is possible to survive them. This understanding is conveyed to the infant by assured holding, and sounds made. Similarly, a therapeutic encounter, using the therapist's mind and experience to help a patient move from overwhelming feelings to thoughts about himself and his life, is a step toward the capacity for self-reflection, and thereby containment.

In this case, Mr. H was able to see a connection between his childhood past and the feelings recreated when he was experiencing rejection from people supposed to help him. He could see that there was no judgment involved in explaining the resultant actions; just a wish to help him change.

Considerable therapeutic work was made by Mr. H with a male therapist over 2 years, which focused on his feelings of fear, and assumptions that he would be rejected by clinical staff. This helped him to accept offers of help as his physical health continued to deteriorate. Later on, this insight offered care staff in a residential home the opportunity for empathy with his situation, and supported them to continue to treat him with kindness and respect.

Psychoanalytic theories helpful to understanding aging

Freud's emphasis was on childhood development. Other analysts have seen development continuing beyond early adulthood. Jung (1931) took on older analysands and elaborated ideas about the second half of life which to him presented different tasks and opportunities from the first half. In the "morning of life" the focus is on nature, instincts, propagation of children, and engagement with the world. The rays of the sun are extending outward. In the "afternoon of life" with the sun's rays being withdrawn, more attention is directed toward the self for self-illumination with an emphasis on culture and spirituality.

Childhood development and experiences do leave their mark, interacting with later development and experiences. In the adult mind and older adult mind are vestiges of all history.

Schemes of development may suggest an ordered sequential journey to maturity but there is not a linear progression, a predetermined path but an interaction between psychological happenings of all ages and with environmental considerations throughout life. Klein (1946) described the shift from the paranoid position to the depressive position in which the infant is able to recognize both the goodness and badness in parental figures. It may only be as an adult that someone gets that balance, not only through therapy but as a consequence of experience and dealings with the world.

Freud's (1905) structural model of the mind (the ego, id, and superego) focuses primarily on the internal world. Later, the Neo-Freudians added a sociological perspective, with more attention given to the external world and how people interact. Out of this tradition Erik Erikson (1959) postulated development continuing throughout the life cycle in the "eight ages of man" with a psychosocial developmental task for each phase, a contention to be negotiated with the solution taken forward to the next and each being dependent on earlier solutions. The child is therefore not only father to the man but also grandfather to the old man. The task in late life is to negotiate between the polarities of ego integrity and ego despair. Development is the result of interaction between the developing individual and his/her environment at that particular time in history. Earlier phases may be activated at times of stress but previous good experiences may exert an intermediary protective effect. The one with a balance of Erikson's concept of ego integrity is someone who reviewing his/her life in old age sees the life as the only one he/she could possibly have had, accepting his/her family of origin as it was and that his/her own life was the only responsibility, accepting life in all its complexities, as it was and now is, including self and others with their positive and negative sides (Garner, 2004b). One takes pleasure in *"having been."* Without emotional integration the individual is beset by despair that time is too short, death is too near to try out another route in life, and he/she faces *"not being."* The patient does not accept his/her life as the only possible one he/she could have had and there are feelings of despair, perhaps disgust, misanthropy, contempt, and displeasure.

Erikson's idea of setting the patient in history is particularly apt in old age psychiatry where patients are seen, whose ages span 40 years. They have lived in different times from the staff and from each other. They may have been influenced by two world wars, poverty, and economic depression and possibly raised by parents born in the Victorian era.

Clinical illustration: Mr. B

Mr. B, a 74-year-old retired hospital engineer with no previous psychiatric history, was referred by his GP (of whom he had been always critical), who was concerned that he had admitted himself prematurely to a residential home. He had decided 3 months after the death of his wife from breast cancer that he could not cope without her, although the GP knew it had been a rather ambivalent relationship. He was verbally sharp and bad tempered with the staff in the home who did not know how to react to him, what to say. He was seen initially by a young male doctor from the local department of Old Age Psychiatry, who also felt overwhelmed by the presentation of this apparently powerful man who had nevertheless put himself in an ostensibly dependent position, admitting himself to the home and loathing it. Should he write a prescription—but for what? He discussed it with the consultant, a middle-aged female who agreed to see the patient, not for a psychiatric interview but for a dynamic assessment and subsequently for treatment in weekly sessions.

Mr. B was born in 1923, father a solicitor, mother a young housewife. A younger brother was born when he was 6, a few months before father was killed in the war. He readily took on some of father's role, seeing himself as caring for mother and being the man of the house. He was clever at school and could have remained after 16 but he chose to leave, taking any job that came along and preferring to study at night school. Brother subsequently went to medical school and became an orthopedic surgeon. In his relationship with his brother and other men, including the GP, he was rather dismissive, as if he needed no one and he always knew the answer. This attitude was repeated with women but laid on top of that was his belief that he could charm them into doing what he wanted. Usually this worked. He had met his wife while on a course in Manchester. She had not really wished to leave the area with which she was familiar, her family, her friends, but she was nevertheless persuaded to join him in London and marry him. He was surprised and irritated that the therapist resisted giving into his request, however charmingly put, to be seen more frequently, at a different time, to speak on the phone, etc. She did not always find that easy, she saw in him elements of her recently dead father: clever, tall, good looking, elegant, essentially untouchable but seductive when he wanted to be, a man to admire but of whom to be wary.

He and his wife had no children, a loss and sadness for them both. He had felt humiliated by the infertility investigations and made his wife agree not to tell his brother. No cause was found and the couple avoided overtly finding fault with each other about the cause. He thought she probably blamed him as he did her. His upset over not having children seemed exacerbated by disappointed rivalry, he having wanted to be a better father than either his own, who left the family by dying and also better than his brother, whose daughter had problems with illegal drug use.

He had engaged with the therapy, initially because he loves puzzles, quizzes, and knowing the answer—he felt at one and the same time that he would already know everything that there was to know about himself, his life, and construing it but also that he may learn something of his own narrative. As well as being the authoritative one with answers, he was also the dependent one who needed assistance.

Mr. B's other interest, particularly with time in retirement had been gardening: planting, tending, watching, growing. This was another theme taken up in therapy—a seed of an idea sown by the therapist could develop over the weeks as he learnt not always to "know" the answer but to make connections, think about relationships, and to share. The therapist was variously the daughter he never had, the doctor sibling/rival, a previous lover.

A couple of years before his wife's death he had developed symptomatic prostatic hypertrophy. It enraged him that he had developed "an old man's complaint." It had not affected his sexual life with his wife but he feared it may. He had always had what he termed "a healthy interest" in women, which had included a few extramarital affairs, about which he thought his wife was ignorant. Now with the prostatism he felt anxious and was testing himself in relation to women, looking and seeing if he was still interested. He had been interested in the curve of the breasts of the cashier at the bank. He arrived home on that day to hear that his wife had been to the GP with a lump. He realized there was no logical connection between his sexual interests and his wife's breast cancer but nevertheless he felt guilty about it.

His self-imposed dependency began to shift slightly over the therapist's scheduled breaks. He understood something about appropriate timing from his experiences of gardening. Initially, he objected fiercely to the breaks, not attending the final session before the holiday. He then came to understand that life had an order to which one needs to adhere and the breaks were also an opportunity to see what it may be like after he had left therapy. It was during the break that he made a friend in the home—a woman who usually dressed in mauve, a color he loathed as it reminded him of an aunt with dementia, a disease which disgusted him. He got over his initial distaste and he realized that they had political and intellectual interests in common. After 10 months of work he was seeing the therapist more positively, less of a rival, more someone with ideas, albeit unusual ones and he began to feel that he had to leave the residential home and return to his own regimen, his own independence, his own home and garden. His house was on the market, not yet sold. He surprised himself by asking his brother (who was willing), to help extricate him from the estate agent, organize a cleaner, and help him with the physical move back home. His garden by this time was a wilderness, beautiful but disorderly. He appreciated the pretty chaos more than he could have imagined but to settle the disorder while endeavoring to keep the untrammeled beauty he employed a gardener while making it very clear he was in charge and would make the decisions. He continued to see the therapist for another 6 months, gradually seeing her as the one who saw and helped him appreciate the beauty among the wilderness of his life.

He regretted his attitude to his brother and the multiple caustic comments he had made about how the surgeon would be no one, nothing without the hospital engineer keeping the buildings running smoothly. He was determined to be different and perhaps even be the "good uncle" his niece had missed out on so far. She now had children so he had another generation with whom to become acquainted, he felt nervous about that but also he had some excitement about the opportunities that may present him. He continued to visit the home where he had temporarily lived to visit "the lady in mauve," he enjoyed her company although the staff continued to find him somewhat acerbic. He regretted his extramarital affairs but on reflection he did wonder whether his wife had actually known but chosen to keep quiet. He admired her for this, feeling he would not have been able to remain silent in those circumstances but appreciated his wife had done so to keep them together. This fueled his new ideas about accepting and tolerating others and maybe they would do the same for you. He continued to see the therapist, understanding more about the intimacy but also the boundary between them, he was pleased that he was offered a follow-up appointment 6 months after discharge.

Case reflections on Mr. B

One of the most important hurdles to overcome when working psychodynamically with older people is the assumption (on the part of therapists as well as patients) that it has been offered too late in the day. Mr. B had closed down his life and by placing himself in a care home, insisted that it was over. He had desperately needed and did use the therapy that was offered. What he was able to do was to come to terms with himself; and with renewed zest for life had made significant changes to his behavior. It is never too late to accept personal responsibility for one's life, if the mind still allows it.

Basic learning points

- Psychoanalytic theory provides a framework for beginning to understand human situations: patients with any diagnosis, their families, and the fears and anxieties of staff caring for them. It emphasizes the uniqueness of individuals. Relatively few patients will be taken on for therapy but psychodynamic understanding may inform usual treatment to the benefit of patients and staff.

- An underlying assumption in psychodynamic work is that there is an area of mental life of which we are usually unaware, the unconscious, which nevertheless may interact with conscious and external experience.

- Psychodynamic theory is a theory of development. Development continues throughout life. There is evidence that the older people who are able to access this therapy do as well as younger ones.

- In later life, dependency issues from infancy and childhood may influence the patient's behavior and mental state.

Conclusions

In this chapter, we have described some of the challenges of aging, most of which are associated with losses of some kind. In addition to the losses of people, health, and sometimes their own orderly minds, older people have to contend with ageist assumptions from a youth conscious culture, and a health and social service that may not be easily accessible to their particular needs. Given these odds, it seems remarkable that most older people manage to negotiate these difficulties reasonably well, until perhaps the balance is so weighed against them. The resilience of the human spirit, along with a good deal of ego-defense mechanisms such as projection and denial, allows most older people to remain willing to engage with the world. Sometimes these defense mechanisms interfere with the ability to get the help needed, or exacerbates a novel loneliness and isolation that has arisen out of physical or mental ill-health or both.

A psychodynamic approach to aging is one that acknowledges that the quality and nature of early experience shapes the psyche and therefore the subsequent experience of later life. In order to use it well, we must interact fully with our patients, gaining information not only about actual past physical and mental traumata, but also how they were perceived, how they were dealt with, and overcome or not. This approach recognizes a non-verbal communication that is based on empathic understanding and listening to the feelings that the patient and his or her own predicament instils in us, the clinicians. This is no less useful, and in fact becomes essential in the realm of dementia, where a severe neurodegenerative disorder eventually robs the patients of their ability to think clearly and to communicate their needs verbally. The responsibility for trying to understand what is being communicated rests with the clinicians, with their intact thinking skills, and their ability to disseminate information about how this might be done. Ensuring that others hear how a psychodynamic framework might offer a way of understanding people's experience, and provide an additional model with which to view illness and illness behavior through teaching is part of this process.

References

Adshead, G. (1998). Psychiatric staff as attachment figures: Understanding management problems in the light of attachment theory. *British Journal of Psychiatry*, *172*, 64–69.

Age Concern (2007). Improving services and support for older people with mental health problems. The second report from the UK Inquiry into Mental Health and Well-Being in Later Life. London: Age Concern England.

Bion, W. (1962). A theory of thinking. *International Journal of Psychoanalysis*, *43*, 306–310.

Byers, A. (1995). Beyond marks. On working with elderly people with severe memory loss. *Inscape*, *1*, 16–22.

Carvarlho, R. (2008). The final challenge: Ageing, dying, individuation. *Journal of Analytical Psychology*, *531*, 1–18.

Darnley-Smith, R. (2004). Music therapy. In S. Evans & J. Garner (Eds.), *Talking over the years: A handbook of dynamic psychotherapy in older adults*. London: Brunner-Routledge.

Davenhill, R., Balfour, A., Rustin, M., Blanchard, M., & Tress, K. (2003). Looking into later life. Psychodynamic observation and old age. *Psychoanalytic Psychotherapy*, *17*, 253–266.

Department of Health (2008). The National Dementia Strategy. London: Department of Health.

Erikson, E. (1959). *Identity and the life cycle: Psychological issues monograph 1*. New York, NY: International Universities Press.

Evans, S. (1998). Beyond the mirror: A group analytic understanding of late life and depression. *Ageing and Mental Health*, *2*, 94–99.

Evans, S. (2004a). Group psychotherapy: Foulkes, Yalom and Bion. In S. Evans & J. Garner (Eds.), *Talking over the years: A handbook of dynamic psychotherapy in older adults*. London: Brunner-Routledge.

Evans, S. (2004b). What works for whom? A survey of provision of psychological therapies for older people in the NHS. *Psychiatric Bulletin*, *28*, 411–414.

Evans, S. (2008). Beyond forgetfulness: How psychoanalytic ideas can help us to understand the experience of patients with dementia. *Psychoanalytic Psychotherapy*, *22*, 155–176.

Evans, S., Chisholme, P., & Walsh, J. (2001). A dynamic psychotherapy group for the elderly. *Group Analysis, 34,* 287–298.

Freud, S. (1905). On psychotherapy. *Standard edition.* Translated and edited by J. Strachey (Vol. 7, pp. 257–268). London: Hogarth Press.

Garner, J. (2004a). Dementia. In S. Evans & J. Garner (Eds.), *Talking over the years: A handbook of dynamic psychotherapy in older adults.* London: Brunner-Routledge.

Garner, J. (2004b). Growing into old age: Erikson and others. In S. Evans & J. Garner (Eds.), *Talking over the years: A handbook of dynamic psychotherapy in older adults.* London: Brunner-Routledge.

Garner, J., & Evans, S. (2000). The institutional abuse of elderly people. *CR 84, Council Report.* London: Royal College of Psychiatrists. Available at: http://www.rcpsych.ac.uk/.

Health Care Commission (2008). 2008 Report. London: TSO.

Hearst, L.E. (1988). The restoration of the impaired self in group psychoanalytic treatment. In N. Slavinsky-Holy (Ed.), *Borderline and narcissistic patients in therapy.* New York, NY: IUP, Inc.

Hess, N. (1987). King Lear and some anxieties of old age. *British Journal of Medical Psychology, 60,* 209–215.

Hess, N. (2004). Loneliness in old age: Klein and others. In S. Evans & J. Garner (Eds.), *Talking over the years: A handbook of dynamic psychotherapy in older adults.* London: Brunner-Routledge.

IAPT (2009). Report from the pathfinder survey-older adults. London: Department of Health.

Jung, C.G. (1931). The stages of life. In H. Read (Ed.), *The collected works* (Translated by R.F.C. Hull) (Vol. 8, pp. 387–415). Princeton, NJ: Princeton University Press.

King, P. (1980). The Life Cycle as indicated by the nature of the transference in the psychoanalysis of the middle-aged and the elderly. *International Journal of Psychoanalysis, 61,* 153–160.

Kitwood, T. (1988). The contribution of psychology to the understanding of dementia. In B. Gearing, M. Johnson, & T. Heller (Eds.), *Mental health problems in old age.* London: John Wiley & Sons.

Klein, M. (1946). Notes on some schizoid mechanisms. Developments in psycho-analysis (Chapter 9). *International Journal of Psychoanalysis, 27,* 99–110.

Knight, B.G. (1996). *Psychotherapy with older adults.* Newbury Park, CA: Sage.

Kohut, H. (1977). *The restoration of the self.* New York, NY: International Universities Press.

Levy, B. (2003). Mind matters: Cognitive and physical effects of aging self-stereotypes. *The Journals of Gerontology Series B: Psychological Sciences and Social Sciences, 8,* P203–P211.

Main, T. (1957). The ailment. Reprinted (1989). In J. John (Ed.), *The ailment and other psychoanalytic essays.* London: Free Association Books.

Martindale, B. (1989). Becoming dependent again: The fears of some elderly persons and their young therapists. *Psychoanalytic Psychotherapy, 4*(1), 67–75.

Morris, A. (2009). A neuropsychological understanding of awareness. Conference Proceedings: Psychological Approaches to Old Age. London: in Press.

Murphy, E. (1982). The social origins of depression in old age. *The British Journal of Psychiatry, 141,* 135–142.

Pollock, G. (1982). On ageing and psychotherapy. *International Journal of Psychoanalysis, 63,* 275–281.

Reich, J., Nduaguba, M., & Yates, W. (1988). Age and sex distribution of DSM-III personality cluster traits in community population. *Comprehensive Psychiatry, 29,* 298–303.

Shakespeare, W. (1971). The complete works. London: Oxford University Press. [King Lear].

Sinason, V. (1992). The man who was losing his brain. In V. Sinason (Ed.), *Mental handicap and the human condition: New approaches from the Tavistock.* London: Free Association Books.

Stern, J.M., & Lovestone, S. (2000). Therapy with the elderly: Introducing psychodynamic psychotherapy to the multi disciplinary team. *The International Journal of Geriatric Psychiatry, 15,* 500–505.

Terry, P. (2008). *Counselling and psychotherapy with older people: A psychodynamic approach.* Second Edition. London: Macmillan.

Violets-Gibson, M. (2004). Dance & movement therapy for people with severe dementia. In S. Evans & J. Garner (Eds.), *Talking over the years: A handbook of dynamic psychotherapy in older adults*. London: Brunner-Routledge.

Waddell, M. (2000). Only connect: Developmental issues from early to late life. *Psychoanalytic Psychotherapy*, *14*, 239–252.

Wesby, R (2004). Inpatient dynamics: Thinking feeling and understanding. In S. Evans & J. Garner (Eds.), *Talking over the years: A handbook of dynamic psychotherapy in older adults*. London: Brunner-Routledge.

Winnicott, D.W. (1947). Hate in the counter-transference. *International Journal of Psychoanalysis, 3*, 69–74.

Chapter 5

Couples coping with cancer

W. Kim Halford, Suzanne Chambers, and
Samantha Clutton

Introduction

I felt well, I try to look after myself—keep fit—and cancer was a bolt out of the blue, a terrible shock.
I didn't hear anything the doctor said after the words 'You have breast cancer.'

(Clare, 81)

I was trying to be strong for her, trying not to show my fear.

(Tom 83)

I didn't know what to say to her, I was trying not to cry myself.

(Kelly, daughter, 51)

My friends kept asking me 'are you sure you're OK?', but I really was doing fine. Cancer was just
something that came along, Dave and I saw we had to deal with it—so we did.

(Cheryl, 73)

Although John and I had a good marriage, I think we had started to take each other for granted. John's
prostate cancer changed all that. As we shared the struggle through the recovery from surgery we talked
more, we got closer. We treasure our time together more now.

(Judy, 71)

After prostate surgery I had 6 weeks at home. I went from working 60 hours per week to spending all
my time at home. I started to feel I was losing who I was.

(Rod, 62)

What I struggled with most was not knowing how to support Rod. The more I tried to talk to him the
more he withdrew.

(Kath 61)

As people age, they are more likely to suffer from physical illnesses and disabilities, which present
significant challenges to the sufferer, partner, and family. One of the most common illnesses
associated with aging is cancer. As the above quotes illustrate, reactions to the diagnosis and treatment of cancers are highly variable among the sufferers, their partner, and family members. This
chapter reviews the psychological effects of cancer diagnosis and treatment on older people, with
a particular emphasis on how couples cope with cancer. The focus is on two of the most common
forms of cancer for older people: breast cancer in women and prostate cancer in men. Aside from
the high prevalence of these forms of cancer, we focus on breast and prostate cancer as each
impact upon parts of the body associated with sexuality and gender identity, and poses particular
challenges to the aging couple.

The significance of cancer

Cancer is a major international public health concern. In 2005, cancer was the second leading cause of death in the world with 12 million new cases and 7.6 million cancer-related deaths (Hall, 2008). Although cancer can occur at any age, it is far more frequent among people over age 65. Internationally, 4.9 million cases of cancer were diagnosed among older adults during 2002—almost 2.9 million in developed countries and over 2 million in developing countries (Boyle & Levin, 2008). The incidence rate was twice as high in developed countries as developing countries, at 1,630 and 781 per 100,000, respectively. The most commonly diagnosed cancers in later life in developed countries were colorectal (16%), lung (15%), prostate (13%), breast (9%), and stomach (7%), while in developing countries the most common types of cancer diagnosed were lung (16%), stomach (14%), esophagus (9%), liver (8%), and colorectal (8%) (Boyle & Levin).

Cancer prevalence is how many people are alive following a diagnosis of cancer, which is a function of both incidence and survival. In developed countries, enhanced screening and treatment procedures have led to earlier detection and effective treatment of many common cancers, which has increased the prevalence of people who have been diagnosed with cancer who are alive (Wingo, Parkin, & Eyre, 2001). Worldwide, it was estimated that at the end of 2002 there was a prevalence of 11.1 million aged people who had been diagnosed with cancer in the last 5 years (Boyle & Levin, 2008). Around 71% (7.9 million) of these people were living in developed countries. By 2020, it is projected that the prevalence of cancer worldwide among older adults will be more than double (Boyle & Levin).

Cancer is a leading cause of burden of disease in later life. The Global Burden of Disease study estimated that in 2004, cancer accounted for 23% of the total disability adjusted life years (DALYs) among aged people in developed countries (World Health Organization, 2004). The burden of cancer is a function both of the direct effects of the cancer and the side effects of medical treatment.

Medical treatments for cancer commonly include surgery, chemotherapy, or radiation therapy, often in combination. The duration and type of treatment are influenced by the site and clinical characteristics of the cancer and the treatment aim (i.e. cure vs. palliation), as well as the person's general health, personal preferences, and accessibility of treatment (Lenhard & Osteen, 2001). In general, more advanced or aggressive cancers require more intensive treatment, and the extent of side effects and physical morbidity experienced are determined in large part by this.

Side effects of surgery relate primarily to the area of the body affected by the procedure. For example, men who undergo surgical removal of the prostate gland for cancer often experience urinary incontinence and erectile dysfunction. By contrast, for women with breast cancer surgical treatment often leads to change in the breast appearance, and lymph gland excision may give rise to lymphedema (fluid retention) in the arm. Men whose prostate cancer is treated by external beam radiation therapy often experience skin irritation on the treatment field, changes in bowel function, fatigue, and a decline in sexual function over time. Women who receive systemic chemotherapy following surgery can experience hair loss, fatigue, cognitive changes, and weight gain. This list of possible side effects is not exhaustive, but illustrates that the physical challenges of cancer treatment are significant and must be taken into account when planning psychological care of persons with cancer. Furthermore, many older patients and their partners have other co-morbid chronic health conditions, such as heart disease or arthritis, which can increase the quality of life (QOL), costs of the disease, and the treatment to the patient and the spouse.

Psychological responses to cancer in patients and spouses

A person diagnosed with cancer faces multiple psychological challenges. Most people diagnosed with cancer experience an initial response of some combination of shock, emotional numbness, hostility, and increased depression and anxiety (Johnson Vickberg, Bovbjerg, DuHamel, Currie, & Redd, 2000; Mehnert & Koch, 2008). Many people report concerns about the possibility of abandonment or death, impaired functioning, and possible threat to finances through treatment costs and lost earnings (Cordova et al., 1995; Moyer & Salovey, 1996; Psychological Aspects of Breast Cancer Study Group [PABCSG], 1987). Other common psychological reactions include concerns about lack of personal control over the treatment, the course of the illness, and uncertainty about the outcome (Silberfarb, 1984); intrusive thoughts about the cancer and the attempt to avoid such thoughts (Palmer, Tucker, Warren, & Adams, 1993); concerns with physical symptoms (PABCSG); and worry about cancer recurrence (Kemeny, Wellisch, & Schain, 1988).

For some patients, the reactions to cancer diagnosis are severe. About 35% of individuals with cancer experience persistent clinically significant distress such as anxiety and depression, adjustment disorders, and post-traumatic stress reactions (Helgeson, Snyder, & Seltman, 2004; Zabora, Brintzenhofeszoc, Curbow, Hooker, & Piantadosi, 2001). In a substantial minority of patients, long-term psychological impairments persist for many (more than 5) years (Mehnert & Koch, 2008; Stein, Syrjala, & Andrykowski, 2008). Many partners of cancer patients also report high levels of psychological distress that can match or even exceed that of the patients themselves (Cliff & Macdonagh, 2000; Omne-Ponten, Holmberg, Bergstrom, Sjoden, & Burns, 1993). The most frequently reported concerns for partners tend to focus on the survival of their spouse (Gotay, 1984), the best ways to be supportive (Kilpatrick, Kristjanson, Tataryn, & Fraser, 1998), and managing the demands of care giving (Zahlis & Shands, 1991). There is a moderate to high concordance between patient and partners on psychological adjustment (Ben-Zur, Gilbar, & Lev, 2001; Dorros, Card, Segrin, & Badger, 2010; Hagedoorn, Sanderman, Bolks, Tuinstra, & Coyne, 2008). That is, the partners of patients coping poorly also tend to be coping poorly.

Cancer in parts of the body associated with sexuality often leads patients to experience problems with body image or sexual identity. Notably, women treated for breast cancer commonly report difficulties with accepting their appearance, feel they are less attractive or feminine (e.g. Andersen, Woods, & Copeland, 1997; Schain, d'Angelo, Dunn, Lichter, & Pierce, 1994), and approximately 50% of women report problems in sexual functioning (Andersen et al., 1997). Common side effects of treatment for prostate cancer include urinary incontinence, and bowel and erectile dysfunction (Eton & Lepore, 2002). In a recent longitudinal study assessing 1,649 men diagnosed with prostate cancer 3 years previously, each of the main treatments led to persistent negative effects on QOL (Smith et al., 2009). Across all treatments, 36–87% of men reported erectile dysfunction; after radical prostatectomy 12% of men had persistent urinary incontinence; and 15% of men who had external beam radiation therapy had moderate to severe bowel problems. Thus, high rates of relationship and sexual difficulties are common even in patients with early stage disease.

Confronting a life-threatening illness such as cancer often leads people to re-evaluate important life priorities and goals (Halldorsdottir & Hamrin, 1996; Pensiero, 1995). This experience may be transient for some, whereas for others it can elicit a considerable range of sustained emotional changes. In addition to the variability in duration of changes, the nature of these emotional changes also varies considerably. Some people report predominantly negative feelings like uncertainty, vulnerability, isolation, and discomfort (Halldorsdottir & Hamrin). However, in some cancer patients the re-evaluation of priorities and goals is associated with positive change, such as increasing attention to highly valued life priorities and intimate relationships, which has been called post-traumatic growth or benefit finding (Manne et al., 2004).

The considerable acute distress experienced by almost all patients after a diagnosis of cancer returns to pre-morbid levels with time in most patients (Grassi & Rosti, 1996; Hoskins, 1997). However, even 5 years after successful treatment for cancer without recurrence, cancer survivors on average report somewhat higher psychological distress, poorer health, and lower QOL than age- and demographically matched controls (Helgeson & Tomich, 2005). About 20–25% of women diagnosed with breast cancer suffer significant depression or anxiety 6 years after the initial cancer diagnosis (Andersen, 1993; Cordova et al., 1995), and 10–15% meet criteria for post-traumatic stress disorder 10 years after diagnosis (Cordova et al.). Some QOL domains are particularly likely to remain impaired in spite of the resolution of mood and other psychosocial outcomes (Andersen, Anderson, & deProsse, 1989). For example, up to 85% of men treated for prostate cancer with surgery have significant long-term impairment in erectile function (Stanford et al., 2000). In summary, although almost everybody diagnosed with cancer experiences some significant immediate distress, there is great variability in how people adjust across the course of cancer treatment and recovery.

Factors mediating adjustment

The stage of cancer, and associated prognosis, both mediate psychological adjustment. People with more advanced stage disease display greater distress, more negative attitudes toward themselves and the future, greater concern with physical symptoms, and more interpersonal difficulties (Cassileth, Lusk, Miller, Brown, & Miller, 1985; Cella & Tross, 1986; PABCSG, 1987). The greater difficulties associated with advanced stage of disease probably are attributable to the need for intensive, invasive, and urgent treatments, which are often distressing (Andersen, 1993; Bremer, Moore, Bourbon, Hess, & Bremer, 1997; Schover et al., 1995). In addition, higher distress almost certainly results from the fact that long-term survival might be unlikely, and increased levels of debilitation or pain are often experienced in later stages of the disease (Andersen). However, the nature of the cancer, its stage, and the treatments received only account for modest variance in psychological adjustment, and other variables moderate psychological adjustment. For example, patient age interacts with stage of disease, so that the most severe distress is evident with advanced cancers in younger patients (Vinokur, Threatt, Caplan, & Zimmerman, 1989). In younger patients, the threat of death seems particularly distressing, possibly because of a perception of a large loss of anticipated life expectancy.

Good long-term coping is predicted by an active, rather than avoidant, coping style (Antoni et al., 2001; Carver, Meyer, & Antoni, 2000). During the acute crisis that often follows cancer diagnosis people often use many active coping strategies (Sorlie & Sexton, 2001), and the number of strategies used reflects total coping effort (Coyne & Racioppo, 2000). Coping effort usually decreases markedly across the first year after diagnosis (Carver et al., 1993; Heim, Augustiny, Schaffner, & Valach, 1993; Scott, Halford, & Ward, 2004). Sustained high coping effort is associated with poor long-term adjustment to cancer (Coyne & Gottlieb, 1996; Parle & Maguire, 1995).

Developing realistic cognition, and active coping with upsetting cognition, predicts improved adjustment to a range of traumatic events (Brewin, 2001; Redd et al., 2001). Negative cognition about the cancer (e.g. unrealistically negative views about prognosis) or the self (e.g. "I should be coping better," "I am a burden to my family"), seems likely to promote poor adjustment. Such negative thoughts also affect specific aspects of adjustment after cancer. For example, holding a negative view of one's sexuality predicts sexual difficulties in women with gynecological cancer (Andersen et al., 1997) and breast cancer (Yurek, Farrar, & Andersen, 2000). In summary, adaptive coping with cancer seems to be characterized initially by active coping, challenging and processing negative cognition, and a subsequent reduction in coping effort.

Social support, and in particular partner support for patients in committed relationships, is a major influence on psychological adjustment to cancer. High perceived support is associated with less depression, anxiety, and general maladjustment to cancer in patients (Grassi & Rosti, 1996;

Hoskins, 1995; Roberts, Lepore, & Helgeson, 2006). Specifically, high emotional expressiveness and cohesion in the couple relationship predicts better adjustment (Ben-Zur et al., 2001). Moreover, as noted earlier spouses of people with cancer often experience significant adjustment difficulties, and the level of social support provided to the spouse by the patient predicts long-term adjustment to the patient's cancer as well as both partners' marital satisfaction (Ptacek, Pierce, Dodge, & Ptacek, 1997). Thus, mutual social support by spouses predicts well-being for both patients and their partner.

Promoting couple coping with cancer

In couples, partners' individual responses to stress interact, and social support is often mutual (Halford, 2006). In fact, many authors suggest that partner interactions are so crucial that, in essence, most couples are conjointly coping with major stresses (e.g. Coyne & Smith, 1991). Effective couple coping is suggested to develop through partners' empathic communication that develops emotional connection and a shared, realistic, and positive appraisal of the stress (Cutrona, 1996). In turn, this shared appraisal is argued to promote conjoint coping and mutual support (Coyne & Smith, 1994; DeLongis & O'Brien, 1990). Couples' reported use of empathic communication is associated with better adjustment to cancer (Manne, Dougherty, Veach, & Kless, 1999). Psychological interventions that promote couple communication and mutual support enhance adjustment to cancer diagnosis and treatment (Manne, Ostroff, Winkel, Grana, & Fox, 2005; Scott et al., 2004), and these effects are mediated by enhanced emotional communication between the partners and development of active coping and positive cognitive appraisal (Manne et al., 2008).

There have been many trials of psychological interventions to promote better adjustment to cancer (see Newell, Sanson-Fisher, & Savolainen, 2002 for a review). Interventions typically include at least one of three components: psychoeducation, coping training, and social support enhancement (Fawzy & Fawzy, 1998; Schneiderman, Antoni, Saab, & Ironson, 2001). Psychoeducation usually provides information about the nature of the cancer, the treatment and likely side effects, and common psychological responses to cancer. Coping training usually teaches active coping skills, such as stress management and realistic cognitive appraisal of stress. Social support enhancement most often involves offering psychoeducation to groups of patients, with the idea that the patients provide each other with mutual support.

Many of the studies of psychosocial interventions to assist cancer patients report few, if any, significant sustained benefits of intervention on mood, coping, or social functioning (e.g. Bultz, Speca, Brasher, Geggie, & Page, 2000; Stanton et al., 2002). Some studies do report significant benefits (e.g. Antoni et al., 2001, 2008; Edgar, Rosberger, & Nowlis, 1992; Helgeson, Cohen, Schulz, & Yasko, 2000), though reviewers have noted that any reported significant effects on mood and coping have generally small effect sizes (Newell et al., 2002). The results have led some reviewers to question the value of current interventions in improving adjustment to cancer (e.g. Lepore & Coyne, 2006; Newell et al.).

The variable and weak effects of interventions might be due to the failure to address couple coping. As argued earlier, mutual partner support seems critical in adjustment to cancer, yet interventions promoting social support have relied on fellow patients to enhance social support (Helgeson & Cohen, 1996). Several published intervention studies have evaluated couple interventions in which the women had early stage cancer, and have produced consistent positive effects in women's adjustment, body image, and sexual satisfaction (Christensen, 1983; Manne et al., 2005; Scott et al., 2004). In the only study that compared individual and couple interventions, the couple program produced significantly larger positive effects (Scott et al.).

Although there is as yet no published randomized controlled trial of couple interventions for cancer in men, there are some promising preliminary results that have been reported (Chambers et al., 2008). In summary, research suggests that the couple-focused approach has the strongest evidence for its effectiveness in enhancing coping with cancer.

Overview of a couple coping approach

When delivering couple-based psychological interventions for people coping with cancer, therapists providing psychological support need a sound understanding of cancer treatments, and how they can impact on psychological functioning. Cancer is a highly heterogeneous disease even within cancer sites, and medical treatment varies according to the clinical features of the disease, the individuals' pre-morbid health states, and personal preferences. For example, radiotherapy and chemotherapy are often provided after surgery in the treatment of breast cancer, and often are associated with a range of side effects like fatigue, edema, and swelling. Assistance in managing these side effects is often an important element of effective psychological care (Lenhard & Osteen, 2001).

Couple intervention needs to address the specific cancer-related stressors that a particular couple are facing. The most salient stressors vary across the course of diagnosis, treatment, and recovery, and also vary between couples. For example, couples in which the man has been newly diagnosed with prostate cancer often prioritize support on managing the initial distress associated with diagnosis, assistance in decision making about what treatment to pursue, and preparation for managing the side effects of treatment (e.g. incontinence). In the months following treatment, sexual dysfunction typically become the pre-eminent therapy focus. However, some men or women know about the likely effects of prostatectomy on erectile dysfunction and want this addressed early in the course of psychological therapy. Other couples have not been sexually active for some time before cancer diagnosis, and erectile dysfunction is not a major focus of their concerns.

Couple interventions for older couples confronting cancer need to be delivered flexibly with respect to the timing, duration, and location of sessions. At least one of the individuals is coping with serious illness, there often are significant time demands from the medical treatments, as well as considerations about the physical health and mobility of older couples need to be taken into consideration. Many of the published support programs provided for cancer sufferers are group programs held at specific times and addressing a relatively fixed curriculum (e.g. Manne et al., 2005; Penedo et al., 2006). If a patient is frequently unwell or lives in a geographically remote area, remote access technologies such as telephone- or Internet-based delivery can be effective in delivering psychological interventions (Chambers et al., 2008).

It is our experience that for couples who do not have significant pre-morbid psychiatric or other relationship problems, five to eight sessions can address major coping challenges couples face with early stage cancers, which tend to have a good prognosis. The aim is to facilitate the couple's adjustment to the diagnosis of cancer and experience of treatment. Table 5.1 shows an outline of a typical course of therapy for a newly diagnosed cancer patient and his/her partner. Based on the research reviewed previously in the chapter, there are four key components of the intervention: psychoeducation; promoting active coping and shared realistic positive cognitions; enhancing effective couple communication, mutual support, and conjoint couple coping; and maintaining or improving intimacy and sexual satisfaction after treatment. A problem-solving approach (Nezu, Nezu, & Lombardo, 2004) is used to guide the couple to define the nature of the couple's specific problems, generate potential solutions, systematically evaluate possible consequences of each option, select an appropriate solution, and evaluate outcomes.

Table 5.1 Suggested timing and content of sessions

Session	Expected issue	Approximate session timing	Session goal
1	Pre-treatment: coming to terms with diagnosis; preparing for treatment; ways to show support.	As soon as possible after diagnosis	◆ Establish rapport with the couple and engage them in the intervention. ◆ Assess each partner's level of distress and identify individual and shared concerns. ◆ Provide psychoeducation about individual and couple adjustment to cancer. ◆ Provide a rationale and strategies to facilitate support between the couple.
2	Pre-treatment: as for session 1 and managing treatment after effects.	1–2 weeks following session 1	◆ Assess couples level of distress and identify individual and shared concerns. ◆ Review and consolidate strategies to manage distress and show support. ◆ Provide a rationale and strategies to facilitate couple communication. ◆ Provide treatment education to assist the couple to prepare for treatment and recovery at home.
3	Post-treatment: recovery from treatment including pain, fatigue, and site-specific effects.	3–4 weeks post-treatment	◆ Re-assess the couple's level of distress and identify current concerns. ◆ Normalize concerns and progress through treatment or recovery. ◆ Review and encourage the use of stress management strategies. ◆ Teach a problem-solving approach to manage cancer-related challenges. ◆ Review specific strategies to assist in managing treatment side effects and other concerns such as fatigue and sleep disturbance where relevant.
4	Managing acute side effects and resumption of normal activities. Potential increase in couple-related distress due to reduction in physical intimacy and usual ways of showing care and concern.	6 weeks post-treatment	◆ Re-assess levels of distress and identify current concerns. ◆ Review and encourage the continuing use of stress management strategies to manage current and future challenges. ◆ Review strategies to manage treatment side effects. ◆ Teach activity planning skills to increase energy and motivation and improve QOL.

(Continued)

Table 5.1 (continued) Suggested timing and content of sessions

Session	Expected issue	Approximate session timing	Session goal
5	Reduction in or loss of intimacy and/or sexual activity; fear of cancer recurrence; adapting to changes in physical function/body image.	8 weeks post-treatment	◆ To re-assess levels of distress and identify current concerns. ◆ Review and encourage the use of stress management and activity planning to manage current and future cancer challenges. ◆ Review specific strategies to assist in the management of persistent side effects. ◆ Identify concerns and provide strategies to improve sexual function and intimacy. ◆ Teach strategies for managing fear of cancer recurrence that may include cognitive restructuring or mindfulness techniques. ◆ Introduce goal-setting strategies to work toward meaningful goals.

Our intervention model includes flexibility in the delivery of individual components with the intention that therapy will be tailored to each couple's needs and situation. Agenda setting is undertaken at the start of each session to ensure clarity is achieved regarding goals in the context of the couple's agreed priorities and the intervention components identified as important at various phases of the treatment process. Agenda setting is guided by utilizing a "concerns sheet" in which clients are encouraged to note down any problems or concerns that arise between sessions, which can be reframed as goals to achieve within the intervention. We illustrate these principles in the two case studies that follow.

Chris and Jill coping with prostate cancer

Chris (aged 77 years) and Jill (aged 75 years) are both retired, have been married 50 years, and live in an outer suburb of a large city. They have an adult son and daughter, who both live interstate. Chris is a former small business owner and the couple are financially secure but do not have private health insurance. Chris was diagnosed with early stage prostate cancer 3 weeks ago after blood tests as part of a routine medical checkup. Chris's doctor has explained that there are four treatment options: no immediate treatment with close monitoring of disease progression with possible treatment in the future; external beam radiation therapy which entails daily visits for treatment over a 6-week period, which is available through the public hospital system and so is inexpensive; brachytherapy which entails surgical insertion of a small radioactive implant in the prostate gland, and can be done in one day with an overnight hospital stay, but is only available through private health care providers and not as part of the Australian national health system; or surgery to remove the prostate gland. The doctor advised Chris that there was no hurry to decide, that Chris should carefully consider his options and come back for a further appointment in a month.

Chris was shocked when the doctor confirmed that he had prostate cancer but felt much better once he was told that the cancer was treatable. He is keen to "get rid of the cancer" but is very concerned about the possibility that treatment might affect his continence and sexual function. The closer it comes to having to make a decision, the more difficult it has been for Chris to think through the issues. Lately, Chris has found that the only time he finds any real peace is when he is busy with jobs around the house. Chris failed to keep his last hospital appointment and is yet to make a new appointment time.

Chris's urologist referred him to see a hospital psychologist following a telephone call from Jill who was very concerned about Chris' failure to keep his follow-up appointment. Chris was reluctant to attend the appointment with the psychologist and agreed only because he felt that this might help Jill to feel a bit better about his situation. Chris admitted that he was feeling very confused about treatment options, and, although he denied feeling anxious or depressed he acknowledged that he had become increasingly withdrawn and irritable. When asked about his reluctance to make a treatment decision, Chris explained that he felt distressed by the possible outcomes of all of his treatment choices. He had a strong feeling that surgery to remove the prostate gave the best chance of cure, as leaving the cancer inside meant that it could "take hold," and he reported a close friend had died of advanced prostate cancer shortly after diagnosis. On the other hand, Chris found the idea of not being able to get an erection—which is very common after prostatectomy—almost unbearable. Although his erections were not as firm as they used to be, he was having intercourse regularly (about once a fortnight) and prided himself on the fact that he and Jill still enjoyed sex as a couple. He was worried about how erectile dysfunction might impact on how Jill saw him as a man. Chris explained that it is difficult for him to talk to Jill lately as she seeks to talk with him about the cancer, which often made him feel distressed, and he did not want to distress Jill by telling her about his concerns.

Jill was highly distressed about Chris's cancer and wanted him to have treatment as soon as possible. She was terrified of him dying and his cancellation of his last appointment increased her anxiety. Chris had always taken care of their finances, while Jill looked after the children and the house. She did not drive and felt very anxious about being left alone. At the same time Jill felt that Chris consistently underestimated her ability to cope, and she resented that they rarely sat down and talked about big decisions. Jill reported that Chris had refused to allow her to come to doctors' appointments, and seemed to avoid talking with her about his cancer, which made her feel that—once again—he did not value her input.

Jill was aware that Chris placed a lot of importance on their sex life and suspected that this might be part of the reason behind his refusal to make a treatment decision. However, Jill had not really enjoyed sex for some years and—although she enjoyed the cuddles that they have after sex—she was not particularly concerned about not being able to have intercourse in the future. Jill felt frightened and alone and had gone to her doctor for tablets to try and calm herself down.

Conceptualization, treatment, and outcome

The key presenting problems for Chris and Jill were their distress following the recent diagnosis, the difficulty in reaching a decision about what treatment option to pursue, and the strain in the couple relationship around discussing the cancer and how to manage treatment and its potential side effects. Several predisposing factors seemed relevant to the presenting problems. First, Chris had negative beliefs about cancer treatment and prognosis, and negative views about the potential impact of impotence on his relationship with Jill. Second, Chris and Jill had a long-standing pattern of responding to life challenges with Chris making major decisions in their relationship, and Jill being both reliant on Chris and somewhat resentful of being reliant. Third, the couple often did not engage in effective communication and misunderstood each other's views on important issues. The immediate precipitant of the presenting problems was the diagnosis of prostate cancer, and the difficult treatment choices confronting Chris and Jill. In response to these challenges, the problems were maintained by Chris avoiding contact with the medical team, distracting himself, and thereby temporarily reducing his anxiety. Jill ruminated on her concerns but was unable to effectively engage with and challenge her negative cognitions. The couple had a pattern of Jill attempting to initiate conversation about the cancer with Chris, he then felt increasing anxiety and withdrew from the conversation. This pattern frustrated both partners, failed to help them resolve how to proceed, and resulted in each being anxious.

The psychological intervention with Chris and Jill involved six face-to-face sessions and had five key components. First, empathic listening, psychoeducation, and gentle cognitive restructuring by the therapist were used to help each partner develop more realistic and helpful beliefs about the treatment options, and their likely side effects. In particular, it was emphasized that the cancer was detected at an early stage, that there was a good prognosis with several of the treatment options, and that there were strategies that could be employed to attempt to reduce and manage treatment side effects. Psychoeducational materials were used that involved the couple watching a DVD recording of other prostate cancer patients talking about how they had managed treatment and its side effects. Second, psychoeducation through use of educational recordings and discussion was used to illustrate how the distress experienced by both Chris and Jill was quite common in prostate cancer patients and their spouse. Both partners were assisted to develop their stress management skills with the use of relaxation training to reduce arousal associated with distress, development of present moment awareness to reduce avoidance, and scheduling of shared positive activities to enhance mood. Third, the couple was assisted to develop their positive communication skills, and to reduce the Jill approach-Chris withdraw pattern, by active listening to each other. The therapist used prompting and modeling to assist the partners to listen empathically to each other. Fourth, the therapist used a structured problem-solving approach to have the couple discuss the treatment options available to Chris, and their perceptions of the advantages and disadvantages of each option. These first four steps culminated in Chris deciding, in consultation with Jill, to proceed with surgery.

The fifth component of therapy focused on enhancing psychological and sexual intimacy in the couple. Approximately 4 weeks after surgery the couple began discussing their feelings about their sex life, and exploring ways that they could express affection and sexual interest to each other. The therapist advised the couple on the use of sensate focus, which is a series of sensual and sexual exploration exercises. This included education on how sexuality could be expressed without intercourse.

Across the course of therapy Chris and Jill reported substantial declines in their distress, Chris made the decision he had been avoiding and the couple began to discuss the important challenges they confronted. After surgery, Chris was able to regain some erectile functioning and while the firmness of his erections did not always allow intercourse, the couple was sexually active and enjoyed the sense of intimacy from the physical closeness. Their enhanced couple communication allowed the couple to develop a greater sense of mutual understanding, not just about the cancer and its effects, but also other important issues in their life.

Pam and Ken coping with breast cancer

Pam (aged 69 years) had been married to Ken (aged 72 years) for 15 years; they were partially retired farmers who lived on a property just outside a small rural town. The farm was managed by Ken's son. Pam also bred Labrador dogs as a business. This is the second marriage for both Pam and Ken and they have four adult children from previous marriages. Pam was diagnosed with early stage breast cancer 14 months ago following routine breast screening, and underwent a mastectomy and chemotherapy. At the time of presentation she had recently completed her chemotherapy.

Pam rang a Cancer Helpline requesting help for her low mood and anxiety since the end of her chemotherapy. It was not feasible for Pam to attend face-to-face counseling in the city, so therapy consisted of seven telephone counseling sessions with a specialist cancer psychologist. The first two sessions were assessment sessions, the first with Pam and the second with her husband Ken. Five couple therapy sessions followed, conducted using a speaker telephone so the therapist could speak to the couple.

Pam reported that she had been feeling particularly distressed since the end of cancer treatments approximately 2 months ago. She had lost her enthusiasm for previously enjoyable activities and noticed that she was starting to "makes excuses" to avoid spending time with friends and family. This was particularly upsetting for Pam who had set her sights on the end of treatment as a time when she would be able to start really enjoying her life again. Pam had also noticed that she has become preoccupied with the possible recurrence of the cancer, and thinking that something else might go wrong with her health. These thoughts had persisted despite Pam being advised by her surgeon at a recent 12-month follow-up that there was no evidence of the cancer and her prognosis is good.

Pam was particularly upset about her relationship with her husband, which she felt had deteriorated significantly in the preceding months. She reported they had not had sex in many months and that, although they rarely argued, it felt as if they were distant like "two strangers living under the same roof." Ken had not initiated sex and did not seem to be interested. Pam reported some reduction in libido compared to before the chemotherapy, and she was reluctant for Ken to see her naked. At the same time she missed the emotional closeness and reassurance that came with sexual contact. Pam worried whether Ken still loved her in the way that he did before.

Pam reported her initial reaction to her cancer diagnosis was shock and numbness, and thought "this is not happening to me." This was followed by several weeks of intense anxiety and despair, mixed with some relief and gratitude when she learned that the cancer had not spread. Despite feeling periodically overwhelmed with fear, Pam was aware that Ken lost his first wife to cancer and made a point of not talking to him about her negative thoughts. Pam was worried about the loss of her breast but she and Ken both agreed that it was easier to have a mastectomy than to contemplate the alternative of 6 weeks of daily radiation therapy in the city. She recovered well physically from the surgery but hated that her breast was missing and had not properly looked at her chest area since the surgery.

Despite feeling increasingly tired over the course of her chemotherapy Pam felt that she "coped well all the way through treatment." She was in regular contact with her family doctor and the breast cancer nurses at the local hospital, and felt reassured that the medical treatment of the cancer was well managed. Despite her fatigue she managed to take care of her dog breeding business and rarely had to ask others to help out.

Of particular concern to Pam was her relationship with Ken, which she felt had deteriorated markedly over several months leading up to the time of her presentation to the Helpline. Pam reported that Ken provided lots of practical support for Pam across the time of her cancer diagnosis and treatment, however she felt that he had not really connected with her "journey with cancer." She reported she had tried to talk with Ken about her feelings and often became teary, and Ken had then looked uncomfortable and tried to distract her, telling her to "think positively" or making an effort to "solve the problem." Frustrated by what she experienced as a lack of understanding of her feelings, Pam had gradually given up trying to talk with Ken about how she felt about herself and the effects of the cancer on her.

Ken reported that he loves Pam deeply, and was very concerned about her well-being over the weeks leading up to her presentation to the Cancer Helpline. He was devastated at her diagnosis and was determined to do "whatever it took to get her better." Ken encouraged Pam to get the mastectomy done because he felt that this would improve her chances of cure. Ken had steered clear of reminders of the cancer throughout treatment and had tried to make sure that Pam did the same, believing that they "needed to avoid their emotions getting on top of them." He helped her out as much as he could and made a point of not burdening her with his concerns about money and the farm. Ken felt it was wrong to even think about sex when Pam was so ill, and he avoided physical contact that might arouse him. After the end of chemotherapy and the lack of cancer recurrence at the 12-month follow-up, Ken had expected that their "life would return to normal." However, he saw Pam as more emotionally fragile than before and easily upset. Ken was feeling exhausted and unsure what more he could do to make things better.

Conceptualization, treatment, and outcome

The main presenting problems were the depression and anxiety evident in Pam, and the relationship strain between Ken and Pam including the lack of sexual and emotional closeness. One key predisposing factor for the onset of the problems was Ken's experience of the death of his former wife of cancer, and the negative beliefs and expectations that set up for both spouses about cancer treatment. Another predisposing factor was the fatigue and physical changes Pam had experienced through the cancer treatments. The couple had ongoing financial stress, which they had not discussed and which was worrying each of them. Finally, there was a pattern of both spouses avoiding discussing emotionally charged issues due to competing demands on their time and energy, and because of fear of upsetting the other.

The immediate precipitant of Pam's distress seemed to be the end of active cancer treatment, when the support for Pam from the health care system was withdrawn. In addition, with the end of the time demands associated with active treatment Pam had increased time to process the thoughts and feelings associated with her cancer diagnosis and treatment. Both partners experienced negative thoughts about cancer that were triggered by ongoing cancer reminders (particularly Pam's physical appearance, media stories about cancer, and comments by friends and family about the cancer diagnosis and treatment), and maintained by avoidance of difficult thoughts and feelings. Depressed mood was maintained by a reduction in rewarding activities since the diagnosis. Pam's low self-image was triggered by negative thoughts about her attractiveness and maintained by avoidance of thoughts about her physical appearance, looking at herself in the mirror, and physical intimacy with Ken. Relationship strain was compounded by the reduction in intimacy and mutual avoidance of discussing key problems. A reduction in engagement in pleasurable and rewarding activities also was eroding the sense of pleasure and closeness in the couple's relationship.

The first couple session consisted of psychoeducation about the impact of serious illness on relationships, and the common, understandable pattern of avoiding discussing difficult issues in an attempt to protect themselves from negative thoughts and feelings. The couple and the therapist discussed the dangers inherent in these well-intentioned behaviors, including the potential for increased misunderstanding and reduced feelings of closeness that comes about by not sharing difficulties. Pam and Ken were encouraged to talk openly and honestly about the impact of the cancer within the session, even though that discussion initially might be upsetting. Pam became very upset when talking about her feelings. Ken was encouraged just to listen without interrupting or trying to make her feel better. Ken found it difficult to share his experiences and stated that he had never previously fully acknowledged the grief that he felt over the loss of his first wife. Across the first two sessions the couple did gradually open up to each other, and were encouraged to have further conversations between sessions. Both Pam and Ken reported an enormous sense of relief at being able to share these thoughts and feelings.

The second and third sessions consisted of identifying reinforcing activities and gradually having Pam build up positive activities, and to monitor and begin to challenge negative thinking about the chance of cancer recurrence and her body image. By the fourth session, Pam and the therapist had developed a hierarchy of situations in which Pam would allow Ken to see her naked, and she was encouraged to use positive coping self-statements to manage her anxiety in these situations. This then moved into the use of sensate focus in which the couple massaged each other in sensual and then increasingly sexual ways.

The last session focused on the couple applying their recently refined communication skills and problem solving to discuss their financial difficulties, and how they might manage these more effectively. Ken and Pam reported a greatly increased sense of closeness through sharing more positive activities, discussing long-standing problems, and recommencing their sex life together. Pam also reported that, while she still was concerned about the possible recurrence of cancer, the frequency of worrying about that had decreased markedly, and she was sleeping much better.

Conclusions and reflections

The cases of Chris and Jill, and Pam and Ken, illustrate the diversity of patterns of onset of psychological distress associated with cancer diagnosis and treatment. For Chris, his distress emerged at the time of diagnosis, and challenges related to his fear about the efficacy of treatment and the potential side effects of treatment. In contrast, although Pam found the initial diagnosis and long course of treatment very challenging, it was 12 months after successful treatment that she felt she needed help.

The two cases also illustrate challenges that are common in couples confronting cancer diagnosis and treatment. As cancer occurs predominantly in older persons, many couples who experience cancer in one of the partners have been together for considerable periods. As is common, both case example couples described themselves as happily married, yet the spouses found it hard to support each other effectively. A significant contributor to the lack of mutual support was avoidance of discussing difficult issues. Such avoidance is understandable. Discussing fear of one partner dying is not easy, nor is it easy talking about insecurity about whether you will still be loved or desired if you have lost a key aspect of your sexuality (e.g. losing a breast or the capacity to attain erections). Avoidance of discussion can (temporarily) ease one's distress, and reduce obvious signs of upset in one's spouse. However, avoidance also fails to develop understanding of the other, and prevents effective development of shared coping strategies.

Another issue evident in both these cases are gender differences in how people cope with the stress of cancer diagnosis and treatment. On average women tend to respond to stress by emotional disclosure to those close to them more than men do, whereas men are more likely to attempt to do things to try to change the situation or solve a problem (Taylor et al., 2000). Each of these approaches to stress has utility when coping with cancer. Women are more likely than men to self-disclose about their feelings in response to the cancer and its treatment, which is associated with better adjustment. Men are more likely than women to seek out information to inform action, and information seeking is also associated with better adjustment. A challenge for couples is to be able to draw upon these different approaches to coping and address the couple's individual and conjoint needs.

In our work with couples we seek to develop a conceptualization of how each partner and the couple are adapting to the challenges of cancer diagnosis and treatment. We draw upon the general principles of what are the most common challenges couples confront to guide these individual conceptualizations, focusing upon psychoeducation to facilitate informed decisions, identifying and challenging unhelpful cognitions, promoting active coping, and encouraging empathic communication and mutual support between spouses. In addition, with breast and prostate cancer impacting on areas of the body closely associated with body image and sexuality, there is a need to assess how the couple are functioning sexually. The assessment is used to negotiate the goals of therapy with the couple, and to develop an individually tailored intervention to assist couples.

Diagnosis and treatment for cancer is confronting for the sufferer and those closest to them. Advances in early detection and treatment mean that the medical prognosis for patients has improved significantly. However, the psychological experiences across the course of diagnosis, treatment, and thereafter are often harrowing, and a substantial minority of patients and their spouses experience long-term problems in adjusting. Effective couple-based psychological education and therapy helps couples to make the required treatment-related decisions and reduce their cancer-related distress. Moreover, the process of the spouses working effectively together to manage the challenges often brings an enhanced sense of closeness and intimacy to the couple's relationship. One cancer survivor expressed it this way:

> I would never say I was glad to have cancer. Yet somehow going through it all made me cherish my life, my marriage. Lots of little things have changed. My husband and I go for walks, we talk more, I spend more time with my grandkids. And my house is quite a bit messier (laughs).

Reflective questions

1. How might men and women differ in the support they seek and provide when confronting cancer diagnosis? What implications does this have for assisting cancer patients and their spouse?

2. How might previous experience and beliefs about cancer diagnosis and treatment influence people's adjustment to cancer?

3. What knowledge about cancer diagnosis, treatment, and side effects is needed to assist men diagnosed with prostate cancer or women diagnosed with breast cancer?

4. What enables some people diagnosed with cancer to cope effectively with the rigors of treatment, while others struggle to cope?

Acknowledgment

Preparation of this chapter was supported by a National Health and Medical Research Council of Australia project grant entitled "A randomized controlled trial of early intervention to improve sexual and couple functioning after prostate cancer" to S. Steginga (Chambers), L. Schover, W.K. Halford, S. Occhipinti, R. Gardiner, and J. Dunn.

References

Andersen, B.L. (1993). Predicting sexual and psychologic morbidity and improving the quality of life for women with gynecologic cancer. *Cancer, 71*, 1678–1690.

Andersen, B.L., Anderson, B., & deProsse, C. (1989). Controlled prospective longitudinal study of women with cancer: I. Sexual functioning outcomes. *Journal of Consulting and Clinical Psychology, 57*, 683–691.

Andersen, B.L., Woods, X.A., & Copeland, L.J. (1997). Sexual self-schema and sexual morbidity among gynecologic cancer survivors. *Journal of Consulting and Clinical Psychology, 65*, 221–229.

Antoni, M.H., Lehman, J.M., Kilbourn, K.M., Boyers, A.E., Culver, J.L., Alferi, S.M., et al. (2001). Cognitive-behavioral stress management intervention decreases the prevalence of depression and enhances benefit finding among women under treatment for early-stage breast cancer. *Health Psychology, 20*, 20–32.

Antoni, M.H., Pereira, D.B., Marion, I., Ennis, N., Andrasik, M.P., Rose, R., et al. (2008). Stress management effects on perceived stress and cervical neoplasia in low-income HIV-infected women. *Journal of Psychosomatic Research*, 65(4), 389–401.

Ben-Zur, H., Gilbar, O., & Lev, S. (2001). Coping with breast cancer: Patient, spouse and dyad models. *Psychosomatic Medicine*, 63, 32–39.

Boyle, P., & Levin, B. (2008). World Cancer Report 2008. Geneva, Switzerland: World Health Organization.

Bremer, B.A., Moore, C.T., Bourbon, B.M., Hess, D.R., & Bremer, K.L. (1997). Perceptions of control, physical exercise, and psychological adjustment to breast cancer in South African women. *Annals of Behavioral Medicine*, 19, 51–60.

Brewin, C.R. (2001). A cognitive neuroscience account of posttraumatic stress disorder and its treatment. *Behavior Research and Therapy*, 39, 373–393.

Bultz, B.D., Speca, M., Brasher, P.M., Geggie, P.H.S., & Page, S.A. (2000). A randomized controlled trial of a brief psychoeducational support group for partners of early stage breast cancer patients. *Psycho-oncology*, 9, 303–313.

Carver, C.S., Pozo, C., Harris, S.D., Noriega, V., Scheier, M.F., Robinson, D.S., et al. (1993). How coping mediates the effect of optimism on distress: A study of women with early stage breast cancer. *Journal of Personality and Social Psychology*, 65, 375–390.

Carver, C.S., Meyer, B., & Antoni, M.H. (2000). Responsiveness to threats and incentives, expectancy of recurrence, and distress and disengagement: Moderator effects in women with early stage breast cancer. *Journal of Consulting and Clinical Psychology*, 68, 965–975.

Cassileth, B., Lusk, E., Miller, D., Brown, L., & Miller, C. (1985). Psychosocial correlates of survival in advanced malignant disease. *New England Journal of Medicine*, 312, 1151–1555.

Cella, D.F., & Tross, S. (1986). Psychological adjustment to survival from Hodgkin's disease. *Journal of Consulting and Clinical Psychology*, 54, 616–622.

Chambers, S.K., Schover, L., Halford, W.K., Clutton, S., Ferguson, M., Gorden, L., et al. (2008). ProsCan for couples: Randomized controlled trial of a couple based sexuality intervention for men with localized prostate cancer who received radical prostatectomy. *BMC Cancer*, 8, 226.

Christensen, D.N. (1983). Postmastectomy couple counselling: An outcome study of a structured treatment protocol. *Journal of Sex and Marital Therapy*, 9, 266–275.

Cliff, A.M., & Macdonagh, R.P. (2000). Psychosocial morbidity in prostate cancer II: A comparison of patients and partners. *British Journal of Urology International*, 86, 834–839.

Cordova, M.J., Andrykowski, M.A., Kenady, D.E., McGrath, P.C., Sloan, D.A., & Redd, W.H. (1995). Frequency and correlates of posttraumatic stress disorder-like symptoms after treatment for breast cancer. *Journal of Consulting and Clinical Psychology*, 63, 981–986.

Coyne, J.C., & Smith, D.A. (1991). Couple coping with myocardial infarction: A contextual perspective on wives' distress. *Journal of Personality and Social Psychology*, 61, 404–412.

Coyne, J.C., & Smith, D.A. (1994). Couples coping with myocardial infarction: Contextual perspective on patient self-efficacy. *Journal of Family Psychology*, 8, 43–54.

Coyne, J.C., & Gottlieb, B.H. (1996). The mismeasure of coping by checklist. *Journal of Personality*, 64, 959–991.

Coyne, J.C., & Racioppo, M.W. (2000). Never the twain shall meet? Closing the gap between coping research and clinical intervention research. *American Psychologist*, 55, 655–664.

Cutrona, C.E. (1996). Social support as a determinant of marital quality. In G.R. Pierce, B.R. Sarason, & I.G. Sarason (Eds.), *Handbook of social support and the family* (pp. 173–194). New York, NY: Plenum Press.

DeLongis, A., & O'Brien, T.B. (1990). An interpersonal framework for stress and coping: An application to the families of Alzheimer's patients. In M.A.P. Stephens, J.H. Crowther, S.E. Hobfoll, & D.L. Tennenbaum (Eds.), *Stress and coping in later life families* (pp. 221–239). Washington, DC: Hemisphere.

Dorros, S.M., Card, N.E., Segrin, C., Badger, T.A. (2010). Interdependence in women with breast cancer and their partners: An interindividual model of distress. *Journal of Consulting and Clinical Psychology*, *78*, 121–125.

Edgar, L., Rosberger, Z., & Nowlis, D. (1992). Coping with cancer during the first year after diagnosis: Assessment and intervention. *Cancer*, *69*, 817–828.

Eton, D.T., & Lepore, S.J. (2002). Prostate cancer and health-related quality of life: A review of the literature. *Psycho-oncology*, *11*, 307–326.

Fawzy, F.I., & Fawzy, N.W. (1998). Psychoeducational interventions. In J. Holland (Ed.), *Textbook of psycho-oncology* (pp. 676–693). New York, NY: Oxford University Press.

Gotay, C.C. (1984). The experience of cancer during early and advanced stages: The views of patients and their mates. *Social Science and Medicine*, *18*, 605–613.

Grassi, L., & Rosti, G. (1996). Psychosocial morbidity and adjustment to illness among long-term cancer survivors: A six-year follow-up study. *Psychosomatics*, *37*, 523–532.

Hagedoorn, M., Sanderman, R., Bolks, H.N., Tuinistra, J., & Coyne, J.C. (2008). Distress in couples coping with cancer: A meta-analysis and critical review of role and gender. *Psychological Bulletin*, *134*, 1–30.

Halford, W.K. (2006). Strength in numbers: The couple relationship in adult therapy. *Behaviour Change*, *23*, 87–102.

Hall, D. (2008). World Cancer Report with 2012 Forecasts. Lionchase holdings. Accessed on line November 18, 2009.

Halldorsdottir, S., & Hamrin, E. (1996). Experiencing existential changes: The lived experience of having cancer. *Cancer Nursing*, *19*, 29–36.

Heim, E., Augustiny, K.F., Schaffner, L., & Valach, L. (1993). Coping with breast cancer. *Journal of Psychosomatic Research*, *37*, 523–542.

Helgeson, V.S., & Cohen, S. (1996). Social support and adjustment to cancer: Reconciling descriptive, correlational, and intervention research. *Health Psychology*, *15*, 135–148.

Helgeson, V.S., & Tomich, P.L. (2005). Surviving cancer: A comparison of 5-year disease-free breast cancer survivors with healthy women. *Psycho-oncology*, *14*, 307–317.

Helgeson, V.S., Cohen, S., Schulz, R., & Yasko, J. (2000). Group support interventions for women with breast cancer: Who benefits from what? *Health Psychology*, *19*, 107–114.

Helgeson, V., Snyder, S.P., & Seltman, H. (2004). Psychological and physical adjustment to breast cancer over 4 years: Identifying distinct trajectories of change. *Health Psychology*, *23*, 3–15.

Hoskins, C.N. (1995). Adjustment to breast cancer in couples. *Psychological Reports*, *77*, 435–454.

Hoskins, C.N. (1997). Breast cancer treatment-related patterns in side effects, psychological distress, and perceived health status. *Oncology Nursing Forum*, *24*, 1575–1583.

Johnson Vickberg, S.M., Bovbjerg, D.H., DuHamel, K.N., Currie, V., & Redd, W.H. (2000). Intrusive thoughts and psychological distress among breast cancer survivors: Global meaning as a possible protective factor. *Behavioral Medicine*, *25*, 152–162.

Kemeny, M.M., Wellisch, D.K., & Schain, W.S. (1988). Psychosocial outcome in a randomized surgical trial for treatment of primary breast cancer. *Cancer*, *62*, 1231–1237.

Kilpatrick, M.G., Kristjanson, L.J., Tataryn, D.J., & Fraser, V.H. (1998). Information needs of husbands of women with breast cancer. *Oncology Nursing Forum*, *25*, 1595–1601.

Lenhard, R.E., & Osteen, R.T. (2001). General approach to cancer patients. In R.E. Lenhard, R.T. Osteen, & T. Gansler (Eds.), *Clinical oncology* (pp. 149–158). Atlanta, GA: American Cancer Society.

Lepore, S.J., & Coyne, J.C. (2006). Psychological interventions for distress in cancer patients: A review of reviews. *Annals of Behavioral Medicine*, *32*, 85–92.

Manne, S.L., Dougherty, J., Veach, S., & Kless, R. (1999). Hiding worries from one's spouse: Protective buffering among cancer patients and their spouses. *Cancer Research, Therapy, and Control*, *8*, 175–188.

Manne, S., Ostroff, J., Winkel, G., Goldstein, L., Fox, K., & Grana, G. (2004). Posttraumatic growth after breast cancer: Patient, partner, and couple perspectives. *Psychosomatic Medicine*, *66*, 442–454.

Manne, S., Ostroff, J., Winkel, G., Grana, G., & Fox, K. (2005). Partner unsupportive responses, avoidance and distress among women with early stage breast cancer: Patient and partner perspectives. *Health Psychology, 24*, 635–641.

Manne, S.L., Winkel, G., Rubin, S., Edelson, M., Rosenblum, N., Bergman, C., et al. (2008). Mediators of a coping and communication-enhancing intervention and supportive counseling among women diagnosed with gynecological cancers. *Journal of Consulting and Clinical Psychology, 76*, 1034–1045.

Mehnert, A., & Koch, U. (2008). Psychological morbidity and health-related quality of life and its association with awareness, utilization, and need for psychosocial support in a cancer register-based sample of long-term breast cancer survivors. *Journal of Psychosomatic Research, 64*, 383–391.

Moyer, A., & Salovey, P. (1996). Psychosocial sequelae of breast cancer and its treatment. *Annals of Behavioral Medicine, 18*, 110–125.

Newell, S.A., Sanson-Fisher, R.W., & Savolainen, N.J. (2002). Systematic review of psychological therapies for cancer patients: Overview and recommendations for future research. *Journal of the National Cancer Institute, 94*, 558–584.

Nezu, A.M., Nezu, C.M., & Lombardo, E.R. (2004). *Cognitive-behavioral case formulation and treatment design: A problem-solving approach.* New York, NY: Springer.

Omne-Ponten, M., Holmberg, L., Bergstrom, R., Sjoden, P.O., & Burns, T. (1993). Psychosocial adjustment among husbands of women treated for breast cancer: Mastectomy vs. breast-conserving surgery. *European Journal of Cancer, 29A*, 1393–1397.

Palmer, A.G., Tucker, S., Warren, R., & Adams, M. (1993). Understanding women's responses to treatment for cervical intra-epithelial neoplasia. *British Journal of Clinical Psychology, 32*, 101–112.

Parle, M., & Maguire, P. (1995). Exploring relationships between cancer, coping, and mental health. *Journal of Psychosocial Oncology, 13*, 27–50.

Penedo, F.J., Molton, I., Dahn, J.R., Shen, B.J., Kinsinger, D., Traeger, L., et al. (2006). A randomized clinical trial of group-based cognitive-behavioral stress management in localized prostate cancer: Development of stress management skills improves quality of life and benefit finding. *Annals of Behavioral Medicine, 31*, 261–270.

Pensiero, L. (1995). Stage IV malignant melanoma: Psychosocial issues. *Cancer, 75*(S2), 742–747.

Psychological Aspects of Breast Cancer Study Group (PABCSG) (1987). Psychological response to mastectomy: A prospective comparison study. *Cancer, 59*, 189–196.

Ptacek, J.T., Pierce, G.R., Dodge, L., & Ptacek, J.J. (1997). Social support in spouses of cancer patients: What do they get and to what end? *Personal Relationships, 4*, 431–449.

Redd, W.H., DuHamel, K.N., Johnson Vickberg, S.M., Ostroff, J.L., Smith, M.Y., Jacobsen, P.B., et al. (2001). Long-term adjustment in cancer survivors. In A. Baum & B.L. Andersen (Eds.), *Psychosocial interventions for cancer* (pp. 77–97). Washington, DC: American Psychological Association.

Roberts, K.J., Lepore, S.J., & Helgeson, V. (2006). Social-cognitive correlates of adjustment to prostate cancer. *Psycho-oncology, 15*, 183–192.

Schain, W.S., d'Angelo, T.M., Dunn, M.E., Lichter, A.S., & Pierce, L.J. (1994). Mastectomy versus conservative surgery and radiation therapy. Psychosocial consequences. *Cancer, 73*, 1221–1228.

Schneiderman, N., Antoni, M.H., Saab, P.G., & Ironson, G. (2001). Health psychology: Psychosocial and biobehavioral aspects of chronic disease management. *Annual Review of Psychology, 52*, 555–580.

Schover, L.R., Yetman, R.J., Tuason, L.J., Meisler, E., Esselstyn, C.B., Hermann, R.E., et al. (1995). Partial mastectomy and breast reconstruction. A comparison of their effects on psychosocial adjustment, body image, and sexuality. *Cancer, 75*(1), 54–64.

Scott, J.L., Halford, W.K., & Ward, B. (2004). United we stand? The effects of a couple-coping intervention on adjustment to early stage breast or gynaecological cancer. *Journal of Consulting and Clinical Psychology, 72*, 1122–1135.

Silberfarb, P.M. (1984). Psychiatric problems in breast cancer. *Cancer, 53*, 820–824.

Smith, D.P., King, M.T., Egger, S., Berry, M.P., Stricker, P.D., Cozzi, P., et al. (2009). Quality of life three years after diagnosis of localised prostate cancer: Population based cohort study. *British Medical Journal, 339*, 4817.

Sorlie, T., & Sexton, H.C. (2001). Predictors of the process of coping in surgical patients. *Personality and Individual Differences, 30*, 947–960.

Stanford, J., Feng, Z., Hamilton, A.S., Gilliland, F., Stephenson, R., Eley, J.W., et al. (2000). Urinary and sexual function after radical prostatectomy for clinically localized prostate cancer: The Prostate Cancer Outcomes Study. *Journal of the American Medical Association, 283*(3), 354–360.

Stanton, A.L., Danoff-Burg, S., Sworowski, L.A., Collins, C.A., Branstelter, A.D., Rodriguez-Hanley, A., et al. (2002). Randomized, controlled trial of written emotional expression and benefit finding in breast cancer patients. *Journal of Clinical Oncology, 20*, 4160–4168.

Stein, K.D., Syrjala, K.L., & Andrykowski, M.A. (2008). Physical and psychological long-term and late effects of cancer. *Cancer, 112*(S11), 2577–2592.

Taylor, S.E., Klein, L.C., Lewis, B.P., Gruenewald, T.L., Gurung, R.A.R., & Updegraff, J.A. (2000). Biobehavioral responses to stress in females: Tend-and-befriend, not fight-or-flight. *Psychological Review, 107*, 411–429.

Vinokur, A.D., Threatt, B.A., Caplan, R.D., & Zimmerman, B.L. (1989). Physical and psychosocial functioning and adjustment to breast cancer. Long-term follow-up of a screening population. *Cancer, 63*, 394–405.

Wingo, P.A., Parkin, D.M., & Eyre, H.J. (2001). Measuring the occurrence of cancer: impact and statistics. In R.E. Lenhard, R.T. Osteen, & T. Gansler (Eds.), *Clinical oncology* (pp. 1–20). Atlanta, GA: American Cancer Society.

World Health Organization (2004). *The global burden of disease: 2004 update.* Department of Health Statistics and Informatics in the Information, Evidence and Research Cluster of World Health Organization; Geneva, Switzerland: World Health Organization Press.

Yurek, D.L., Farrar, W.B., & Andersen, B.L. (2000). Breast cancer surgery: Comparing surgical groups and determining individual differences in postoperative sexuality and body change stress. *Journal of Consulting and Clinical Psychology, 38*, 697–709.

Zabora, J., Brintzenhofeszoc, K., Curbow, B., Hooker, C., & Piantadosi, S. (2001). The prevalence of psychological distress by cancer site. *Psycho-oncology, 10*, 19–28.

Zahlis, E.H., & Shands, M.E. (1991). Breast cancer: Demands of the illness on the patient partner. *Journal of Psychosocial Oncology, 9*, 75–93.

Chapter 6

Think family: systemic therapy in later life

Susan M. Benbow and Gillian Goodwillie

The personal context

We have come to this chapter by different routes and from different backgrounds but have been working together in an all-age family clinic for 3 years. One of us (Susan) is an old age psychiatrist who first encountered family therapy as a trainee in child psychiatry and then trained in general psychiatry in a community mental health placement where family therapy was routinely offered. After moving into old age psychiatry, it seemed even more important to work with families, and a supportive employer funded a Diploma in Family Therapy at the Cardiff Family Institute. Family work has continued throughout changes in job (from central Manchester to Wolverhampton and Staffordshire University) and into life post-Wolverhampton. Harlene Anderson (2007a) uses the term "philosophical stance," a "way of being" in relationship and conversation which she sees as the heart and spirit of collaborative therapy, and, although I didn't know those phrases at that time, it was this that sustained me through life as a consultant old age psychiatrist in the National Health Service, being privileged to walk alongside and learn from lots of older adults and their families at times in their lives when they needed someone alongside and with them. Family therapy wasn't something that happened in the clinic on a Thursday or Friday morning, it was something that underpinned and sustained the whole of my practice, and still does: I commend it to others working with older adults.

> The therapist wants to learn and understand the client from the client's perspective and preferences. The therapist wants to learn the client's lived experience and the meanings and understandings associated with it.

> (Anderson, 2007a, p. 47)

The other one of us (Gillian) was a locum in a Geriatric Unit and this brief experience transformed my thinking and practice. Length of admission seemed to correlate closely with the relational context of the patient as well as their medical condition or prognosis. A patient with a supportive family could often achieve earlier discharge than someone whose family was unavailable or disinterested. It seemed that unresolved conflicts had the potential to resurface and this could influence whether a partner or close relative was willing to support a discharge plan. I recall a 70-year-old man who appeared ready for rehabilitation following a stroke. His wife told me that for 50 years she had put up with her husband's abuse of her and that she saw no reason now to become his carer. Their adult daughter, whom I also interviewed, shared her mother's view, having witnessed his violence from childhood. The history of family relationships had the capacity to affect whether a patient could return home and how he/she might adjust to the changes in health. Later I went to work in a Child Psychiatric Department where I joined a weekly Family Therapy workshop. The importance of working with families underpinned working practice within the team and I subsequently trained as a systemic psychotherapist at The Kensington Consultation Centre in London. Since then I have worked in a range of different work settings as a systemic psychotherapist and I first met Susan when I was teaching on the Family Therapy Training programme at Manchester University. Our paths met again when we both were working in Wolverhampton, in Child and Adolescent Mental Health and Older Adult Mental Health, respectively. We realized that we could collaborate and provide a service which could offer families a treatment approach across the life cycle.

Useful concepts for practitioners

This chapter will describe three ideas that are important to systemic practice when working transgenerationally with a special focus on implications for work with older families. These are:

1. The concept of the family life cycle.
2. The idea of using "Social Graces" to inform clinical practice and help professionals respond sensitively to clients whose lived experience and identities may be different to their own.
3. The use of a genogram or family tree.

These concepts are some that are used within the practice of systemic therapy. In systemic therapy over the past 20 years or so there has been a move away from a preoccupation with techniques, which tended not to address issues of professional power and control (Hoffman, 1993). There is now much greater emphasis on the relationship between therapists and those they work with, and the development of ideas about collaboration (Anderson, 2007a) and dialogue (Anderson, 2007b). Alongside this there is debate about "not-knowing" and "client-as-expert" (Anderson, 2005), concepts which involve respect and dignity for family members and a recognition that they hold expertise regarding their own/their family member's illness and/or circumstances. This is coupled with the acknowledgment that the therapist doesn't necessarily know best. This philosophy involves the expertise of the therapist being made available in partnership with the knowledge and experience of family members in order to make space for the family to develop new ways of understanding current difficulties. Dallos and Draper (2005) give an authoritative overview of these developments and their book offers source references for those who wish to follow these ideas up.

We describe here a total of five case studies: four case studies will briefly illustrate the issues that can arise when working with later life families and the fifth demonstrates the value of consulting across professional agencies, utilizing the knowledge and skills that family therapists bring to this work.

Concept of the family life cycle

The concept of the family life cycle is an important systemic idea (Carter & McGoldrick, 1999) which considers how families can manage the transitions that occur within relationships at different life stages. Birth, death, and the formation or dissolution of partnerships may inform complex interactional processes involving cultural, societal, family, and individual factors shaping how these events are negotiated within a family. This perspective suggests that there are likely to be times that the family may be more vulnerable to managing successfully challenges to the family, both internal and external.

Social graces

The idea of "Social Graces" (Roper-Hall, 1993) is a useful construct for practitioners delivering services within the diverse communities they serve. The word is an acronym to invite connection and reflection regarding inequalities that may be more or less visible to the professionals working with any client family. Gender, race, religion, age, abilities, class, culture, ethnicity, and sexual orientation need to be considered and conceptualized as active constituents which will contribute to the outcomes of professional involvement in any context. Ethnocentric professional practice can contribute significantly to clinical failure. We will explore the issues of agism that can surround the work with later life families.

The use of a genogram

The genogram (McGoldrick, Gerson, & Petry, 2008) is a useful tool with later life families (Benbow et al., 1990), both in therapy and in routine practice, but, with a multigenerational family in particular, it can be large, complex, and a lengthy exercise, although often engaging, sometimes very enjoyable for families, and highly relevant in opening up conversations. It can be a good way of starting to talk about cross-generational life cycle issues. However, even sheets of flipchart paper may not be large enough to accommodate the different generations when a couple are in their 80s or 90s. The genogram is also a way of engaging with the history of the family and talking about history that is still alive in the present.

The family in later life

One of the images of later life that produced a lasting impression was a diagram of the family life cycle with later life represented as a coffin on a dead end off the main cycle (Fig. 6.1—modified from Turnbull, 1989). This image fails to acknowledge the important contributions that older adults make to the life of families. It perpetuates an agist view of later life, implying that work and bringing up children are the important roles of families, and that retirement starts at a fixed age which defines the start of later life, after which it's downhill until death. In the twenty-first century, it is not appropriate to see retirement as the "hub" of the later life cycle (Mouratoglou, 1991). Many people undergo several so-called "retirements," develop portfolio careers, or end their paid work at an earlier stage in life and make a transition to other ways of contributing to society and spending their time. There is no longer a single milestone age which determines the distinction between work and pension, and indeed concepts of what the future holds and how long the future might be have also radically altered with increases in life expectancy and the altered population profile. Rarely is there recognition of the contribution that older adults may make to families: acknowledging the role of grandparent, maybe great grandparent; of carrying, sharing, and bequeathing the family's history; of advising, nurturing, and supporting younger generations (perhaps even contributing to childcare); perhaps offering financial support or shared housing to younger family members; of demonstrating how to live with illness, disability, and loss; and of continuing to contribute as citizens to society. All these contributions are evolving and successive cohorts of older adults may have differing views on them, while differing generations of therapists will also have their own perspectives. A coffin doesn't quite symbolize the many ways in which older adults contribute to families and all aspects of family life. Froma Walsh (1999) writes about "challenges and opportunities" confronting later life families, highlighting the wide variety of pathways through later life, the transitions faced at this stage, and the cross-generational interplay of life cycle stages and issues within families: the developmental needs of one generation may occur at a time which brings conflict with the needs of another generation within the family. Walsh argues for a resilience-based approach to practice with later life families.

An alternative model to the life cycle is the family life spiral (Fig. 6.2) (Combrinck-Graham, 1988). The family life spiral is distorted to signify that at some times in family life family members tend to be close and intricately involved with one another: the forces within the family may be

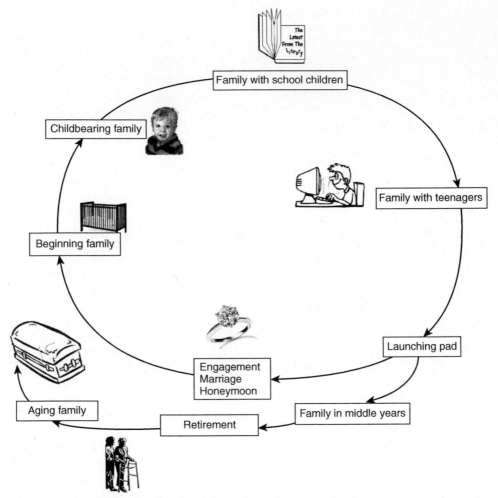

Fig. 6.1 A misrepresentation of the family life cycle.

regarded as centripetal—pulling people together. At other times family members are focussed more outside the family and the forces within the family may be regarded as centrifugal. This can be a useful concept when looking at cross-generational issues: for example, the eldest generation of a family may be coping with issues that commonly require families to focus energy in supporting one another, such as chronic illness, disability, and a need for care, while a younger generation might be experiencing a period of growing interests and activities outside the family such as early retirement with its freedom from paid employment. Dealing with these differing needs brings the potential for cross-generational conflicts and misunderstandings.

McGoldrick (1999) pointed out that the final phase of life might be considered to be "for women only" as women tend to outlive men and rarely have younger partners. Gender issues can be a major theme for families (Benbow, 2005). Men and women may have differing ideas and expectations about later life and the challenges it brings (e.g. retirement from paid employment, becoming a grandparent, losing a partner). A married Irish woman, now disabled by Parkinson's disease, said in the family clinic that "men can enjoy themselves." She described how, in her family and in her marriage, men come home from work, put their slippers on, and sit relaxing

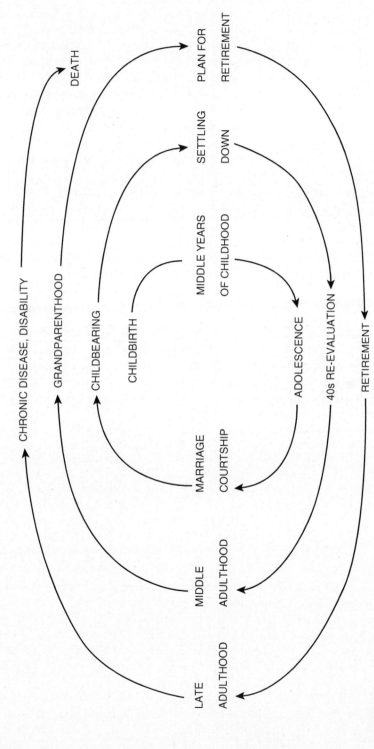

Fig. 6.2 The family life spiral.

while their wives cook supper for them: then, after eating, the men go down to the pub and meet their friends while their wives clear up the house. After she and her husband retired, this pattern continued: her husband still met his friends in the pub for a few drinks in the evening and she continued to do the household chores. Parkinson's disease was diagnosed, she became disabled, and her husband grew to regard himself as her carer. Yet despite this, he continued to go to the pub, while his wife grew increasingly angry: her last chance of enjoying herself appeared to have slipped away. His requests for respite care only served to fuel her anger further.

There are particular challenges in working with people who are in the later stages of their own lives. Oates Schuster (2001) writes about researching a Writing Group in a nursing home, saying how she is motivated to "look for examples of alternative ways of being old, frail, and dependent, ways that might provide greater opportunity for self-expression and that might enhance one's dignity and integrity" (p. 203). This is a challenge for families, as well as for the professionals who work with them.

Agism remains an important issue to consider in working with people in later life. Ivey, Wieling, and Harris (2000) found that relational and mental health concerns experienced by elder couples are perceived less seriously by practising marriage and family therapists than the same concerns experienced by younger couples. Older adults themselves are not immune to agism and may expect to be treated differently themselves because of their age. Therapists' different expectations of older adults may influence the conversations they have with later life families.

Issues of later life

There are some issues that will recur in later life therapy, including loss and grief, chronic illness and disability, retirement and the adjustment to stopping paid employment, and moving into sheltered accommodation or care home. None of these is exclusive to later life but the meanings associated may be different from those in younger families. Cognitive impairment or dementia is also more common in later life, and, like any other chronic illness, it can be an appropriate focus in therapy (Benbow, Marriott, Morley, & Walsh, 1993).

Case study 1 illustrates some of these issues in the large and close family of a relatively young man.

Case study 1: the A family

Mr. A was in his late 60s, married with 10 children, all living locally and in regular contact. Eighteen months before referral to the family therapy clinic he had a stroke that left him with speech difficulty, cognitive impairment, unable to walk, and needing total nursing care. On the advice of medical staff he moved into a nursing home after a lengthy period of rehabilitation. At first he was going to visit his wife, who moved into a ground floor flat near the Home, three times a week but he became persistently low in mood, tearful, indicating that he was fed up of his disabilities and felt life was not worth living. He was treated with several antidepressant drugs but showed no improvement. For the 4 months before referral he was reluctant to get out of bed and didn't want to engage in any activities or go out of the home. If he was persuaded to go to visit his wife, he would stay in bed all day and take no interest in any visitors or activities. The social worker and psychiatrist both felt that the interaction between him, his family, and the nursing home was a major factor in his low mood and withdrawal, but a series of meetings in the Home had not led to any change.

Mr. A, his wife, and all 10 children were invited to the family clinic. It was standard practice at the time to invite families to bring along any other family members who they felt should be present. Mr. A attended with his wife, eight children, and one adult grandchild. Two therapists met with the family. The two eldest daughters and Mrs. A did most of the talking for the first 15 minutes.

They described how Mr. A was going home 3 days per week ("we all thought it was a good idea"—"no way are we leaving him there 7 days a week"). They said "we all decided it." Regarding the nursing home, they said "we don't think it's really that good"; "it's very depressing"; "we don't visit him in the nursing home because it depresses the family and there's too many of us." Mrs. A was unable to care for her husband on his visits home because of arthritis, so the eldest daughter explained: "we have a rota—it's in my kitchen on the wall." The rota set out which family member would care for Mr. A during his home visits. At first no one dissented from the views expressed, most family members nodding and appearing to agree. When the opportunity arose the therapists asked the two quietest members of the family for their views and the facade of unity cracked: "I don't think it does work"; "lots of problems with the rota"; "there's people that won't go on it"; "it's not fair."

An animated discussion followed and it became clear that there was a range of views in the family about how the situation should be dealt with, and considerable disagreement with the idea of the rota that the two eldest daughters had imposed in an attempted solution. "There's nothing but trouble—all the family's falling out all the time." "For a family that used to be dead close–it's fell apart." "We're all raving at one another."

Three main areas of discussion dominated the rest of the meeting: how do decisions get made in a big family; how do differences get resolved; how do people show they care/show affection; and how can family members care for older and younger generations when their needs appear to conflict? The concluding theme was loyalty. The therapists observed that the children were committed to one another, loyal, and loving, but they were loyal and loving to older and younger generations that pulled them in two directions. They observed that "raving" might not be a bad thing if it kept members of the family talking and asked them to reflect on whether there might be other ways of showing care and concern apart from being on a rota.

The family were invited back to the clinic and on the second occasion, about 4 weeks later, Mrs. A and four of the children came. They reported that the family had decided to cut down Mr. A's visits home to once weekly and family members now had a loose rota (not on the kitchen wall) for visiting him in the Home during the week: "so that we don't all go at once." Mr. A was staying up during the day in the Home (and on his visits to his wife) and spending time with other residents. He also was described as brighter, more interested in what was going on, and enjoying the family's visits. The family didn't feel that they needed a further appointment but it was left that they could return to the clinic if they felt it would be helpful in future.

Reflections on working with the A family

The two meetings with the family were perceived as very helpful by all concerned, and this case study highlights the following:

- Families can have a powerful impact on what might be regarded as medical or nursing issues (major stroke, nursing home care, etc).

- Family interventions can address issues which might be perceived as psychiatric illness (in this case Mr. A was treated for a depressive illness but the symptoms of depression responded to the family intervention).

- It is important to invite all those who might wish to be involved—the family team had some qualms about inviting all 10 of Mr. A's children but went ahead and did so. It may be indicative of how much people care that most of the family attended and all took part actively in the conversation.

- A small number of sessions (in this case two) can sometimes have significant impact on the situation.

This illustrates a brief and effective intervention. The role of the two eldest daughters in the decision-making process was interesting and shows younger siblings (although themselves adult) may become locked into patterns of relating: perhaps reflecting their childhood experience in a big family of eldest daughters acting as surrogate parents to their younger siblings.

Family and systemic therapy in later life

One definition of systemic therapy is:

> Systemic therapy (whether treating individuals, couples or families) focuses on the relational context, addresses patterns of interaction and meaning, and aims to facilitate personal and interpersonal resources within a system as a whole. Therapeutic work may include consultation to wider networks such as other professionals working with the individual or the family.

> (Department of Health, 2001, p. 45)

Gergen and Kaye (1992) wrote that therapy could be thought of as "the forging of meaning in the context of collaborative discourse" and Rober (1999) quotes a definition of psychotherapy from Goolishian and Winderman "a linguistic activity in which conversation about a problem generates the development of new meaning." Thus, there is no reason why this shouldn't be as important (or perhaps even more important) in later life as in early life, but somehow the weight of interest still rests on the early stages of the life cycle. The recent initiative Improving Access to Psychological Therapies (CSIP Choice and Access Team, 2007) openly ascribes to an emphasis on addressing social exclusion through employment, thereby marginalizing older people. Similarly, although psychological therapies are often considered in relation to mental ill-health, they have relevance and importance in the management of physical ill-health, particularly the management of chronic disease (Martire, Lustig, Schulz, Miller, & Helgeson, 2004), and this is more common in later life.

When people have quieter voices than others (perhaps because of agism), it is important that they are given a context where their voice can be heard. Hoffman (1993) writes about reflexivity as "a mutually influenced process ... as opposed to one that is hierarchical and unidirectional" (p. 127). Lax (1992) uses the term co-construction to describe how the story a person tells in therapy is told in conjunction with a therapist and is therefore "neither the client's nor the therapist's story, but a co-construction of the two" (p. 73).

In the United Kingdom, there is a drive to improve access to psychological therapies (Department of Health, 2008) but this is based on providing services for people with mental health problems. We believe that good practice would involve integrating family approaches across the whole range of older adult services.

Some work with older adults has clear links with therapies and developments in older adult physical and mental health services. Hargrave (1994) described video life reviews which used ideas from reminiscence to make videos of older adults undertaking life reviews. He describes these as "re-storying" past events with new narratives and new meanings.

Some of the current ideas in family therapy fit well into work with later life families. Andrews (2007) has described honoring elders in conversations about their lives, which she believed had meaning and therapeutic value for the people involved. In families, conversations about long lives and connections between the generations can honor the older generations, both present and absent. Anderson's (2005) concepts of not-knowing, client-as-expert, mutual/shared inquiry, and conversational partnership may be eminently appropriate to later life therapy, often allowing a slower pace, accepting of life review, respectful of an elder's life experience and expertise, and fitting situations where the therapist will almost inevitably come from a younger generation than the clients.

Case study 2 illustrates the use of family therapy in a setting of chronic physical illness and the importance of understanding how relationships impact on illness.

Case study 2: the B family

A man with Parkinson's disease in his late 80s was referred to the family clinic by a geriatric physician after several admissions to medical care with hypothermia. On the last occasion this had followed a row with his wife that culminated in her locking him out of the house in the winter, despite his poor mobility and despite the fact that they both knew he had been hypothermic in the past.

They came to the family clinic as a couple for several sessions. When they drew up a genogram and talked about how they came to marry, the wife talked about how she married him after his best friend (her fiancé) died in the armed forces during the Second World War. She felt that it kept a link to her fiancé, but she never had great affection for him. He loved her and was aware that he was "second best." He earned a good living as a teacher and they had a comfortable and busy lifestyle. This was curtailed when he became unwell and her life became restricted as his carer. She still resented the fact that he had survived the war and the man she loved had died.

In the sessions they talked about how their marriage had depended on them developing separate interests and spending time apart which was no longer practical given Mr. B's disabilities. They considered a range of options which might help to improve the situation they found themselves in and decided to separate. Mr. B moved into a residential home. This was socially acceptable to both of them because of his physical health although they had not seriously considered living apart in the past, and meant that he could be supported by staff to pursue his interests in books, reading, and writing in a way that his wife had not been able to do. Mrs. B continued to visit her husband and both felt that they could accept the outcome, which left each free to develop their interests.

Reflections on working with the B family

- The history of relationships may be relevant and important to understanding and dealing with current difficulties presented by older adults.
- Existing relationship difficulties may affect the management of physical illness in later life.
- The therapy enabled the couple to voice and seriously consider options which they would previously have been unable to contemplate.
- Separation may be paradoxically more acceptable in later life because it may be legitimized/made more acceptable by physical illness or disabilities.
- Unresolved conflicts within long-term relationships may be alleviated by the couple separating.

Case study 3 illustrates the complexity of issues raised by work with a couple in their 60s, with an intermingling of themes perhaps more typical of earlier life stages with more traditional themes associated with later life.

Case study 3: the C family

Mr. C, a married man in his 60s, was admitted to an in-patient old age psychiatry bed to be withdrawn from addictive opiate drugs which he had been given for some years at an increasing dosage for chronic pain. He had been doing less and less at home, taking more and more pain killers, spending most of his time on his bed sleeping, and complaining of feeling very low with fleeting thoughts of suicide. His wife felt that they had little relationship left and resented having to care for him.

This was Mrs. C's second marriage; they met when she was a single parent raising two small children, married, and had three daughters together. The youngest daughter had left home 12 months before the referral to go to University in the South of England. The middle daughter was married with children and living a short distance away, and the eldest had limited contact because of her "high-powered job." Mr. C had been more withdrawn and increasingly unhappy for about 12 months and referral was precipitated by his wife telling him she was thinking about leaving.

The first two meetings with the couple took place while Mr. C was an in-patient. A genogram was drawn up with them (see Fig. 6.3) and highlighted a number of themes. Mr. C was born after an older and much-loved brother died and was given the same name as his dead brother. He had been ill for much of his childhood and vividly described how his mother took him to a succession of doctors in an attempt to find out what was wrong. He now had very little contact with his siblings and knew little about their lives. Despite his health problems he had managed to establish a successful business and worked hard despite treatment including operations (culminating in a stoma) for ongoing physical health problems. His wife had been adopted and didn't know anything about her family of origin. She had recently and unsuccessfully been attempting to get information from social services about her mother. She believed that her adoptive mother had known more about her background than she had shared with her, and resented the fact that she might now never know. The stoma had impacted on their sexual relationship, but Mrs. C said that this wasn't an issue for her, although she described how she now regarded herself as her husband's carer rather than his partner. Both talked about how Mr. C's illness had ruined their retirement plans. They had intended to sell up and move to live in Spain for a "life in the sun," but both felt that this was no longer an option because of Mr. C's illness. Mr. C's multiple roles as businessman, husband, father, grandfather, patient, and addict to pain killers was a strong theme, alongside his wife's roles as adoptive daughter, daughter of unknown parents, wife, mother, grandmother, and carer.

Following Mr. C's discharge from the ward, his withdrawal from drugs continued at home and the couple attended for three more meetings in the family clinic. The couple talked about their expectations and hopes for the future, given Mr. C's illness. Both wanted him to "do more" but had different views regarding what he should aim to do and how quickly he might try to do so. In the clinic a major theme was to talk about how people often changed their interests, ideas, and activities as they grew older, and perhaps in response to illnesses and events. The couple planned (and successfully carried out) some modest trips out to visit their married daughter and grandchildren and to go to places of interest in the locality. Mr. C took up bowling, an interest which he felt he could pursue despite his physical problems and established a routine of bowling twice weekly. His wife accepted that there had been improvements but remained rather negative about progress and continued to raise the possibility of a new life in the sun although both husband and wife now appeared to see this more as a fantasy rather than a realistic plan. From time to time one of the couple still wondered whether Mr. C should see another specialist or try a different medication but this became less prominent in later meetings and was not acted upon. The couple was discharged from the clinic after five sessions as they felt that they had established a new routine which was working well for both of them, but with the offer that they could request to be seen again if they wished in future.

Reflections on working with the C family

The work with the C family illustrates a number of important points in later life family therapy:

+ The intermingling of physical, psychological, relationship, family of origin, and age-related issues.

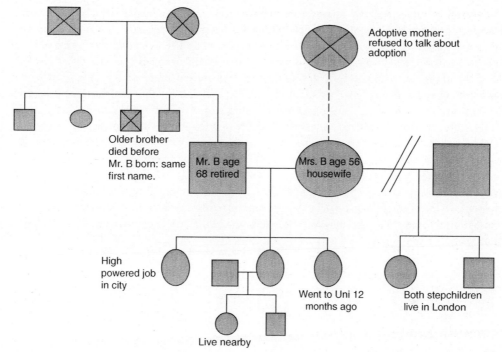

Fig. 6.3 Genogram of the C family (case study 3).

- How themes which are often seen as more characteristic of work with families earlier in the life cycle may still be important in later life families, for example adoption, addiction to drugs. However, it also illustrates how these themes become entangled in issues more specific to later life, for example loss of paid employment, post-retirement planning, adapting to the restrictions of physical illness, being a grandparent.

- How psychological therapies commonly take place alongside other physical and psychiatric interventions—this may need flexibility in how the work is carried out and may raise communication issues within services.

- The use of a formal family clinic (with use of a team working with two therapists) in combination with less formal sessions when the two therapists saw the couple in a quiet room in the in-patient unit.

- Issues of identity and transition. The wife's narrative of identity was disrupted in this case and her husband's personal identity had changed abruptly, moving from a strong identity as a family provider to becoming unproductive and a recipient of care.

Case study 4 illustrates some of the themes more commonly associated with later life in work with a couple who both had multiple medical problems and who were placing considerable demands on physical health care services.

Case study 4: the D family

The D family, a couple in their early 70s, were referred after repeatedly presenting to the Accident and Emergency Department, usually following an incident when Mrs. D. had phoned an ambulance saying she thought her husband was having a heart attack. Mr. D. was described as always full of nerves, and had angina, chronic obstructive airways disease (which caused some breathlessness but didn't significantly limit his lifestyle), and a duodenal ulcer. He complained to his family doctor that he was agitated, couldn't sleep, and felt that his nerves were bad. He described anxiety symptoms, but went on to say that of his "problem": "actually it's the wife." Mrs. D had been in hospital shortly before the problems started after losing her eyesight. When asked what the doctors had told her about her eyesight she replied: "they said it was nerves." She had her own health problems; diabetes, a hiatus hernia, and a recent slight stroke. She said she felt upset all the time, often wanted to cry, was constantly worried about Mr. D and kept thinking he's having a heart attack. Their family doctor made the referral saying: "they wind each other up and cannot cope with each other. They are turning up in Casualty all the time."

They attended the family clinic together for four meetings. It emerged that they had married fairly late and had no children because Mr. D had cared for his mother until her death. Before she died Mr. D's mother had made a will leaving the house to Mr. D's nephew (his sister's son and his mother's only grandchild) although with the requirement that Mr. D could live in the house until his death.

Reflections on working with the D family

◆ Some of the major themes in the family sessions were common to people in late life: physical health, death, where to live if the couple couldn't cope in the home or if one of them should die, how could one of the couple cope without the other.

◆ Money was an issue; in relation to the house and Mr. D's mother's will.

◆ The first two family meetings were canceled and then rearranged because one of the couple was ill and unable to attend. This is not uncommon in working with older adults who have chronic illness, and can stretch therapy out over a longer timescale than might be expected.

◆ There may also be issues of making sure that there is easy access for people with a disability to the clinic base. For some older people going by public transport to a clinic might be impossible and the practicalities of ensuring people can get to the clinic and into the building need to be addressed. We have offered some family meetings in the home where this was felt to be appropriate.

◆ Most of Mr. and Mrs. D's worries had been unspoken and the opportunity to talk about them and plan openly paralleled a decrease in panic calls to the medical services. The couple declined the suggestion of inviting their nephew to a joint meeting in the clinic.

Case study 5 illustrates consulting across complex professional systems and multi-agency work, demonstrating how systemic therapists can undertake a helpful role without seeing the family at the center of concerns.

Case study 5: the E family

The E family was referred to us from learning disability services. One daughter (DE) had been admitted to an in-patient bed under the Mental Health Act with violent aggressive behavior in the context of an illness described as schizophrenia in association with mild learning disability and diabetes. The referring team described the family dynamics as extremely complicated. DE was the fourth of nine children of Mr. E's second wife. Mr. E was originally from India and had lived in the United Kingdom for many years. When it became clear that his first wife was unable to have children, he married a second wife who then came to the United Kingdom but never learned to speak any English. His second wife had a total of nine children, who ranged in age from late teens to early 30s at the time of referral (five boys and four girls). Four of the children were given to

Mr. E's first wife in infancy to raise as her own. DE and four of her younger siblings remained with their birth mother and all were on the at-risk register at some point during childhood as a result of neglect or physical abuse. The two families lived separately in neighboring streets and Mr. E divided his time between them. After a long period of ill-health, Mr. E died about 12 months before referral leaving the two women to bring up the now adult children. The children living with the birth mother, who herself had several long-standing health problems, were forbidden from having contact with their stepmother and their siblings who lived with her.

The problem which led to referral was that staff felt that DE's mother's attitude was exacerbating their difficulty in managing both her mental health and her diabetes. Her mother was said to refuse to accept that DE had a mental illness and described her violent aggressive behavior as being silly or playful. Similarly, she did not accept that DE needed treatment for diabetes. She also was reported to have been telling DE not to take her medications as they would poison her. The staff caring for DE on the in-patient unit felt that the reason for her lack of progress was her mother's attitude and that even if she did respond to treatment in hospital she would be likely to relapse once she returned to her family.

After reviewing the referral information the family team arranged a consultation with the team caring for DE. Prior to that meeting a number of staff members involved in DE's care sent letters with their views to the team. The consultation meeting was held in a conference room and involved the psychiatrist, ward doctor, social worker, key nurse, ward manager, and clinical psychologist, all of whom were involved in DE's care. The family team opened the consultation by asking for some basic information about the family, for example we had not been able to understand how many children were in the family as different letters had given different numbers. It emerged that each member of the team held some information about the family but that information had not been shared across the team. Some team members had established good working relationships with individual family members (in particular the social worker had seen DE's birth mother on several occasions and had useful information about her, but this fact was not generally appreciated).

Everyone at the meeting had chance to contribute what they knew and what they thought might be helpful and the meeting concluded with agreement that the social worker and psychiatrist (together with an interpreter) would visit DE's birth mother to clarify a number of points and talk with her about future management. The family team left open an offer to meet with the family together with members of the team managing her care if necessary in future but acknowledged the combined expertise of the team caring for her.

Reflections on consultation to the team working with the E family

◆ This was a complex case involving a large family with well-established splits and alliances.

◆ The cultural aspects introduced problematic dilemmas for the professionals attempting to engage sensitively with this family. Medical approaches associated with modern western practice can sometimes be viewed with suspicion by ethnic groups which place faith in traditional methods. This would give an explanation for DE's mother's apparent lack of co-operation with the medication regimes required to manage her daughter's mental and physical health.

◆ The team caring for the referred patient had a wealth of knowledge about the family and expertise to draw on but, possibly because of the complexity of the situation, cultural differences, and the challenge of key family members being unable to speak English, had been unable to share their knowledge and produce an action plan.

◆ The family team reviewed the referral and found the information presented by the team patchy and contradictory. They decided to offer a consultation to the team as a first step, and the consultation revealed that the information held by team members was similarly patchy. The consultation offered a setting where information and views were brought together, and this helped the team to feel more confident and to formulate a plan of how to move DE's care forward by working with key family members, who seemed to have previously been marginalized in terms of their involvement in care planning.

Conclusions and points for reflection

Families are at least as important in later life as they are earlier in the family life cycle and those working with older adults need to be sensitive to the impacts that both physical and mental illnesses have on all family members. Unfortunately, in settings where the emphasis is on physical and/or mental ill-health and its treatment/rehabilitation family issues sometimes are neglected, despite the fact that work with the family can powerfully complement other forms of treatment.

In reflecting on how services are provided, it may be helpful to think about three aspects of systemic therapy:

◆ First, how can ideas and techniques from systemic therapy be employed in work with older adults, for example how are families kept involved in the assessment and treatment of relatives with physical ill-health? How is their expert knowledge about their relative accessed and used to inform care planning?

◆ Second, is there access to systemic consultation in relation to complex family situations which would benefit from this?

◆ Third, is there access to formal family and systemic psychotherapy when the need arises?

It is also useful to reflect on the four challenges set out below:

◆ How might services and individual practitioners work differently with older adults?

When seeing someone in an individual setting there will still be opportunities to ask about family involvement, attitudes and beliefs, and to reflect on their impact on the individual's illness or circumstances.

◆ How might services and staff members work differently with the families of older adults?

Not uncommonly families feel excluded from the care of relatives in the health/social care system. They often have a great deal of knowledge and understanding about their relative and their illness. How can families be more involved? How can their knowledge and concern be brought into the support of developing and implementing an effective treatment plan? Sometimes confidentiality is cited as a reason for excluding families or carers and this can adversely impact on a person's care (Wynaden & Orb, 2005). If professionals are themselves persuaded of the importance of involving families in care and feel confident in their own expertise, this will help them to negotiate ways of ensuring that involvement.

◆ How might services and individual staff members work differently with colleagues from their own and other agencies?

Collaboration with families is important but collaboration across the whole of the support system is important in managing chronic disease and complex co-morbidity. Ideas and approaches from family therapy can be used to bring teams from different agencies together and harness the expertise of all involved.

◆ How can services be delivered in a way which appreciates the role and significance of the relational system and recognizes that this creates a context for each individual?

Services are often organized by client group or diagnostic category, which can lead to a narrow focus, blind to the roles of older adults as family members and important influences on the life cycle of the family as a whole. In the United Kingdom, health and social services have been moving over recent years to shift the balance of power toward the client or service user (Department of Health, 2000); this should lead to respect and recognition for the client's roles within the family and community.

How can a broader perspective be encouraged which would recognize the importance and centrality of the family in policy objectives? How can an approach be encouraged which would "Think Family" and place the relational system as a partner in the commissioning and delivery of services across the family life cycle?

In this chapter, we have suggested three useful concepts for practitioners, which we have set within the context of the philosophy, theory, and approach of systemic therapy. The use of these concepts and of systemic therapy is illustrated using five case studies. Readers are encouraged to reflect on the use of systemic therapy in settings where older adults and their families present with physical or mental health problems or for rehabilitation, and to consider the challenges posed for individuals, services, and organizations by thinking systemically.

References

Anderson, H. (2005). Myths about 'not-knowing'. *Family Process, 44*, 497–504.

Anderson, H. (2007a). The heart and spirit of collaborative therapy: The philosophical stance—'a way of being' in relationship and conversation. In H. Anderson & D. Gehart (Eds.), *Collaborative therapy relationships and conversations that make a difference* (pp. 43–59). London: Routledge.

Anderson, H. (2007b). Dialogue: People creating meaning with each other and finding ways to go on. In H. Anderson & D. Gehart (Eds.), *Collaborative therapy relationships and conversations that make a difference* (pp. 33–41). London: Routledge.

Andrews, J. (2007). Honoring elders through conversations about their lives. In H. Anderson & D. Gehart (Eds.), *Collaborative therapy relationships and conversations that make a difference* (pp. 149–166). London: Routledge.

Benbow, S.M. (2005). Gender issues in therapy with later life families. *Context, 77*, 3–6.

Benbow, S.M., Egan, D., Marriott, A., Tregay, K., Walsh, S., Wells, J., et al. (1990). Using the family life cycle in later life families. *Journal of Family Therapy, 12*, 321–340.

Benbow, S.M., Marriott, A., Morley, M., & Walsh, S. (1993). Family therapy and dementia: Review and clinical experience. *International Journal of Geriatric Psychiatry, 8*, 717–725.

Carter, B., & McGoldrick, M. (Eds.) (1999). *The expanded family life cycle. Individual, family and social perspectives*. London: Allyn and Bacon.

Combrinck-Graham, L. (1988). Adolescent sexuality in the family life spiral. In C.J. Falicov (Ed.), *Family transitions continuity and change over the life cycle* (pp. 107–131). London: Guilford Press.

CSIP Choice and Access Team (2007). *Commissioning a brighter future. Improving access to psychological therapies. Positive practice guide*. Retrieved from http://www.dh.gov.uk/prod_consum_dh/groups/dh_digitalassets/@dh/@en/documents/digitalasset/dh_074821.pdf (accessed 18 June 2010).

Dallos, R., & Draper, R. (2005). *An introduction to family therapy: Systemic theory and practice*. Second Edition. Buckingham: Open University Press.

Department of Health (2000). *The NHS Plan: A plan for investment. A plan for reform*. London: Department of Health. Retrieved from http://www.dh.gov.uk/en/Publicationsandstatistics/Publications/PublicationsPolicyandGuidance/DH_4002960 (accessed 26 September 2008).

Department of Health (2001). *Treatment choice in psychological therapies and counselling. Evidence based clinical practice guideline*. Retrieved from http://www.dh.gov.uk/prod_consum_dh/groups/dh_digitalassets/@dh/@en/documents/digitalasset/dh_4058245.pdf (accessed 18 June 2010).

Department of Health (2008). *Improving access to psychological therapies implementation plan: National guidelines for regional delivery*. Retrieved from http://www.iapt.nhs.uk/wp-content/uploads/2009/04/nat-guidelines-regional-delivery.pdf (accessed 18 June 2010).

Gergen, K.J., & Kaye, J. (1992). Beyond narrative in the negotiation of therapeutic meaning. In S. McNamee & K.J. Gergen (Eds.), *Therapy as social construction* (pp. 166–185). London: Sage Publications.

Hargrave, T.D. (1994). Using video life reviews with older adults. *Journal of Family Therapy, 16*, 259–268.

Hoffman, L. (1993). A reflexive stance. In *Exchanging voices. A collaborative approach to family therapy* (pp. 111–133). London: Karnac Books.

Ivey, D.C., Wieling, E., & Harris, S.M. (2000). Save the young—the elderly have lived their lives: Ageism in marriage and family therapy. *Family Process, 39*, 163–175.

Lax, W.D. (1992). Postmodern thinking in a clinical practice. In S. McNamee & K.J. Gergen (Eds.), *Therapy as social construction* (pp. 69–85). London: Sage Publications.

Martire, L.M., Lustig, A.P., Schulz, R., Miller, G.E., & Helgeson, V.S. (2004). Is it beneficial to involve a family member? A meta-analysis of psychosocial interventions for chronic illness. *Health Psychology, 23*(6), 599–611.

McGoldrick, M. (1999). Women and the family life cycle. In B. Carter & M. McGoldrick (Eds.), *The expanded family life cycle. Individual, family and social perspectives* (pp. 106–123). London: Allyn and Bacon.

McGoldrick, M., Gerson, R., & Petry, S. (2008). *Genograms assessment and intervention*. Third Edition. London: WW Norton & Company, Inc.

Mouratoglou, V. (1991). Older people and their families. *Context, 3*, 10–15.

Oates Schuster, E. (2001). Compelled to honor privacy: Reflections from researching in a nursing home. In A.L. Cole & J.G. Knowles (Eds.), *Lives in context. The art of life history research* (pp. 202–207). Lanham, MD: AltaMira Press.

Rober, P. (1999). The therapist's inner conversation in family therapy practice: Some ideas about the self of the therapist, therapeutic impasse, and the process of reflection. *Family Process, 38*, 209–228.

Roper-Hall, A. (1993). Cited in Burnham, J. (1993). Systemic supervision: The evolution of reflexivity in the context of the supervisory relationships. *Human Systems, 4*, 349–381.

Turnbull, J. (1989). Violence, families and society. *Psychiatry in Practice, 8*, 10–13.

Walsh, F. (1999). Families in later life: Challenges and opportunities. In B. Carter & M. McGoldrick (Eds.), *The expanded family life cycle. Individual, family and social perspectives* (pp. 307–326). London: Allyn and Bacon.

Wynaden, D., & Orb, A. (2005). Impact of patient confidentiality on carers of people who have a mental disorder. *International Journal of Mental Health Nursing, 14*, 166–171.

Chapter 7

Clinical supervision for psychotherapy with older adults

Bob G. Knight

Introduction

A key part of any training in psychotherapy is clinical supervision. Although a thorough knowledge base regarding both normal aging and late-life psychopathology, as well as assessment and psychotherapy with older clients, is necessary to become a skilled therapist with older adults, it is not sufficient. Supervised clinical experience is the training method that assures that the knowledge base is applied in the clinical setting. Duffy and Morales noted (1997, p. 373): "Although important knowledge about aging processes may be efficiently provided in academic courses, effective learning is often limited by lack of clinical experience." They further noted that (p. 374) "… there is a vast difference between supervised experience and experience alone." As will be explored in this chapter, there are numerous ways that trainees can fail to use what they know, and know well, when in the therapy room with an older client.

It is useful to start with a definition of clinical supervision. The now classic definition by Bernard and Goodyear states (2009, p. 7): "Supervision is an intervention provided by a more senior member of a profession to a more junior member or members of that same profession. This relation is evaluative and hierarchical, extends over time, and has the simultaneous purposes of enhancing the professional functioning of the more junior person(s); monitoring the quality of professional services offered to the clients that she, he, or they see; and serving as a gatekeeper for those who are to enter the particular profession." The literature on clinical supervision in psychotherapy with older adults is not extensive, but suggests the centrality of clinical supervision to learning to do psychotherapy and other psychological services with older adults (e.g. Knight, Karel, Hinrichsen, Qualls, & Duffy, 2009).

The small literature on supervision in clinical geropsychology suggests a couple of potential modifications to the Bernard and Goodyear definition. Qualls, Duffy, and Crose (1995, p. 124) noted, "The scope of supervision may be broader in geropsychology than in other specializations within psychology because the clients are so diverse, the supervisees often come from several disciplines with several levels of competence and expertise, and the settings are diverse." To expand on their second point: psychotherapists often come to focus on working with older adults after becoming well-established in their own careers. Although there certainly are trainees who are young and not yet licensed as independent practitioners, there is also a need for supervised clinical experience on the part of therapists who are experienced independent practitioners of psychotherapy, but have minimal training and experience with older clients (Qualls et al., 1995; Duffy & Morales, 1997). This circumstance can change the meaning of the terms junior and senior in the above definition in ways that affect the supervisory experience for both participants.

Second, mental health and aging is a broadly interdisciplinary field. It is likely that some and perhaps even most of the supervisory experiences will take place across disciplinary lines

(Duffy & Morales, 1997). When supervising trainees or practicing professionals of another discipline, conversations about what is shared and what is different in disciplinary practices, viewpoints, and cultures are an important part of the supervision process. In many ways, these discussions can be as useful in understanding disciplinary identity as having role models from one's own profession.

Since the main basis of this chapter is my own experience as a clinical supervisor, I will begin by describing some of the elements of that experience. For the past 30 years, I have provided clinical supervision to trainees and fairly frequent consultation to colleagues on clinical cases involving older adults. For the first decade, my training experience was in the context of a community mental health center where I supervised clinical psychology interns, clinical social work interns, MSWs (master's degree in social work) getting hours toward their clinical license, and also consulted with licensed colleagues in those disciplines and with psychiatrists and family practice physicians in the associated medical surgical hospital. For the past two decades, the supervision has been with doctoral level clinical psychology students and master's level students in social work and gerontology. Many, but not all, of those students have elected to specialize in work with older adults. I have continued to consult with licensed professionals, mainly with clinical psychologists.

Throughout this experience, my supervision of trainees has largely depended on ample opportunities to observe the trainee's work, either by co-therapy or by use of audio and/or video recordings of sessions. Consultations typically do not allow for this direct observation. In general, my belief is that direct observation of the trainee's work is essential to effective training to work with older clients. Put simply, people virtually never self-report ageism as an influence on what they are doing. This failure to report can be due to simple lack of awareness as well as a desire to appear competent in front of the clinical supervisor. I have used both group and individual methods of supervision, and have some preference for group supervision. I think the greater span of clinical exposure is useful. I also believe that students who pay careful attention to the supervision of others learn lessons for themselves about therapy that may be easier to take in when not "in the hot seat" oneself and also can learn about the supervisory process by observation.

In the sections that follow, I first address some general issues in supervising assessment. Next a variety of relationship issues in therapy with older adults are addressed. Finally, issues in doing therapy with older adults are explored.

Supervising psychological assessment

In this section, the intent is not to go into detail regarding training in specifics of assessment methods, but to discuss general issues in helping students learn to overcome common problems in the assessment process. The focus is on assessment as an initial stage of the psychotherapy process, rather than assessment for its own sake.

When the assessment occurs as part of an ongoing psychotherapy relationship, it is important to keep trainees keenly aware of the hypothetical nature of initial assessments and diagnosis. There is also a need to help students integrate testing information and especially the use of cut off scores with what is constantly being learned about the client's functional abilities. Novice trainees may attribute too much significance to a client being on one side or the other of the cut off score for a mental status exam or a brief depression scale. In one case I supervised, the client had no errors on the Mini-Mental State Examination, but it became obvious over the first few sessions that there was significant forgetting of session content. Exploring the client's personal history, including repetitive questioning over the course of an hour long interview, revealed that the client knew that she had recently moved from another state, but she gave different answers at different points in the interview as to what state she was from. She knew she had been a college professor but could not remember the names of colleges where she had taught.

In the opposite direction, I have supervised a case where the client had been diagnosed with dementia by a licensed psychologist with a good reputation for assessment. The diagnosis had been made based on current IQ score and an assumption that the score must have been higher in middle age when the client was working as an accountant. The client had restricted functioning in various ways, but after a few sessions of therapy, it seemed plausible that this was due to depression, dependent personality traits, and the dynamic of his relationship with his wife. Retesting revealed no change in IQ score over the 7-year period since the diagnosis, more than adequate reason to rule out a progressive dementia.

With depression scales, the issues that arise often are based in the nominal fallacy that a high score on an instrument called a depression screen must indicate a diagnosis of depression. Screens by their very nature cannot stand alone in determining a diagnosis, although several are commonly (mis)used in just this way. Combined with heightened awareness of dementia and depression as important psychological diagnoses in later life, this can blind trainees to the possibility that the high score is due to situational crisis, to marital distress, to clinical anxiety, to chronic schizophrenia, or reflects long-term dysphoria related to personality disorders. In our training clinic, we not infrequently see low income older adults living in single room occupancy hotels in downtown LA or on Skid Row. All get high scores on simple depression measures. Most come in with diagnoses of depression from primary care physicians or community-based mental health or homelessness programs. Trainees often find it difficult to get past this prima facie evidence for depression to explore for longer-term mental health history and evidence of severe mental illness. With appropriate guidance in building rapport and doing the needed clinical interviewing for history, most report lifelong histories of marginal social and occupational functioning and many acknowledge histories of psychotic symptoms and prescriptions for antipsychotic medications. Some have current hallucinations or paranoid delusions that they have learned over the decades to reveal only to people that they can trust.

The larger context of psychological assessment in later life is also a challenge for trainees. Medical co-morbidities are normative with older clients. Learning to sort out physical versus psychological causes of problems and symptoms can be an attractive element of working with older clients, especially for trainees with interest in health psychology. Confronting the realities of medical care, especially for lower income and minority older adults can be an important professional development experience, albeit not always a pleasant one. One trainee saw an older African American woman who had significant levels of depression and anxiety. Over the course of the therapy, we became concerned about a widely fluctuating mental status that seemed independent of her anxiety levels, and unlikely to be due to anxiety in any case. The client's physician was in a group clinic in her neighborhood. He proved nearly impossible to reach by telephone and unresponsive to our input conveyed by letter or to the client's requests for evaluation that included our concerns about what the causes of her transient confusional states might be. His responses to her and to us indicated that he saw her reports of physical problems as entirely due to anxiety, and was unimpressed that psychologists did not see anxiety as a potential explanation. The client got some relief after a neighbor took her to the hospital where her medical treatment was adjusted.

Age stereotypes and assessment

A common problem in accurate assessment of older adults, and one that is especially common in trainees choosing to specialize in working with older adults, is the influence of positive age stereotypes. Even trainees who have had significant experience and skills in working with people who are already identified as having dementia can have problems recognizing the onset of dementia in a client that they first knew as having normal cognition. In *Older Adults in Psychotherapy* (1992), I shared an early experience of my own in which it took an embarrassingly long time for me to recognize dementia in a client I had worked with for several years (Sophia). In one supervision case, the client had been referred from a dementia assessment clinic at which the supervising neurologist was especially concerned about false positive diagnoses of dementia. The client was reporting several memory and cognitive problems, which the trainee therapist ascribed to depression. The client was convinced that he could no longer do the type of thinking that he did as a working engineer prior to retirement. He also reported that he could no longer follow bridge games and was quitting because he knew his partners were "carrying him." After considerable prompting from myself, we got the records of repeated testing from the research center, which showed deficits in a couple of areas related to the client's complaints. More importantly, there was a clear pattern of ongoing decline over the repeated testing. The client was relieved to have some confirmation of his subjective experience of decline, and was also quite pleased to have the opportunity to discuss the decline with his therapist. The trainee therapist, on the other hand, was quite saddened by the realization of the client's cognitive impairment and the likely prognosis of progressive decline. We discussed her feelings in the supervision, and the importance of handling one's own reactions outside of the therapy sessions.

In my experience, it is not unusual for trainee therapists to be slow to recognize substance abuse in clients of any age, and this does seem to be even more difficult with older adult clients. With one recent supervisee, the client had recently left a rehab facility in another state for alcoholism treatment and moved to our area to be near children and away from an ex-husband. Although she was somewhat motivated for therapy, she was resistant to going to the 12-step meeting recommended as follow-up from the rehab facility. The trainee therapist kept finding reasons to conceptualize the case as "really being about depression" and seemed to have issues of her own about 12-step groups. In supervision, it appeared that this was a mix of reluctance to see older adults as alcoholic and the reported negative experience of some family members with 12-step programs, along with a research- and theory-based opposition to the idea of abstinence as the only path to sobriety. These issues were handled fairly quickly in supervision. However, it soon became obvious that the client was drinking heavily in response to stress and calling the answering service to contact the therapist in between weekly visits.

Although not the only types of examples, these instances of difficulty recognizing dementia and substance abuse illustrate the way in which essentially positive and well-motivated stereotypes about older adults can interfere with accurate assessment, and therefore with appropriate treatment. In the next section, we turn to issues related to the therapeutic relationship.

Relationship issues with older clients

Cohort competency

Building rapport and accurately understanding older adult clients can depend on one's ability to get outside of one's own cohort perspective and to understand the point of view of people born and raised in another time and place. This requires some sense of historical changes over time, but more particularly it requires the ability to learn the client's perspective on what it has been like to be a member of that cohort. Transcending the values and perspectives of one's own cohort can be as difficult as becoming aware of cultural biases and unquestioned assumptions. Earlier born cohorts can have very different typical life histories. In understanding how a client's life has been normative or differs from the usual experience of that cohort, it is helpful to know, for example, whether most women of that cohort married in very early adulthood or later, how common it was for women to work, and what the social attitudes were to the children of divorce. It can be diffi-cult for therapists born during or after the 1970s to understand the extent to which traditional gender roles were both socially enforced and personally desired by some women who came of age in the 1940s and 1950s. A big surprise for me personally was the felt realization that every cohort perceives itself as modern and blazing new ground when they are in their 20s. I had implicitly assumed that earlier born traditional people had understood all their lives that they were old fashioned.

One of the most common issues that supervisees have found difficult in work with older adults is dealing with the openly expressed prejudices of older clients. For later born cohorts who have grown up in multicultural environments and with social mores that tend toward the assumption that the differences are unimportant, it can be difficult to work with clients who openly express bias toward a range of ethnic groups, including some subgroups of whites that many later born therapists no longer think of as ethnically separate, or at least not as the target of discrimination and bias. We then discuss in supervision whether the bias is relevant to the client's clinical issues. Usually, it is not and the clinical conversation can be steered elsewhere and the frequency of the comments declines somewhat if not responded to at all. There are occasions when the prejudice can be clinically relevant. I supervised a case once that involved an older man with a paranoid personality style and a wide range of biases that clearly came across in his daily conversation and behavior. This was leading to conflicts with his Asian American landlord and with the African American and Latino students at schools where he substitute taught. With support in supervision, the student was able to guide the client to change his overt behavior, if not his underlying attitudes, with some improvement in his living and working situations.

The therapist's own discomfort with expressed racism can also be an issue and the trainee can be guided to understand the very different social context in which the earlier born client was raised. The therapist then has to decide whether her personal reaction is strong enough that it needs to be discussed with the client, the client needs to be referred to another therapist, or whether work can continue.

Another example of large and clinically relevant cohort differences comes from the radically different experiences of growing up gay or lesbian for individuals who were middle aged or older in the 1970s when bias, discrimination, and persecution of gay and lesbian individuals began to be reversed. The secretiveness, internalized bias, and discomfort of being "out" or sometimes even with socializing with other gay and lesbian people can come as a real surprise to later born trainees (gay and straight) who have grown up in a more accepting social environment.

Cultural competency

One of the best cross-cultural interactions I have supervised was between an older African American client who was very steeped in Los Angeles area African American history, culture, and politics (including some affiliation with the Black Panthers in her youth) and a white female therapist from an upper middle class background. The therapist had the graceful ability to be open and non-defensive when told she was completely different and could not understand what it meant to grow up and grow old black in the United States. The therapist openly acknowledged that this was true and asked the client to share her experience. The therapist was also non-reactive to the client's stereotyping and occasional derogatory remarks about white people as group, including some generalizations that could easily be heard as including the therapist.

One example of unskillful handling of cultural differences that did not involve felt bias involved a trainee who was working with an Asian American family with an older member who had dementia. Much of the interaction had been with a daughter who had primary caregiving respon-sibility and who was fluent in English. At one point in the therapy, a family meeting seemed like an important strategic step, and the trainee made arrangements to set up the meeting and to involve another trainee who was Korean American and fluent in Korean. This turned out to be not especially helpful when the meeting occurred and the second trainee realized that the family was Filipino. As we discussed the situation later, the trainee insisted convincingly and with feeling that she had no bias against any Asian group, but clearly there was a striking lack of cultural competency in the misidentification of the culture the clients were from. More generally, I think many therapists feel that their lack of emotional bias against various groups is equivalent to cultural competency.

Working in a multicultural environment, we not infrequently have client-therapist pairs in which the client is an older African American and the trainee is Asian American or an Asian international student. Much of what is written and taught about cross-cultural interactions appear to assume that the therapist is white. It is interesting to explore with trainees the potential stereotypes and biases of their experience with regard to African American clients and also to encourage them to find out what the clients' assumptions about Asian heritage people are. In many instances, this has lead to discovery of positive stereotypes (e.g. "I assume we both place a higher value on family than white people do."), whether accurate or not.

Who is the client?

There is a tendency among many people working with older adults, including therapists, to identify with and start to work on behalf of someone else in the family other than the older adult client. This is typically someone closer in age to the therapist than the client is. This tendency can be encouraged by the fact that it is often a younger family member who arranges the first visit and may accompany the older client to appointments. The approach here is straightforward and directive: the supervisee is directed to focus on the older adult, and we explore in supervision why there was an impulse to do otherwise. It can help to have the supervisee think through how he/she would feel if a relative accompanied him/her to therapy and the therapist worked on issues identified by the relative rather than by himself/herself.

Handling comments on one's youth

One of the most common questions that I get both in supervision and during lectures on therapy with older adults is how to handle questions about the therapists' age. A lot of the impact of such questions comes from the therapists' anxiety about working with older adults and their own concerns about what they have to offer someone who is further along in the life cycle than oneself. The answer to this is that we have psychotherapeutic skills and process to offer. I have come to believe over the years that one advantage of working with clients older than oneself is that it keeps the focus on the psychotherapy and provides some protection against any tendency to assume that one is sharing one's own life experience and wisdom, which is generally not especially useful to the client.

Older adults are generally quite used to relying on professionals of all sorts who are younger than themselves. I often find that what is really being asked is what stage of training the trainee is at. Because many people are not great at judging the age of those much different than themselves in age, older adults can be quite relieved to discover that the therapist is not as young as they thought. Generally, I suggest that trainees stay calm, clarify the question (e.g. age vs. training or experience), and explain non-defensively what they have to offer the client. Once the question is answered, it can be helpful to explore what the client feels that he or she has learned about the therapist by knowing his or her age.

It is also worth noting that some clients ask about the therapist's age exactly because they suspect the question will make the therapist anxious and distract him/her from whatever was being discussed before the question is asked. It is always worth checking what the topic was changed from and thinking about whether the question was strategic resistance on the client's part.

Issues for older trainees

Although younger therapists and trainees are often more concerned about the influence of their youth on the therapy and the therapeutic relationship, middle-aged and older therapists are often overly convinced that their age will be an asset. In general, this is most often the case with those whose understanding of older clients is based entirely on their own clinical and personal experiences, not uncommon among therapists who age in place along with their clients and referral sources. Frequent referencing of personal experience of one's own aging or of caring for parents as guidance for understanding older clients and knowing what they need to do are key signs of this type of problem. If the older therapist is open to input, a combination of acquiring a broader knowledge base about aging through coursework or independent study and some consultation on older adult cases from a trained geropsychologist can go a long way toward correcting many of the problems that arise from an overly narrow personal understanding of the aging process and of older adults.

The supervision issues become more complicated if the older therapist being supervised has difficulty separating his/her own issues, and the family's issues, regarding aging from those of his/her clients. In my experience, concurrent experience with major chronic illness and caregiving issues at home can render even therapists with considerable expertise and skill in aging issues paralyzed on the job. Many of the problems that are a focus of therapy with older adults are among the toughest that people face and handling them personally and professionally at the same time is often emotionally overwhelming. I once worked with a geropsychiatrist teammate who was among the very best I have known. However, when her husband became quite ill and needed care, she found client's problems overwhelming and had difficulty with diagnoses and treatments that would have been quite routine otherwise. The rest of us on the team provided support during these months by being available to listen and also by pointing out when her feelings seemed to be getting in the way of thinking about her clients. We also worked with her on shifting a few clients whose problems were most similar to her own to having medications continued by the client's primary care physician or by another psychiatrist. Being aware of the impact of familial or personal current issues with aging, being willing to admit it, and working out ways to assure that clients get the service that they need are important personal skills to have for therapists working with older adults. Ideally, handling these intersections of personal experiences with aging-related problems and work can include ensuring that the therapist has support from colleagues or in her own therapy. In some instances, it may be necessary to refer out clients whose presenting problems are quite similar to those being experienced by the therapist.

Being older can raise the likelihood of the therapists feeling that their own experience of aging or their experience helping family members is directly relevant to their clients' problems. This feeling can lead to the therapists being too quick to identify with the person in a family system who is most like them. It can also lead to therapists settling on one type of solution to a problem as fitting all clients: "Frail older adults should be put into long-term care settings because it's too much of a strain on the family to care for them at home." Or "Frail older adults should be kept at home because it's the right and loving thing to do." Any such "one size fits all" solution is indication of the therapist's personal values intruding into the therapy.

Older therapists who have negative thoughts and feelings about their own aging can be hampered in recognizing problems in older clients and in expressing appropriate empathy and engaging in active problem solving. Their negative feelings can lead to denial on the client's behalf as well as their own and the taking of an inappropriately positive stance toward age-related changes and problems: denying or minimizing changes in vision, hearing, cognition, physical appearance, etc. For example, I have had middle-aged trainees who were quite attractive who would change the subject in therapy when a female client would begin to express sadness over no longer being seen as physically attractive or no longer attracting admiring glances from men.

For many therapists and trainees, simply having these issues brought to their attention may be enough to reduce their influence on the therapy. In general, these personal feelings seem to have the strongest influence on the therapy when they operate outside of explicit conscious attention. When that does not work, the supervisor will need to work on changing these perceptions of aging as part of the ongoing work of supervision and may need to consider encouraging therapy for the trainee if the work in supervision seems to cross the boundary between supervision and therapy for the trainee.

Supervising therapeutic intervention

Interrupting clients and staying on topic

Many older adults are somewhat digressive in conversational style. As we get older, we have an increased number of life experiences and also a growing interconnectedness among those experiences, and it is easy to move from one to another and get fairly far away from the original topic by a series of connected steps. In general, many of us are taught in our younger years that it is impolite to interrupt our elders. The combination of these two tendencies means that supervision often involves giving direction to trainees about the need to interrupt clients and keep them on topic and some skills for doing so. Rehearsing polite verbal interruptions can be quite useful. With particularly verbose clients or shyer trainees, having them set up hand signals with the client that indicate when the therapist wants to speak can be helpful; if introduced in a diplomatic way, this can lead the client to see it as amusing rather than annoying. In general, my experience has been that clients appreciate the structure and the idea that the therapist is actively working with them to find clear resolution of confusing issues and solutions to problems.

A related issue, from the therapist's viewpoint, is how to handle repetitive story telling. First, it is important to know whether the repetition may be due to significant cognitive decline. If so, the major supervision issue is likely to be helping the therapist find ways to handle the annoyance that people often experience at listening to repeated stories and/or having to repeat oneself multiple times. Depending on the severity of the cognitive impairment, it may also raise the question of whether verbal psychological intervention is going to be useful.

For other clients, a good first step is to have the therapist point out the repetition and ask the client why the story is repeated, including the suggestion that perhaps the repetition means that the therapist is not understanding the meaning of the story. In general, I find that older clients respond positively to learning that someone is paying enough attention to what they are saying to notice repetition. From time to time, the clients' response also includes their perception that the therapist has not gotten the point of the story, and this becomes quite important to the progress of therapy.

Confronting older clients

Although much of therapy can be explorative and collaborative, sometimes therapeutic change depends on having clients talk about topics they prefer to avoid and which may be emotionally painful, or pointing out to clients how their behavior is causing some of their problems. Both trainees and experienced therapists seem to fairly frequently experience more difficulty in confronting older clients than younger clients. For example, in one case that I supervised, the client was an octogenarian who had focused on needing more social contact and support as one of her main themes for improving her mood. It became clear over the course of therapy that she was isolated in large part because of tendencies to be very critical in virtually all social interactions and to hold on to grudges with family and long time friends for years and decades. The trainee therapist built up a very strong rapport with the client. With the rapport established, the therapist was coached and encouraged in ways to continually point out to the client how this behavior resulted in people contacting her less and being less willing to spend time with her. Change was slow, but noticeable and important.

With a male client in his late sixties, it became obvious to both the therapist and supervisor that the high level of conflict and criticism in his marriage was a major source of his chronic depressed mood. He was very reluctant to discuss how he felt about his wife or the marriage, parallel to his reluctance to talk with her about his feelings while being nearly constantly criticized. The therapist was also reluctant to move into this domain, partly fearing what would happen if the marriage broke up as a result of the therapy and the client ended up on his own. With encouragement, coaching, and support from the supervisor, the therapist was able to get the client to talk about his feelings, including exploring in sessions the pros and cons of leaving his wife, and it became clear he did not want to do so. In the near term, the exploration helped the client become a bit more assertive in his relationship and also reminded him that he loved her deeply. His wife responded fairly well to the combination of assertiveness and increased affection from him. Later, we saw the client after his wife died, and the therapist was surprised at the client's resilience and improvement in mood following a brief period of grieving.

The motivations for avoiding successful confrontations like these can be varied, but often share the same roots as the unwillingness to interrupt older clients and direct the therapeutic conversation: it seems impolite to insist on older clients' confronting issues that they prefer not to talk about. It can also be complicated by an unexamined assumption that older adults are too frail to handle the emotional material or that it is too late in life to expect actual therapeutic change. Regardless of the rationale, the end result is that the older client is not permitted the opportunity for meaningful therapeutic change and the relief that it would bring.

Because psychotherapists and other helping professionals would virtually never actually conceptualize a case as withholding of active treatment, the rationale is often expressed in terms of the client needing support rather than therapeutic intervention. The same assumptions regarding the client's frailty and emotional neediness are often used to rationalize never ending support. In general, the supervisee should be challenged to explore whether these beliefs are realistic and to consider what the treatment recommendation would be if the client were middle aged or younger, and then asked to explain why, in this particular instance, that recommendation needs to be changed. There can be specific reasons for modification, but there are virtually no reasons not to pursue active treatment and change. More often than not, the rationale for modification is driven by the trainee's stereotypes about aging rather than by the actual needs of the client.

Termination

Therapists seem to have even more problems approaching termination with older clients than with younger ones. There seems to be an underlying, widespread assumption that older clients need the therapy even more than younger clients. The idea that the client will feel hurt or rejected is also often expressed. In 30 years of experience doing and supervising therapy with older clients, the modal reaction from the client to being told that therapy is nearing an end is a kind of happy surprise that the therapist agrees that progress has been made and that goals of therapy have been accomplished. Early in my career a few clients phrased this as "graduating from therapy," and I have come to use the term frequently.

Some significant minority of older clients may in fact experience a fairly high degree of isolation and come to rely on therapy as a substitute for friendship. This is not a majority of older clients, but is certainly experienced by some. When this is actually the case, it is useful to spend a few weeks with building up social support as the goal of the therapy. Psychotherapy is not a substitute for support from friends and family, and in most settings, psychotherapy is not allowed to go on indefinitely in any case. By working with clients to find more authentic sources of ongoing social support, the supervisee can learn much about the role of therapy in clients' lives and also reappraise his/her own concepts about the nature of therapy and about being supportive of clients.

There are, of course, some exceptions to this generally easy acceptance of termination by older clients. In my experience, these have generally been clients with lifelong dependency issues or personality disorders. It then becomes a question whether the goals of therapy shift to include work on the personality disorder.

Conclusion

A valuable goal for clinical supervision in psychotherapy is one articulated by Duffy and Morales (1997, p. 375): "Learning to 'meet the person' without being preoccupied with age differences and disability allows an intense 'personalized' psychological relationship that is necessary in being therapeutic with any client." Later in the same paragraph they note that "Without this, the 'differentness' and related stress of the geriatric practicum experience can have the effect of alienating and discouraging trainees." How are we doing as a field with supervision in clinical geropsychology?

The simple answer is that we do not know. There is simply no empirical work evaluating clinical supervision in cases involving older adults. In this we lag behind other areas of professional psychology primarily in the quantitative sense. Reviews of the clinical supervision literature more generally are very critical of methods (e.g. an extensive reliance on self-report measures and the satisfaction with the experience of the participants in supervision) and what is really known, especially with regard to the seemingly key question of how supervision affects client outcomes (Bernard & Goodyear, 2009; Fallendar & Shafranske, 2004).

Also in common with much of the field, there has been relatively little attention to the gatekeeper functions of supervision in geriatric mental health. In part, this is driven by a desire to see more people working with older adults, but greater concern with the monitoring roles of clinical supervision with regard to both client care and with whether the supervisee has really become competent to work with older adults is in order. In the language of clinical supervision trainers, clinical geropsychology has tended to be more focused on the formative evaluation of trainees than on summative evaluation (Bernard & Goodyear, 2009; Fallendar & Shafranske, 2004). My observation is that while we are by no means unique in this (Bernard & Goodyear discuss this issue for the whole field), we in clinical geropsychology have tended to avoid discussion of gatekeeping, much less to act on it. With an expanding public focus on psychological services for older adults, greater attention is needed to the quality of such services for the older adult consumer of psychotherapy.

In this chapter, I have focused mainly on common elements across supervision experiences in teaching psychotherapists to work with older adults. These shared themes have included common errors in assessment and case formulation, including those related to positive stereotypes of aging and positive attachment to older clients. Relationship issues including cohort competency, cultural competency, focus on the older adult as the real client, and handling comments on one's relative youth are also important and frequent issues in supervision in professional geropsychology. Finally, therapists new to working with older clients often experience difficulties interrupting clients and keeping them on topic, confronting older clients, and terminating the therapy relationship.

Working with clients who are further along in the life cycle than oneself is personally challenging in ways that can lead to considerable professional and personal growth. As noted by Qualls et al. (1995, p. 125), "The clinician's beliefs about his or her own future, aging, and death create a relationship dynamic with the older client that is ripe with countertransference possibilities." They list potential themes of relationship problems that can arise for the supervisee, including: (a) feeling overwhelmed by the client's multiple problems and the need to gain knowledge from other health disciplines; (b) anxiety about the need to collaborate with de facto interdisciplinary teams caring for an older client; (c) blaming others in the client's support system for not caring enough as the therapist sees herself as "the good child" in the system; (d) resisting taking on unfamiliar roles like case management; and (e) handling issues related to death and grief. These are not only the bane of young professionals; the middle-aged and older therapist can be even more vulnerable to identification with the client and wanting the client to handle issues in the way that the therapist would.

The goal of clinical supervision is to assure that the therapy remains the client's therapy. Good geropsychological supervision is essential to having active therapy that is focused on the older client's issues. Nonetheless, through supervision on such cases therapists also learn important lessons about the nature of therapy and about their own aging: future, present, or recent past.

References

Bernard, J.M., & Goodyear, R.K. (2009). *Fundamentals of clinical supervision.* Fourth Edition. Upper Saddle River, NJ: Merrill.

Duffy, M., & Morales, P. (1997). Supervision of psychotherapy with older patients. In C.E. Watkins (Ed.), *Handbook of psychotherapy supervision* (pp. 366–380). New York, NY: John Wiley & Sons.

Fallendar, C.A., & Shafranske, E.P. (2004). *Clinical supervision: A competency-based approach.* Washington, DC: American Psychological Association.

Knight, B.G., Karel, M.J., Hinrichsen, G.A., Qualls, S.H., & Duffy, M. (2009). Pikes Peak Model for training in professional geropsychology. *American Psychologist, 64,* 205–214.

Qualls, S.H., Duffy, M., & Crose, R. (1995). Supervision in community practicum settings. In B.G. Knight, L. Teri, J. Santos, & P. Wohlford (Eds.), *Mental health services for older adults: Implications for training and practice in geropsychology.* Washington, DC: American Psychological Association.

Chapter 8

Treating late-life anxiety in chronic medical illness and cognitive impairment: two case studies

Inger H. Nordhus and Minna J. Hynninen

Introduction

Estimated prevalence rates of anxiety in older individuals range greatly, primarily as a function of the heterogeneity of the older population, and are often confounded by medical co-morbidity, medication use, and functional health status. Community prevalence rates of diagnosable anxiety disorders range from about 2% to 19% (Flint, 1994). In a recent study, community prevalence estimates were found to be 14%, and even higher in medical settings (Bryant, Jackson, & Ames, 2008). According to the criteria of the *Diagnostic and Statistical Manual of Mental Disorders* (DSM), anxiety disorders in later life are classified similarly to those in adult life and include panic disorder with and without agoraphobia, generalized anxiety disorder (GAD), social phobia, specific phobia, obsessive-compulsive disorder, and post-traumatic and acute stress disorder (American Psychiatric Association, 2000). Pure anxiety disorders in later life are rare, and are often found in conjunction with another psychiatric disorder like depression and/or a medical condition (Flint, 2005). GAD seems to be most prevalent in community samples, but anxiety disorder not otherwise specified (ADNOS) is the diagnosis most often assigned in primary care settings where older adults with anxiety typically seek treatment (Stanley, Roberts, Bourland, & Novy, 2001). Patients suffering from anxiety have an increased risk of becoming depressed, and left untreated, anxiety disorders tend to become chronic (Larkin, et al., 1992). Prospective research involving older adults has demonstrated that anxiety symptoms are associated with medical illness such as coronary heart disease and self-reported mobility limitations (Mehta et al., 2007). Furthermore, anxiety disorders in later life have been found to be prospectively associated with an increased mortality rate (Brenes, et al., 2007).

Patients suffering from anxiety disorders and subclinical anxiety symptoms disproportionately complain of as well as demonstrate tension or restlessness; they may exhibit anxiousness, autonomic hyperactivity and vigilance, insomnia, distractibility, shortness of breath, numbness, apprehension, worry, and rumination. These symptoms are often conceptualized in terms of three components: affective, cognitive, and somatic symptoms. Affective symptoms refer to the emotional feelings associated with anxiety (e.g. anxiousness, nervousness), cognitive symptoms of anxiety reflect thoughts and worries, while somatic symptoms of anxiety refer to bodily symptoms such as racing heart, sleep problems, or shortness of breath. The development of insomnia, either in terms of sleep-onset difficulties, problems maintaining sleep or early morning awakening, and/or impaired daytime functioning may contribute to the maintenance of anxiety as part of the worry-rumination-somatic symptoms vicious cycle.

It has generally been maintained in the clinical literature on late-life psychiatric disorders that specific symptoms measured by an anxiety scale are important because anxiety may present more frequently as somatic symptoms among older adults. When reviewing age differences in self-reported affective, cognitive, and somatic components of anxiety in recent literature, Brenes (2006) found that anxious older adults reported less worry than their younger counterparts; however, no differences emerged with respect to measures of affective or somatic symptoms. Although the research on the relation of anxiety and age has produced inconsistent findings, the main lesson to be learned is that we need to be aware of how we assess anxiety in older patients. In fact, older adults may not attribute symptoms of anxiety to an anxiety problem, but rather misattribute them to an anticipated or a co-morbid physical illness. The assessment instruments chosen as well as the complexity of the health status of the older patient are, therefore, crucial for interpreting the clinical presentation of the patient (Nordhus, 2008). The more recent attention given to anxiety symptoms in dementia amplifies this issue.

One important question regarding anxiety symptoms in persons with dementia is whether they should be considered as a separate clinical entity or as part of a broader syndrome. It has been suggested that there is a strong overlap between anxiety and agitation, and that agitation may be a symptom of generalized anxiety (Mintzer, Brawman-Mintzer, Mirski, & Barkin, 2000). According to a recent review by Seignourel, Kunik, Snow, Wilson, and Stanely (2008), evidence so far provides more support for the distinctiveness of anxiety and agitation than for their equivalence, implying that one should add questions about anxiety as part of the dementia workup. Another possibility is that agitation is confounded with depression in patients suffering from dementia. Between 68% and 75% of individuals with dementia and GAD also meet the criteria for a Major Depressive Disorder (Starkstein, Jorge, Petracca, & Robinson, 2007), and GAD is associated with greater depressive symptoms in Alzheimer's disease. From these findings, it seems evident that we should expect that depression and anxiety are highly co-morbid in individuals with dementia, in terms of diagnosable disorders or as subclinical syndromes, and the latter position may in turn develop into clinically diagnosable problems.

But how can we best assess affective symptoms in dementia, and anxiety in particular? The option of asking the patient may not always be optimal, primarily as a consequence of the current occurrence of difficulties communicating and remembering their symptoms. It is now commonly recommended to collect information from multiple sources, including caregiver, patient, staff, and medical records as a basis for measuring anxiety as well as depression in dementia, and for the former, the Rating Anxiety in Dementia scale (RAID; Shankar, Walker, & Frost, 1999) is widely used and will be further presented in connection with one of the cases described below.

According to the recommended guidelines, the first line of treatment for anxiety disorders consists of psychological treatment or antidepressant drugs (NICE, 2007). It has been demonstrated that older adults with anxiety disorders most often do not receive appropriate treatment, with only about 5% receiving psychological treatment and below 4% being prescribed an antidepressant (de Beurs et al., 1999). A major problem concerning psychological treatment is the fact that older adults in general have lower access to psychological interventions as compared to younger adults. Both patient and psychotherapist characteristics have been cited and discussed for decades as contributing causes to the scarcity of older patients in psychological treatment. Furthermore, general practitioners may also be reluctant to prescribe drugs for anxiety symptoms, being wary of increased side effects in later life, among them the increased risk of falling, memory complaints, and dependency associated with the use of benzodiazepines (French et al., 2006), as well as being concerned about adverse drug interactions in an age group known for an extensive polypharmacy (Yuan, Tsoi, & Hunt, 2006). Consequently, anxiety may for various reasons go unattended or at least not being optimally addressed.

Cognitive behavioral therapy (CBT) has gained prominence as the psychological treatment of choice for anxiety disorders (APA, 2002). Recent reviews generally conclude that psychological treatment is effective for anxiety disorders in late life, but also emphasize that there is a need for rigorous controlled trials for different anxiety disorders, in various care settings, as well as more deliberate inclusion of patients aged 65 years and above (Ayers, Sorrell, Thorp, & Wetherell, 2007; Nordhus & Pallesen, 2003; Pinquart & Duberstein, 2007). Although CBT has demonstrated some benefits for late-life anxiety according to these reviews, the samples involved have typically been homogeneous and restricted to young-old, active, healthy, and well-educated individuals recruited from the community. Therefore, less is known about treating older patients who do not fit this profile, thus limiting the generalizability of findings to settings where older adults typically receive medical care. In the past few years, treatment studies focusing on GAD in primary care have been conducted (e.g. Stanley et al., 2009), clearly demonstrating the potential for doing effective treatment research in clinically relevant contexts.

When doing CBT research and treatment in clinical settings, strong arguments have been made for inclusion of learning and memory aids to deal with age-associated cognitive impairment in patients suffering from anxiety (Mohlman et al., 2003). This is often referred to as *augmented* CBT, leaning on intensive cognitive training, proposing that sound executive skills should be considered necessary for the successful use of CBT. This includes a set of cognitive operations like allocation and control of attention, inhibitory control, metacognition, self-monitoring, and other goal-oriented skills (Mohlman, 2008). It is further maintained that through repeated practice, executive skills can be improved in otherwise relatively healthy and well-functioning older individuals (no organic brain disease), implying that patients suffering from severe cognitive illnesses, such as Alzheimer's disease, are not the primary aim of augmented CBT as described by these authors. An obvious value of this perspective is that by bolstering or tailoring the treatment to specific symptoms and cognitive needs of the older patient one can contribute to ensuring that the therapeutic process is perceived as responsive and clinically relevant, thus reducing attrition and enhancing engagement. Hopefully, future clinical trials will identify more precisely how cognitive training may facilitate CBT outcomes (Mohlman, 2008).

Although recent clinical trials involving older adults remain inconclusive on whether age-related adaptations of efficacious psychological treatment techniques are necessary for anxiety disorders in later life (Stanley et al., 2003; Wetherell et al., 2005), an intriguing development is the more recent small-scale trials demonstrating promising adaptations for doing CBT for anxiety in patients suffering from cognitive decline consistent with dementia (Kraus et al., 2008, Paukert et al., 2010). Based on (a protocol and) findings from their previous anxiety treatment studies on older cognitively intact patients (Stanley et al., 2003), modifications are made in terms of the content, structure, and learning strategies of CBT to adapt skills to patients with co-existing anxiety and dementia; this approach has been termed as cognitive behavioral therapy for anxiety in dementia (CBT-AD; Kraus et al., 2008). Basically, these adaptations build on the same cognitive processes described in Mohlman's approaches focusing on identifying type of impairment, but additionally, collaterals (family members, friends, or other caregivers) are involved in treatment as "coaches" to facilitate learning and memory as well as encouraging ongoing practice. The latter thus brings in an element of a co-therapist to the treatment process.

In terms of providing insight into best practice in managing complex cases, we find the development of the standard CBT protocols briefly reviewed above highly relevant. The augmented treatment manuals give us practical as well as empirically informed guidance for therapeutic approaches in clinical contexts. Based on established treatment models, these adaptations bring us ideally closer to the understanding of the mechanisms involved in therapeutic change, and should therefore be addressed in clinical science as well as in clinical practice.

Case formulation

There is a general consensus among practicing clinicians across therapeutic paradigms that a case formulation is an essential step to providing effective treatment, particularly for complex presentations (Tarrier, 2006). Complex cases may involve multiple different presenting problems, and clinicians are often required to oscillate between the complaints offered by the patient and/or the patient's significant others. A case formulation is basically the summation of the clinician's understanding of how the patient's problem (psychopathology) develops, perpetuates, and evolves over time. Based on this understanding, interventions aimed at reducing the impact of causal and/or maintaining factors are planned. Furthermore, case formulations are based on established theoretical frameworks, and may potentially enhance therapeutic outcomes, by suggesting more specific, precise interventions (Bieling & Kuyken, 2003; Kuyken, Padesky, & Dudley, 2009). Thus, they may represent an approach to the development of an *individualized treatment plan*.

Current cognitive behavioral treatments for anxiety disorders draw on empirically based theoretical models to support the use of specific treatment techniques and processes. Some models may emphasize symptom reduction, while other models may focus on acceptance and mindfulness learning, or a combination of these. Common for all anxiety disorders are varying manifestations of subjective, physiological, and behavioral symptoms of anxiety in addition to distortions in cognitive content and processes (Beck, 1976).

In the following case studies, a cognitive behavioral case formulation on anxiety will be based on these common elements in anxiety and the development of a treatment plan.

Case study 1: co-morbid anxiety in a chronically ill man

John was a 65-year-old male with chronic obstructive pulmonary disease (COPD), which is a serious and progressive condition that is mostly irreversible. COPD causes symptoms such as dyspnea and fatigue due to reduced lung capacity. As a systemic disease, COPD also produces multiple structural and functional effects that may lead to co-morbid conditions. Anxiety and depression are two of the most common co-morbidities in COPD.

John was interviewed in connection with intake to a 10-week CBT in a group format for COPD patients with symptoms of anxiety and depression. He had stopped working 3 years ago, 1 year after the lung disease was diagnosed, and was receiving a disability pension. He reported that he could not work anymore as a taxi driver because of frequent attacks of dyspnea and shortness of breath. According to his description, the attacks usually started with feelings of not getting enough air and having pressure against his chest, and soon escalated into a full-blown panic with feelings of suffocation and a paralyzing fear of dying. John was very anxious of the attacks and wanted to avoid them by all means. Thus, he had started avoiding all situations and activities during which he had experienced an attack, such as going to restaurants, movie theatres and shopping malls, driving in tunnels, and taking buss or train. Although he had never been very active physically, John was now restraining himself from all activities that could cause physical exertion, as he believed it would make his condition worse. Although he believed that this was necessary, he also expressed irritation because of his current passive lifestyle. Lately, he had isolated himself more and more, because, as he expressed it, he did not want to slow others down or be a burden to others. He also admitted being ashamed of having COPD, as it is known as a "smokers' disease," and he was trying to hide the symptoms from others. From time to time, John was feeling depressed and thought that he was a hopeless case.

Assessing and interpreting the symptoms

A medical assessment indicated that John's COPD was relatively mild and he did not have any additional physical co-morbidity. He completed the Beck Anxiety Inventory (BAI; Beck & Steer, 1993) scoring 38, indicating severe anxiety, and the Beck Depression Inventory-II (BDI-II; Beck, Steer, & Brown, 1996) scoring 26, indicating moderate depression. The symptoms that he reported on the BAI and the BDI-II were discussed further in the assessment interview and a structured diagnostic interview was conducted.

Due to an overlap or close association in symptoms, anxiety and depression are often hard to distinguish from symptoms of COPD. The diagnostic criteria are the same for patients with a medical illness as for those without, but special care must be taken to distinguish between symptoms that are a direct consequence of the disease and those that are unrelated. The clinician should know the degree to which the medical condition is known to cause anxiety, and assess the timeline for onset of the co-morbid conditions. John's symptoms were consistent with panic attacks and he also seemed to suffer from agoraphobia. However, it was less clear to what extent his panic attacks were actually cued by COPD symptoms. The DSM-IV criteria for panic disorder require recurrent panic attacks that do not occur in the presence of an identifiable trigger. Thus, a patient who has panic attacks only when experiencing COPD-related dyspnea or other symptoms does not meet the criteria for panic disorder. John had no history of previous psychological disorders and his first panic attack had occurred after the COPD diagnosis was made. However, the assessment revealed that although the panic attacks were initially triggered by breathing difficulty, he was now having attacks that were not preceded by respiratory symptoms. Also, since John's COPD was mild, it seemed that his breathing problems were somewhat out of proportion for his actual physical health and that his medical condition could not completely account for his psychological distress. He was diagnosed with *panic disorder with agoraphobia*. Although he also reported several depressive symptoms, his episodes of low mood and feelings of hopelessness did not last long enough to be consistent with the criteria for depressive disorders.

John was motivated to join the CBT group and hoped to get help with managing his anxiety. He said that since there is no cure for the lung disease, he had believed that nothing could be done to improve his situation, but he was certainly willing to try anything.

Case formulation

According to the cognitive model of panic disorder, catastrophic misinterpretations of internal events, bodily sensations, or mental experiences, lead to a panic attack (Clark, 1986). Even though the first attack may be due to biological factors, in later attacks effects of normal reactions such as tiredness, stress, or excitement may be misinterpreted (Wells, 2006). The disorder is maintained by an interaction among safety behaviors, avoidance, and selective attention to sensations that may trigger misinterpretations (Clark; Salkovski, 1991; Wells, 1997).

In John's case, his anxiety may have initially been created by the unpredictable and fear-arousing symptoms of the respiratory disease. The breathing difficulty triggered the interpretation "I can't breathe, I'm going to suffocate and die," which again elevated his anxiety and panic. Later on, anxiety and panic were likely to contribute to his sensation of breathlessness and make it more acute and excessive relative to his disease severity. Although his interpretation of the breathlessness was not completely inaccurate, the catastrophic thoughts were not helping him to cope with the symptoms. Also, his avoidance of all strenuous activities and potentially stressful situations made him increasingly passive and isolated, which was likely to further lower his mood and contribute to further deterioration in his physical condition. His guilt-driven rumination about the role of smoking in the development of COPD also led him to deny himself social support from friends and family.

The treatment goals for John were to reduce his avoidance behaviors through graded exposure, with the help of effective coping skills and mindfulness-based skills, and to increase his tolerance for physical symptoms.

Treatment and outcome

Cognitive behavioral therapy treatment for persons with chronic obstructive pulmonary disease

The treatment comprised components from efficacious CBT interventions for late-life anxiety and depression (Stanley et al., 2003) and from mindfulness-based interventions (Kabat-Zinn, 1990; Segal, Williams, & Teasdale, 2002). Rather than focusing specifically on any diagnostic category, the wide breadth of coping skills included the intervention-targeted symptoms of both anxiety and depression. The attitude of acceptance and here-and-now orientation of mindfulness were integrated within a cognitive framework and understanding of the maintenance factors of anxiety and depression. The main components included psychoeducation of the role of anxiety and depression in COPD, diaphragmatic breathing to manage shortness of breath, graded exposure and behavioral activation, and mindfulness practice to promote here-and-now orientation and acceptance of one's present experience.

The CBT treatment was adapted for COPD patients, in order to take into account the real limitations and adversities they face. In contrast to traditional CBT for anxiety in healthy individuals (Salkovski, 1991; Wells, 1997), the focus was not so much on reducing safety behaviors as on teaching effective coping skills. COPD is a severe illness with increasing dyspnea on physical exertion and during respiratory infections, and although breathing techniques and activity pacing may be characterized as safety behaviors, they are an important method for self-management of dyspnea (Livermore, Sharpe, & McKenzie, 2008). The aim was to seek a balance between some degree of control over breathlessness, while also increasing tolerance and reducing the fear of dyspnea.

With mindfulness-based techniques, the impact of the feared stimuli (e.g. breathlessness, pain) may be altered by teaching patients to reduce avoidance of experiencing anxiety rather than attempting to reduce anxiety *per se* (e.g. Teasdale, Segal, & Williams, 1995). Mindfulness may function much like a reciprocal inhibition/behavioral exposure, as it changes a response tendency from avoidance to observation of one's present experience (Lynch & Bronner, 2006). With repeated practice, patients learn to experience previously avoided emotions, thoughts, and sensations non-reactively and without judgment. The attitude of acceptance and non-judgment inherent in mindfulness automatically changes the appraisals of feared stimuli without direct attempts to modify or restructure associated thoughts; one's present experience is allowed to be "just what it is." The emphasis on detached attention to self can also help patients to perceive patterns of thought, feeling, and behavior more clearly.

Thus, it was hypothesized that for COPD patients such as John, who respond to physical symptoms with anxiety and panic, mindfulness skills would help him disengage from distressing thoughts and feelings evoked by them, and alter the response tendency from avoidance of anxiety-provoking situations to observation of the present experience with acceptance. It was also assumed that by developing the capacity for self-regulation of attention, mindfulness would help to change his focus from regrets or rumination about past choices that may have contributed to the development of COPD, or from worry for future and fear of death, to a here-and-now orientation. Learning new ways of relating to thoughts, feelings, and events can also alter patients' perceptions of themselves and promote an attitude of self-compassion in contrast to guilt and shame. (A summary of key elements in the case formulation for case study 1 is outlined in Table 8.1.)

Cognitive behavioral therapy treatment for John

John's group had eight participants, all with COPD and symptoms of anxiety and/or depression. The group had 10 weekly sessions that lasted 2 hours, led by one therapist. In between the sessions, the participants practiced the skills and completed homework exercises daily.

Table 8.1 Key elements in the case formulations for the presented cases

Presented problem	Feared stimulus	Perception	Attempts to cope	Treatment focus
Case study 1: Anxiety and chronic, somatic illness • Panic disorder • COPD	Breathing problems, dyspnea	Catastrophic cognitions about dying and losing control	Avoidance of situations and activities that may cause breathing problems, safety-seeking behavior	**CBT + mindfulness skills:** • Exposure/inhibition • Arousal management • Attention management • Acceptance
Case study 2: Anxiety and cognitive impairment • Worry, restlessness • Agitation • Alzheimer's disease	Signs of physical and cognitive decline	Cannot trust own ability to cope, world is an unpredictable and dangerous place, future is hopeless and frightening	Seeking reassurance from daughter and checking that everything is "ok," withdrawal and isolation	**Modified CBT supported by strategies to enhance learning and memory (CBT-AD):** • Exposure/inhibition • Behavioral activation • Arousal management • Attention management

The homework assignments were modified to match the goals and problem formulations of each participant.

Psychoeducation and anxiety monitoring

The psychoeducation in the initial therapy session involved an explanation of the role of avoidance and passivity in the maintenance of anxiety and depression, and how anxiety and depression may add to the burden of COPD and alter one's perception of physical symptoms. Prior to beginning treatment, John had some insight into the impact of anxiety on breathlessness and other respiratory symptoms, but the psychoeducation helped him to modify his beliefs about the dangers of being physically active and also made him more aware of the downsides of coping through avoidance. The participants were also asked to monitor symptoms and signs of anxiety and depression during the coming weeks and identify associated thoughts, feelings, and sensations.

Exposure and managing physical symptoms

Diaphragmatic breathing was introduced as a coping skill to manage breathing problems, and the participants were asked to practice it daily and use it whenever they experienced respiratory distress. The participants also devised a list of activities or situations that they either avoided or wished to do, and created an activity hierarchy with easy activities or situations on the top of the list and more difficult ones at the bottom. The therapist helped them to choose activities and make concrete plans for homework assignments, breaking more complex or difficult tasks into more manageable components with short-term goals. Since John's main problem was panic anxiety and agoraphobic avoidance, but as he also suffered from depressive symptoms, he was encouraged to include exposure tasks on his list in combination with pleasurable activities that would improve his mood. His list included eating a meal at a restaurant with his wife and going shopping as relatively easy tasks to begin with, and starting to exercise at a pulmonary rehabilitation center twice a week as a moderately difficult goal that he would work on later. His most difficult long-term goal, which also was the most important goal, was to start working again. This goal was modified and broken into several smaller subtasks, starting with driving a car alone at first, then driving in tunnels, then taking shifts for his previous employer.

Mindfulness practice

In addition to encouraging the participants to manage breathing problems in connection with the activity assignments with diaphragmatic breathing, mindfulness-based exercises were introduced concurrently. In the exercises, the participants were asked to direct their attention to various aspects of their present experience, such as thoughts or bodily sensations, and observe these events non-judgmentally as they arise and eventually change or pass, bringing the attitude of openness and curiosity to discomfort or unpleasant experiences. The exercises were followed by a discussion and exploration of the participants' experiences, while the therapist modeled friendly curiosity and an accepting stance toward all experiences. The discussions were also used to clarify the characteristics of a mindful stance, and to explore how it differs from being on "autopilot."

Progress

John learned to pay attention to and identify catastrophic thoughts, and to recognize the bodily reactions that followed them. He found the diaphragmatic breathing to be helpful when he experienced respiratory distress, and used it frequently at home and while he was working with exposure assignments. He also found the mindfulness exercises pleasant, and appreciated them as "moments of silence and calm" that allowed him to see his own reactions more clearly and observe them, instead of feeling overwhelmed. Toward the end of the treatment, he started working occasionally for his previous employer, which he perceived as a major improvement in his quality of life. However, at the end of the intervention he was still avoiding a number of feared situations and had not managed to establish a regular exercise routine, as he had planned. He also believed that he could have benefited from some additional sessions with continued work on the activity assignments.

Group experience

John expressed a great appreciation for the other group members and the opportunity to share experiences with others who could really understand him. He said that it was a relief simply to hear that he was not the only one struggling with anxiety, and he also learned a lot from the others by hearing how they coped with the challenges of the disease. Although the formal change theory of CBT focuses on the specific technique components, there is today an increasing acknowledgment of the role of process factors and relational components also in CBT group interventions (Bieling, McCabe, & Antony, 2006). Bringing together individuals sharing the same diagnosis on a weekly basis quickly resulted in a cohesive group, in which the members provided each other with social support, shared practical advice, and were able to talk about their emotional reactions to their life-changing disease.

Outcome

By the end of the treatment, John's BAI score was reduced to 17 and BDI-II to 13. His panic attacks were reduced gradually in frequency and intensity. When John was followed up 6 months later, he was mostly free from panic attacks, although he still showed some agoraphobic avoidance. However, John himself said that he was now much more satisfied with his life, and even though he was anxious from time to time, he was more capable of accepting and tolerating the anxious feelings and bodily sensations without feeling overwhelmed by them.

Case study 2: anxiety in a cognitively impaired woman

Lise was an 85-year-old woman who was referred to a clinic for old age psychiatry. She was divorced and living alone, but had a son and a daughter living close to her. The referral letter from her general practitioner described an increasing impairment in memory and activities of daily living after a hip fracture 1 year ago, as well as symptoms of anxiety and depression.

During the first appointment at the clinic, Lise was somewhat disoriented and had difficulty remembering recent events and conversations. She stayed at home most days and had stopped going for walks because of pain in her hip and fear of falling. Her daughter explained that she was having trouble managing at home by herself and had almost set the house on fire once when she forgot to turn off the stove. She also said that Lise was anxious about being alone, had difficulty with sleep, became easily stressed and worried, and called her on the phone multiple times each day and sometimes also during the night. Lise herself said that she worried about falling at home and not being able to get help.

According to the clinician who met with them initially, Lise seemed to be overmedicated. After her medication was adjusted, there was some improvement in her level of functioning and memory, and she became less confused. However, it seemed that she also became more distressed about her memory problems, and sometimes cried in frustration. She was anxious much of the time and reluctant to leave her apartment and engage in social activities with her friends. Her daughter was showing signs of distress and also expressed her despair at the clinic, saying that she did not know how much longer she could cope with the situation. Lise was offered place at a day center for persons with dementia, which she refused. Instead, it was decided that she would get more assistance at home, and she would also go through a treatment program at the clinic together with her daughter, which could help her to cope with stress and anxiety and improve her quality of life.

Assessing and interpreting the symptoms

A complete medical and psychiatric assessment was conducted at the clinic, including a detailed medical history, physical and neurological examination, CT scan, neuropsychological testing, and a psychiatric assessment. Lise was diagnosed with mild dementia of the Alzheimer's type, and her anxiety was examined further by interviewing both Lise and her daughter, together and separately. On the Neuropsychiatric Inventory (NPI; Cummings et al., 1994), Lise's daughter reported significant symptoms (a score of 4 or higher) of anxiety, depression, agitation, and sleep problems. She also reported severe distress over Lise's anxiety and agitation on the NPI Caregiver Distress Scale. Lise's anxiety was assessed further with the RAID (Shankar et al., 1999), a 20-item inventory that addresses signs and symptoms of anxiety such as worry, sleep disturbance, irritability, as well as a number of physical symptoms, in a 2-week period. Information is gathered from all available sources, including patient, caregiver, and clinical observations, and the clinician determines a single score for each item. The items are rated on a four-point scale, and the total score is the sum of the first 18 items. The last two items assess phobias and panic attacks. The scale has demonstrated satisfactory psychometric qualities.

Lise did not acknowledge being anxious but reported worries about her cognitive performance and her daughter's well-being, feeling tense and uneasy, lacking energy, as well as somatic symptoms that included frequent headaches, muscle aches, and tingling in her hands and feet. Her daughter confirmed Lise's symptoms and also added that Lise was often irritable and restless. Lise's score on the RAID was 20, indicating clinically significant anxiety (reflected by a score greater than 11). Her symptoms also corresponded to those of GAD. Lise's depressive symptoms were assessed with the Geriatric Depression Scale (GDS; Yesavage et al., 1983), and her score of 7 indicated mild depressive symptoms.

Case formulation

According to the cognitive model, a person's thinking will influence his or her mood and behavior, as well as bodily sensations. In persons with dementia, the processing of information is affected by cognitive impairment, and as the disease progresses, making sense of the world becomes increasingly difficult. In addition, anxiety or depression in persons with dementia may produce other biases that will influence perception, such as catastrophizing or overgeneralizations. James (1999) has suggested that anxiety in persons with dementia can effectively be conceptualized using Beck's notion of the cognitive triad (Beck, 1976). The current beliefs that a person holds about himself or herself, the world and the future will influence feelings and actions. In the case of dementia, the world may become unpredictable and at times chaotic, it becomes more and more difficult to trust oneself and one's ability to cope, and the future also seems frightening as things seem to be only getting worse. Certain caretaking practices may appear patronizing or even aggressive, and thus add to the confusion and exacerbate negative mood (James, 1999). Dysfunctional or "challenging behaviors," such as agitation or withdrawal, may be understood as attempts to cope with an incoherent world and others who may seem to be acting strangely (James, 1999).

As a consequence of the decline in her cognitive abilities, as well as the decline in her physical functioning after the hip fracture, Lise seemed to become more attentive to threats in her environment. Her awareness of and attention to potential threats led her to perceive the world increasingly as a dangerous and unpredictable place, which she no longer felt capable of managing. Initially, she responded by isolating herself to the safety of her apartment. Passivity and lack of physical activity exacerbated her physical decline, and the pain and her experience of frailty frightened Lise so that she also became anxious of being alone and feared that something might happen to her even at home. Since she was to a varying degree aware of her memory problems, she became frustrated as well as more and more worried about her ability to cope, feeling hopelessness and fear for the future.

She tried to relieve her anxiety by checking constantly that everything was as it was supposed to be and by seeking support and assurance from her daughter, who was her primary caretaker. As she became more dependent on her daughter, not only for help and care but also for social contact, she started to worry about her daughter and catastrophize about all the bad things that might happen to her. Lise's daughter, on the other hand, was distressed by the frequent phone calls from her mother, and at times she was abrupt, inpatient, and critical in her communications to Lise, which added to Lise's worry and made her even more frustrated.

In order to break the negative cycle based on the reciprocal relationship between worry, anxiety, depressive mood, and maladaptive coping behaviors (avoidance, isolation, checking), the treatment goals for Lise included teaching her new coping skills to manage her distress, so that she would be able to engage in activities and social contacts, which would also likely reduce the pressure on Lise's daughter and, thus, improve their relationship.

Treatment and outcome

Cognitive behavioral therapy for persons with dementia

The CBT-AD approach involves modifying efficacious CBT protocols for late-life anxiety in terms of content and structure for persons with dementia, according to their individual level of functioning, as well as integrating learning strategies to address cognitive deficits (Paukert et al., 2010). Necessary changes to the content might include choosing relatively simple coping skills and emphasizing more on the behavioral treatment components relative to the cognitive skills.

Structural changes may include shorter sessions, limiting the number of topics covered in order to allow for more time for practice and rehearsal, as well as involving a caregiver in the treatment to help with the practice in between sessions.

Problems with short-term memory and language and difficulties with attention are common from early on in the disease process, and these deficits need to be addressed in CBT for persons with dementia. To ensure and enhance comprehension, the therapist may ask the patient to repeat information and use reflective listening. Restorative and compensatory cognitive training techniques may be used to address the deficits in learning and memory. Asking patients to help generate retrieval cues, creating associations between pieces of information, and using written or visual stimuli may be used as compensatory strategies. Procedural memory remains relatively intact late into the progression of the disease, and this preserved ability may be exploited by using motor activity at the time of encoding. Several studies also indicate that even persons with severe dementia can benefit substantially from interventions that incorporate Spaced Retrieval (SR), a restorative method for improving encoding and retrieval (e.g. Bourgeois et al., 2003). The SR technique involves retrieving target information at increasing intervals of time. When the patient c annot remember the information, he or she is given the correct information and asked to repeat it immediately. (A summary of key elements in the case formulation for case study 2 is outlined in Table 8.1).

CBT treatment for Lise

Lise and her daughter attended 11 sessions throughout 3 months. Each session lasted between 30 and 50 minutes. Lise was also asked to practice the skills learned in therapy at home every day. During each session, a concrete plan for homework was created together with Lise and her daughter, designating regular times for practice and when and how her daughter would help her to complete the exercises. Simple, written instructions for practice were provided together with a calendar that would help Lise to keep track of the exercises. In between the sessions, the therapist also called Lise each week to inquire about the practice and answer any questions she might have about the exercises. Lise's daughter was encouraged to call the therapist in case they encountered any problems with the homework.

Anxiety monitoring and deep breathing

The focus of the first three sessions was anxiety monitoring and relaxation with deep breathing. Lise was asked to keep a daily record of her anxiety by marking a checklist of situations in which she had felt *uneasy* (which was the word she preferred to use for describing her anxiety). She also recorded other signs of uneasiness that she had experienced during the day, such as worrisome thoughts, tingling in her hands and feet, and calling her daughter. The therapist explained to Lise and her daughter that anxiety monitoring was necessary in order to understand her anxiety better, so that later on Lise would be able to identify signs of uneasiness and use appropriate coping skills.

Deep breathing was taught by asking Lise to pay attention to her breathing and take slow, even, deep breaths. SR was used in the sessions to teach Lise to use deep breathing when she felt uneasy. The therapist asked Lise "What can you do when you feel uneasy?" and Lise first gave the answer "I will breathe deeply," and then completed a deep breathing exercise together with the therapist. The same procedure was repeated several times during the sessions, with increasing intervals, interspersed with normal conversation in-between. Lise also received a CD with a relaxation exercise with deep breathing that she could listen to at home.

The anxiety monitoring helped to identify a pattern that occurred frequently: when Lise felt uneasy, she would get restless and start worrying about having forgotten something important such as buying or preparing food, followed by an attempt to relieve the anxious feeling by checking that everything is ok, going through her kitchen cabinets, or by calling her daughter. Notes with the text "*When I feel uneasy, I can take deep breaths*" were taped on her refrigerator and a mirror above the telephone, to remind Lise to use the coping skill in these situations. Lise practiced the breathing daily, two or three times a week together with her daughter, and learned to use the skill in most situations when she felt uneasy.

Coping statements and coping cards

In sessions 4 and 5, the focus was on improving Lise's sleep with the help of deep breathing and coping statements. The therapist and Lise discussed what Lise could say to herself to calm herself down when she woke up during the night and felt anxious. Lise chose two sentences: "*Things will be ok*" and "*Not being able to sleep won't hurt me.*" A coping card with instructions to breathe deeply and say the coping statements out loud to herself was prepared for Lise, and it was agreed that she will place it on her bedside table. Lise's daughter reported that they practiced together daily, either in telephone or when she was visiting. Lise lay down in her bed, and her daughter asked her what she could do when she woke up at night and felt uneasy. Lise said that she could pick up the coping card from the bedside table and read it, and then she practiced the breathing and read the coping statements out loud. Although the breathing skill and coping statements increased Lise's ability to manage anxiety during the night to some degree, she still kept waking up during the night, and her sleep did not improve until her activity level was increased through behavioral activation.

Behavioral activation

Behavioral activation was introduced in session 6, and a list of pleasant activities that Lise liked was created. Some of the easier activities, such as listening to the radio, looking at pictures in a photo album, and reading a magazine were chosen as ways in which Lise could distract herself from worrying when she was alone and felt uneasy. The therapist helped Lise and her daughter to make a plan for completing one or two of the more demanding activities each week. Lise started going for regular walks with either her son or daughter, and as she became more physically active, the pain in her hip was somewhat reduced and Lise gained more confidence in her balance and ability to move around. She was positive about engaging in more activities on her list, and began to attend a weekly meeting at the senior center, with music, exercise, and games. Lise's mood improved and her daughter also noted a marked reduction in her anxiety.

Relationship to daughter and worry postponement

In addition to working on teaching Lise new coping skills to manage her anxiety, another goal of the intervention was to improve the relationship between Lise and her daughter. In the sessions, the therapist modeled how to communicate with Lise and gave praise for the work Lise did, no matter what her performance was on a given task. An extra session alone with Lise's daughter was also scheduled, during which the therapist explained how the disease affected Lise's functioning and practiced with the daughter formulating simple and concrete instructions to Lise. This was helpful in terms of reducing both Lise's and her daughter's frustration, and as Lise's daughter became more aware of how hard her mother was trying, she stopped criticizing her for lack of effort.

The frequent phone calls from Lise to her daughter had been another source of strain in their relationship. Toward the end of therapy, Lise was calling her daughter on the phone less, but she still had the occasional bout with several phone calls during one day. As Lise now had several coping skills in her "toolbox" that she could use to manage her worry and distress, it was decided to use the last 2 weeks before the final session to work on this issue. It was decided that Lise's daughter would phone her everyday after she was home from work, unless she would come for a visit, and Lise would try to postpone whatever worries or matters she wanted to bring up with her daughter until that time. Lise got a notebook to write down the concerns she had or wanted to discuss with her daughter, and a new coping card was taped on her mirror at home, giving instructions for going through her set of coping skills (deep breathing, coping statements, distraction with activity) when she felt worried or uneasy, before calling her daughter.

Final session

In the final session, the progress that Lise had made was reviewed, and the therapist helped Lise and her daughter to plan how to maintain the skills she had learned and continue practicing them. Lise's scores on the RAID were reduced from 20 to 10, and her daughter's ratings on the NPI scales and the caregiver distress scales were decreased to a non-clinical level. Lise herself was very satisfied with being able to get out of her apartment and meet people more often, and she commented that she felt optimistic about continuing the more active life.

Summary

In this chapter, we have outlined an individualized framework for the cognitive behavioral formulation of two older patients presenting with complex and co-morbid anxiety disorders. In presenting the two cases, we have emphasized the need to assess and interpret symptoms within *a multifocus approach*. Symptoms, as they appear in the clinical setting or are presented by significant others, involve a mixture of psychological as well as medical problems, which is an obvious premise in the case illustrations. If we add polypharmacy as another premise, we also need to be aware of the *fluctuations* in the symptom presentation. Understanding what the clinical presentation of co-morbid anxiety is, more often than not, a matter of team-work, and even more so in the older patient with medical and functional problems.

At the same time, when a case is defined as complex, involving cognitive and physical decline, we may be so eager to help that we lose the perspective of *the person*. We need to be aware of our own prejudices of older patients as fragile and helpless, and keep in mind that meeting an older person with multiple health problems represents a challenge that may be influenced by our *a priori* expectations of older people as fragile and helpless. Persons with cognitive impairment have regularly been excluded from clinical research as well as clinical practice. The case of Lise illustrates how in apparently difficult clinical presentations there is the potential to exploit the individual resources of the patient, still utilizing the well-known treatment options.

Throughout the chapter, we have sought to emphasize the importance of using established and well-known treatment models with older adults. At the same time, we have illustrated the importance of using treatment options *flexibly and adapting them to the individual patient and his or her problems*. The phenomenon of safety behavior, that is, the overt or covert avoidance of feared outcomes that is carried out in a specific situation (Salkovskis, 1991), may illustrate this point. It is widely asserted by clinicians as well as researchers, that safety behavior is counter-therapeutic and should be extinguished. Safety behavior generally is conceived of as providing only temporary relief from symptoms, and may eventually be a cause of persisting anxiety. In a patient with COPD and anxiety, such as John, it was not easy to establish whether his overt safety behaviors were appropriate or not, given his respiratory illness. In recent literature, it has been emphasized that anxiety-control strategies such as distraction (e.g. attention management) may not necessarily be conceived of as counterproductive in treating anxiety (Parrish, Radomsky, & Dugas, 2008). Although a thorough discussion of the relevance of various therapeutic mechanisms is beyond the scope of our chapter, it is interesting to note that carrying out psychological treatment in older patients with complex symptomatology may result in more focused attention on what mechanisms lead to a positive treatment outcome and what mechanisms are less productive.

One further aspect deserves mentioning. We know too well that not having access to psychological treatment is a common issue in most countries. Whether we live in Europe, Australia, or the United States, older people have not been a major concern in mental health services. There is reason to believe that psychological treatment for older adults is a slowly growing enterprise. Taking mental health problems into contexts like *primary care and medical settings* should be added to our agenda.

Issues for further reflection

+ The presentation of anxiety in older adults may be complicated by multiple factors, such as co-morbid medical illnesses, cognitive impairment, emphasis on somatic symptoms, and fluctuations in symptoms. Identifying and assessing late-life anxiety provides challenges to the clinician or the researcher, in terms of choosing the right assessment instruments, utilizing information from multiple sources, while simultaneously keeping in mind how one's own prejudices against older adults, may influence the clinical interpretation of symptoms.

+ Therapy with older adults may demand creativity and flexibility when tailoring the treatment to meet the patients' needs, even when manualized treatment protocols are used. Individual case formulations are likely to be helpful for understanding complex cases and planning treatment.

+ To what degree do efficacious psychological treatments need to be modified for older adults? Consider the case of John; would he have benefited more from treatment with a greater focus on the inhibition of safety behaviors? When working with older adults with serious medical conditions or cognitive impairment, there may be a need to reflect upon and differentiate between reasonable precautions and considerations for the patient's health and exaggerated anxieties and worries over the patient's safety—from the point of view of the patient, his or her family members and caregivers, as well as one's own concerns as a clinician.

References

American Psychiatric Association (2000). *Diagnostic and statistical manual of mental disorders.* Fourth Edition (text revision). Washington, DC: American Psychiatric Association.

American Psychiatric Association (2002). *Practice guidelines for treatment of psychiatric disorders compendium.* Washington, DC: American Psychiatric Association.

Ayers, C.R., Sorrell, J.T., Thorp, S.R., & Wetherell, J.L. (2007). Evidence-based psychological treatments for late-life anxiety. *Psychology and Aging, 22,* 8–17.

Beck, A.T. (1976). *Cognitive therapy and the emotional disorders.* New York, NY: International University Press.

Beck, A.T., & Steer, R.A. (1993). *Beck Anxiety Inventory manual.* Orlando, FL: Harcourt Brace.

Beck, A.T., Steer, R.A., & Brown, G.K. (1996). *Beck Depression Inventory-II manual.* San Antonio, TX: Hacourt Brace.

Beekman, A.T., de Beurs, E., van Balkom, A.J., Deeg, D.J., van Dyck, R., & van Tilburd, W. (2000). Anxiety and depression in later life: Co-occurrence and communality of risk factors. *American Journal of Psychiatry, 157,* 89–95.

Bieling, P.J., & Kuyken, W. (2003). Is cognitive case formulation science or science fiction? *Clinical Psychology: Science and Practice, 10,* 52–69.

Bieling, P.J., McCabe, R.E., & Antony, M.M. (2006). *Cognitive-behavioral therapy in groups*. New York, NY: Guilford Press.

Bourgeois, M.S., Camp, C., Rose, M., Blanche, W., Malone, M., Carr, J., et al. (2003). A comparison of training strategies to enhance use of external aids by persons with dementia. *Journal of Communication Disorders, 36*, 361–378.

Brenes, G.A. (2006). Age differences in the presentation of anxiety. *Aging & Mental Health, 10*, 298–302.

Brenes, G.A., Kritchevsky, S.B., Mehta, K.M., Yaffe, K., Simonsick, E.C., Ayonayon, H.N., et al. (2007). Scared to death: Results from the Health, Aging, and Body Composition study. *American Journal of Geriatric Psychiatry, 15*, 262–265.

Bryant, C., Jackson, H., & Ames, D. (2008). The prevalence of anxiety in older adults: Methodological issues and a review of the literature. *Journal of Affective Disorders, 109*, 233–250.

Clark, D.M. (1986). A cognitive model of panic. *Behaviour Research and Therapy, 24*, 461–470.

Cummings, J.L., Mega, M., Gray, K., Rosenberg-Thompson, S., Carusi, D.A., & Gornbein, J. (1994). The Neuropsychiatric Inventory: Comprehensive assessment of psychopathology in dementia. *Neurology, 44*, 2308–2314.

de Beurs, E., Beekman, A.T., van Balkom, A.J., Deeg, D.J., van Dyck, R., & van Tilburg, W. (1999). Consequences of anxiety in older adults: Its effect on disability, well-being and use of health services. *Psychological Medicine, 29*, 583–593.

Flint, A.J. (1994). Epidemiology and comorbidity of anxiety disorders in the elderly. *American Journal of Psychiatry, 151*, 640–649.

Flint, A.J. (2005). Generalized anxiety in elderly patients: Epidemiology, diagnosis, and treatment options. *Drugs and Aging, 22*, 101–114.

French, D.D., Campbell, R., Spehar, A., Cunningham, F., Bulat, T., & Luther, S.L. (2006). Drugs and falls in community-dwelling older people: A national veterans study. *Clinical Therapy, 28*, 619–630.

James, I.A. (1999). Using a cognitive rationale to conceptualize anxiety in people with dementia. *Behavioural and Cognitive Psychotherapy, 27*, 345–351.

Kabat-Zinn, J. (1990). *Full catastrophe living: Using the wisdom of your body and mind to face stress, pain and illness*. New York, NY: Dell Publishing.

Kraus, C.A., Seignourel, P., Balasubramanyam, V., Snow, A.L., Wilson, N.L., Kunik, M.E., et al. (2008). Cognitive-behavioral treatment for anxiety in patients with dementia. *Journal of Psychiatric Practice, 14*, 186–192.

Kuyken, W., Padesky, C.A., & Dudley, R. (2009). *Collaborative case conceptualization: Working effectively with clients in cognitive-behavioral therapy*. New York, NY: Guilford Press.

Larkin, B.A., Copeland, J.R., Dewney, M.E., Davidson, I.A., Saunders, P.A., Sharma, V.K., et al (1992). The natural history of neurotic disorders in an elderly urban population. Findings from the Liverpool longitudinal study of continuing health in the community. *British Journal of Psychiatry, 160*, 681–686.

Livermore, N., Sharpe, L., & McKenzie, D. (2008). Cognitive behaviour therapy for panic disorder in chronic obstructive pulmonary disease: Two case studies. *Behavioural and Cognitive Psychotherapy, 36*, 625–630.

Lynch, T.R., & Bronner, L.L. (2006). Mindfulness and dialectical behavior therapy (DBT): Application with depressed older adults with personality disorders. In R.A. Baer (Ed.), *Mindfulness-based treatment approaches. Clinician's guide to evidence base and applications*. Burlington, MA: Academic Press.

Mehta, K.M., Yaffe, K., Brenes, G.A., Newman, A.B., Shorr, R.I., Simonsick, E.M., et al. (2007). Anxiety symptoms and decline in physical function over 5 years in the health, aging and the body composition study. *Journal of the American Geriatric Society, 55*, 265–270.

Mintzer, J.E., Brawman-Mintzer, O., & Mirski, D.F., & Barkin, K. (2000). Anxiety in the behavioral and psychological symptoms of dementia. *International Psychogeriatrics, 12*, 139–142.

Mohlman, J. (2008). More power to the executive? A preliminary test of CBT plus executive skills training for treatment of late-life GAD. *Cognitive and Behavioral Practice, 15*, 306–316.

Mohlman, J., Gorenstein, E.E., Kleber, M., de Jesus, M., Gorman, J.M., & Papp, L.A. (2003). Standard and enhanced cognitive-behavior therapy for late-life generalized anxiety disorder: Two pilot investigations. *American Journal of Geriatric Psychiatry, 11*, 24–32.

NICE Guideline (2007). Available at: http://www.nice.org.uk/nicemedia/pdf/CG022NICEguidelineamended.pdf.

Nordhus, I.H. (2008). Manifestations of depression and anxiety in older adults. In R. Woods & L. Clare (Eds.), *Handbook of the clinical psychology of ageing* (pp. 97–111). Chichester, West Sussex, UK: John Wiley & Sons.

Nordhus, I.H., & Pallesen, S. (2003). Psychological treatment of late-life anxiety: An empirical review. *Journal of Consulting and Clinical Psychology*, 71, 643–651.

Paukert, A.L., Calleo, J., Kraus-Schuman, C., Snow, L., Wilson, N., Petersen, N.J, et al. (2010). Peaceful mind: an open trial of cognitive–behavioral therapy for anxiety in persons with dementia. *International Psychogeriatrics*, 22, 1012–1021.

Parrish, C.L., Radomsky, A.S., & Dugas, M.J. (2008). Anxiety-control strategies: Is there room for neutralization in successful exposure treatment? *Clinical Psychology Review*, 28, 1400–1412.

Pinquart, M., & Duberstein, P.R. (2007). Treatment of anxiety disorders in older adults: A meta-analytic comparison of behavioral and pharmacological interventions. *American Journal of Geriatric Psychiatry*, 15(8), 639–651.

Salkovskis, P.M. (1991). The importance of behaviour in the maintenance of anxiety and panic: A cognitive account. *Behavioural Psychotherapy*, 19, 6–19.

Segal, Z.V., Williams, J.M.G., & Teasdale, J.D. (2002). *Mindfulness-based cognitive therapy for depression.* New York, NY: Guilford Press.

Seignourel, P.J., Kunik, M.E., Snow, L., Wilson, N., & Stanley, M. (2008). Anxiety in dementia: A critical review. *Clinical Psychology Review*, 28, 1071–1082.

Shankar, K.K., Walker, M., & Frost, D. (1999). The development of a valid and reliable scale for rating anxiety in dementia (RAID). *Aging & Mental Health*, 3, 39–49.

Stanley, M.A., Hopko, D.R., Diefenbach, G.J., Bourland, S.L., Rodriguez, H., & Wagener, P. (2003). Cognitive-behavioral therapy for late-life generalized anxiety disorder in primary care: Preliminary findings. *American Journal of Geriatric Psychiatry*, 11(1), 92–96.

Stanley, M.A., Roberts, R.E., Bourland, S.L., & Novy, D.M. (2001). Anxiety disorders among older primary care patients. *Journal of Clinical Geropsychology*, 7, 105–116.

Stanley, M.A., Wilson, N.L., Novy, D.M., Rhoades, H.M., Wagener, P.D., Greisinger, A.J., et al. (2009). Cognitive behavior therapy for generalized anxiety disorder among older adults in primary care: A randomized clinical trial. *Journal of the American Medical Association*, 301(14), 1460–1467.

Starkstein, S.E., Jorge, R., Petracca, G., & Robisnon, R.G. (2007). The construct of generalized anxiety disorder in Alzheimer disease. *American Journal of Geriatric Psychiatry*, 15, 42–49.

Tarrier, N. (2006). An introduction to case formulation and its challenges. In N. Tarrier (Ed.), *Case formulation in cognitive behaviour therapy: The treatment of challenging and complex cases* (pp. 1–12). Hove, East Sussex, England: Routledge.

Teasdale, J.D., Segal, Z.V., & Williams, J.M.G. (1995). How does cognitive therapy prevent relapse and why should attentional control (mindfulness) training help? *Behavior Research and Therapy*, 33, 25–39.

Wells, A. (1997). *Cognitive therapy of anxiety disorders: A practice manual and conceptual guide.* Chichester, West Sussex, UK: John Wiley & Sons.

Wells, A. (2006). Cognitive therapy case formulations in anxiety disorders. In N. Tarrier (Ed.), *Case formulation in cognitive behaviour therapy. The treatment of challenging and complex case* (pp. 52–80). New York, NY: Routledge.

Wetherell, J.L., Hopko, D.R., Diefenbach, G.J., Averill, P.M., Beck, J.G., Craske, M.G., et al. (2005). Cognitive-behavioral therapy for late-life generalized anxiety disorder: Who gets better? *Behavior Therapy*, 36(2), 147–156.

Yesavage, J.A., Brink, T.L., Rose, T.L., Lum, O., Huang, V., Adey, M., et al. (1983). Development and validation of a geriatric depression screening scale: A preliminary report. *Journal of Psychiatric Research*, 17, 37–49.

Yuan, Y., Tsoi, K., & Hunt, R.H. (2006). Selective serotonin reuptake inhibitors and risk of upper GI bleeding: Confusion or confounding? *The American Journal of Medicine*, 119, 19–27.

Chapter 9

The treatment of challenging behavior in care facilities: Ellen

Ian A. James

Introduction

Many of the people with dementia who display challenging behaviors are among the most complex patients we are asked to treat (Hancock, Woods, Challis, & Orrell, 2006). In addition to their needs related to problematic behaviors, such people are often disorientated, possess a different view of reality to others, may suffer from physical impairments, and frequently have marked cognitive and memories difficulties. They may also be taking a great deal of medication, and many will be relying on others (family or professional carers) to deliver a range of basic and personal needs. Those living in 24-hour care homes may further experience interpersonal difficulties with fellow residents and/or staff, and find their care setting both unsettling and under-stimulating. Thus, even in those situations where the etiology of the behavior is relatively simple (e.g. agitation due to constipation), the manner in which it is communicated and then dealt with by the staff, may make its presentation complex, resulting in the "simple" cause being difficult to detect and treat.

Until recently, this group of patients was not offered any form of psychotherapy; rather, they were frequently overmedicated with major and minor tranquilizers (Dempsey & Moore, 2005; Ballard & Waite, 2006). However, new guidelines advocate the use of biopsychosocial treatments before resorting to powerful antipsychotics and benzodiazepines (Howard, Ballard, O'Brien, & Burns, 2001; Dementia Care Strategy, 2009). The present case study illustrates a non-pharmacological approach that has been used over the last 10 years in Newcastle upon Tyne, UK for this patient group (James, Mackenzie, Stephenson, & Roe, 2006; James, 1999). The approach employed is a formulation-led case-specific method that shares features with the successful non-pharmacological interventions undertaken by Cohen-Mansfield, Libin, and Marx (2007) and Bird, Llewellyn-Jones, and Korten (2009).

The aims of this chapter are to illustrate:

1. A formulation-led, biopsychosocial approach, incorporating cognitive behavior therapy principles, for treating challenging behaviors in residential aged care settings.

2. The key structural and process features of the "Newcastle" framework.

3. The range of psychotherapeutic skills required to work competently with residents and staff in 24-hour care facilities.

The term challenging behavior is used in this paper, but it is recognized that this is an unfortunate term as it implies that the perpetrator of the behavior is the "problem," and that the treatment should be targeted at the behavior. In truth, it is clear that the behaviors are often products of a complex interaction of physical, psychological, environmental, interpersonal, and organizational factors (untreated pain, depression, anxiety; infections; constipation; sensory impairment; psychoses; understimulation, overstimulations, boredom, lack of opportunities to meet basic needs—freedom to walk outside, lack of intimate touch, etc.). In many respects it is surprising, given the poor environmental, organizational, and interpersonal features associated with the care we provide in 24-hour care homes, that we do not encounter more shouting, aggression, protesting, refusing to comply with rules, and sexualized behavior.

The case outlined here is typical of the patients seen by a member of the team from the Newcastle Challenging Behavior Service (NCBS). First, an overview of the case is presented, in terms of the referral letter, assessment, formulation, and treatment. Following this, the structural and process features associated with the case are unpacked and discussed in order to provide greater learning opportunities.

Overview of the case

Referral from the medical practitioner

Dear Challenging Behavior team,

> I would be grateful if you would see Mrs. Ellen Jones, aged 86, a resident at Forest View residential care home. Ellen has a diagnosis of Alzheimer's disease, angina and a history of chronic asthma.
>
> Ellen has been in care for six months, prior to this she lived at home and looked after herself with minimum support. She is an independent individual, and can be short-tempered with her carers. She is an ex-matron, working for 40 years at the local hospital.
>
> The care staff have been struggling to support her for the last three months, and thus asked me to see her with the view of prescribing an antipsychotic for her problematic behaviors. These behaviors are outlined below.
>
> Staff report that Ellen is putting herself on the floor, usually at busy times. They also claim she is attention seeking and demanding, and refusing to do things for herself. For example, she is currently refusing to comply with personal care interventions (e.g. washing, dressing). The manager of the home does not think Ellen is suitably placed in residential care and wants her to be transferred to a higher category care facility.
>
> I have undertaken a physical examination, and all tests have been negative and thus there is no obvious physical reason for her deterioration. I would be grateful for your support in this matter. I have resisted the pressure to prescribe anything thus far for her behavior, with the promise of a speedy intervention from yourselves.
>
> Yours sincerely, Consultant Psychiatrist

Assessment

The referral was discussed at a team meeting and allocated to a member of our service; the therapist subsequently visited the care home. The assessment began with a discussion with the manager and the staff, who stated that Ellen's behavior differed with the level of seniority of the staff. She was usually pleasant with the manager or deputy, but would often refuse to cooperate with junior staff. Carers also reported that Ellen was demanding of them, and frequently insulted them (e.g. "You're a bitch"; "I hope you die"; "You useless slut"). The staff would only attend her in pairs as they felt they needed to give each other both physical and moral support. Most of them felt that Ellen should be transferred to another care facility.

In order to obtain factual information about her various behaviors, a series of monitoring charts were explained and given to the staff. The therapist left some examples of completed charts at the home to provide a template to assist with their completion.

Next the therapist had a one-to-one interview with Ellen. From this meeting it was evident her mood was low. She said: "I used to have a good life. I've got nobody, and nobody cares, I've nothing left to live for." During the interview she acknowledged that she could be nasty to the staff, but complained about their treatment of her. She said, "They just ignore me, ... they make excuses to shut me up." "They tell me lies!"

Information about Ellen was also obtained from both case notes held in the care home and medical notes held at the hospital. She also gave permission for the therapist to consult with her own medical practitioner. Further information was obtained from a nephew, although he was unable to give many details because he had lost contact with his aunt in recent years.

At this stage, the therapist's role was mainly to engage in a fact-finding process in relation to both Ellen's past (biography, health status, etc.) and her present behaviors. The next stage involved putting the information together into a presentation to assist the staff to understand and empathize with Ellen' current experiences of living in care. A specific session was organized to do this; this was called the Information Sharing Session (ISS, see section "Information sharing session and formulation"). It is suggested that armed with this greater level of awareness gained during the ISS, the staff would be able to reconceptualize her behavior and no longer merely see her as a "grumpy, foul-mouthed old woman" (Carer quote).

Information sharing session and formulation

All cases seen by NCBS receive an ISS, which is a 45- to 60-minute meeting coordinated by the therapist and conducted at the care home. At this meeting, all the background information collected is presented, and put together with the data from the behavioral charts. During the session, the therapist helps the staff to make links and reflect on the behaviors in relation to the resident's needs. The therapist always asks that as many of the staff as possible attend the ISS. In Ellen's case, 11 carers attended the initial session, and thus it was evident that emotions were running high. The therapist presented the background information with the aid of a flip chart, placing particular emphasis on the following facts:

+ Ellen was depressed.
+ Ellen had a moderately severe dementia, with frontal lobe deficits (making her disinhibited).
+ Ellen had always been fiercely independent—she was struggling to come to terms with having to rely on the staff for personal care.
+ Ellen rarely received any visitors—she had no one who really cared/loved her.
+ Ellen had numerous physical complaints that prevented her from pursuing the activities she previously enjoyed.

Although the problems Ellen was experiencing were highlighted, the staff who attended the ISS found it difficult to empathize with Ellen's situation. For example, when the therapist asked "Now that we have all this information about Ellen, what do you think we should do?" she was met with a barrage of comments: "Get her out," "We don't get paid enough to put up with that," "You wouldn't put up with the comments she makes, so why should we?" "It's because she used to be a qualified nurse (like you) that you're trying to get us to keep her."

It was clear from the high level of expressed emotion that little could be achieved at this session. Therefore, the therapist told the staff that she would leave them with the background information and return a few days later. If they still wanted Ellen to leave at this point, then it would be appropriate to help initiate a move. However, if the staff changed their minds, the therapist would assist in devising interventions. The therapist returned a few days later and met with the staff. Most staff said that they had probably been "a bit too hard" on Ellen and, having reflected on the background information, they felt they should at least give her a chance. Now that the staff were in a more constructive frame of mind, the therapist helped them devise a set of interventions.

A written summary of the discussions from the ISS was given to the staff on the next visit. This summary is termed the "Formulation," and it provides a concise description of the resident's behavior in relation to background information (Fig. 9.1). Attached to the sheet is a treatment plan (i.e. a care plan), which is a user-friendly synopsis of the interventions suggested by the staff during the ISS.

Treatment plan

Ellen's treatment was informed by a concisely written care plan that included environmental, psychological, and pharmacological interventions. For example, she was provided with a mattress variator to assist her mobility, and her fluoxetine was changed to mirtazapine to address her poor appetite. The remaining interventions involved getting the staff to adopt a consistently civil approach to Ellen. The staff were encouraged to adopt boundaries with her. For example, when she swore at them, it was agreed that they would cease their interaction with Ellen, informing her that they were upset and would return in a few minutes. The staff also agreed to spend more "quality" time with her, encouraging her both to talk about her life story and to help around the home (e.g. folding napkins, assisting table-laying at mealtimes, etc.).

The approach was successful, with the benefits apparent within 2 weeks. Ellen became more approachable, and her self-esteem and morale improved markedly. This improvement was also evident on her psychometric scores on the Neuropsychiatric Inventory (NPI; Cummings et al., 1994), which is a pre-/post-assessment measure routinely used by the team.

Following this overview, the next sections provide a guide and theoretical perspective on using the Newcastle framework. The clinical work undertaken with Ellen is now unpacked to illustrate the change mechanisms underpinning the therapist's approach. It is my view that this approach is consistent with a label of a "psychotherapy." This is a term seldom used in this area, although Bird et al. (2009) have started to describe their interventions in this manner.

Description of the Newcastle Challenging Behaviour Service and philosophy of care

The NCBS was developed because of a gap in the existing clinical services in the area, which meant that some of the most complex people in our communities were not receiving adequate psychological care. Traditionally, the private sector care homes had proven difficult places to gain access to, because they had not previously received sustained attention from health service psychotherapists. Thus, they were rather wary of input when it was offered, preferring medication to therapy, owing to the clinical commitments the latter entailed. This, in turn, had made National Health Service (NHS) therapists reluctant to engage with these settings due to the poor reception they received (James, Powell, & Kendell, 2001). In order to break this negative cycle, the NCBS was established, with the following aims:

- Treat challenging behavior in a competent and person-centered manner.
- Treat challenging behavior in the setting in which it was being exhibited.
- Work collaboratively with care facilities to improve the well-being of people in care.
- Prevent unnecessary admissions to hospital.
- Facilitate easier discharge from hospital to appropriate care settings.

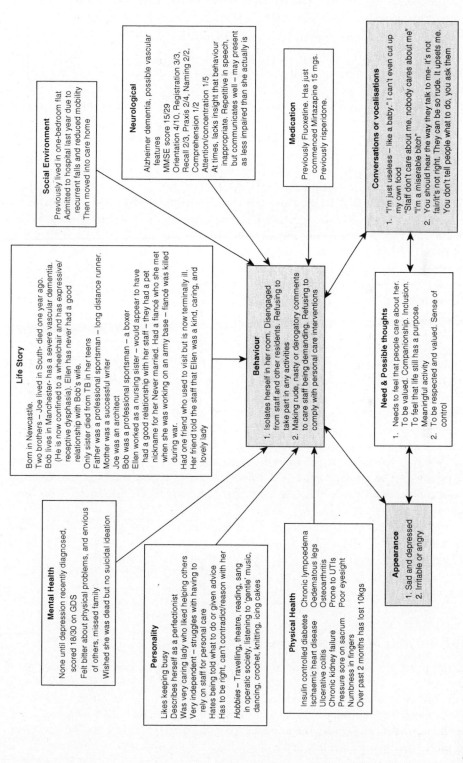

Social Environment

Previously lived in one-bedroom flat
Admitted to hospital last year due to
recurrent falls and reduced mobility
Then moved into care home

Neurological

Alzheimer dementia, possible vascular
features
MMSE score 15/29
Orientation 4/10, Registration 3/3,
Recall 2/3, Praxis 2/4, Naming 2/2,
Comprehension 1/2
Attention/concentration 1/5
At times, lacks insight that behaviour
inappropriate. Repetitive in speech,
but communicates well – may present
as less impaired than she actually is

Medication

Previously Fluoxetine. Has just
commenced Mirtazapine 15 mgs.
Previously risperidone.

Life Story

Born in Newcastle.
Two brothers – Joe lived in South- died one year ago.
Bob lives in Manchester- has a severe vascular dementia.
(He is now confined to a wheelchair and has expressive/
receptive dysphasia). Ellen has never had a good
relationship with Bob's wife.
Only sister died from TB in her teens
Father was a professional sportsman – long distance runner.
Mother was a successful writer
Joe was an architect
Bob was a professional sportsman – a boxer
Ellen worked as a nursing sister – would appear to have
had a good relationship with her staff – they had a pet
nickname for her Never married. Had a fiancé who she met
when she was working on an army base – fiancé was killed
during war.
Had one friend who used to visit but is now terminally ill.
Her friend told the staff that Ellen was a kind, caring, and
lovely lady

Conversations or vocalisations

1. "I'm just useless – like a baby. I can't even cut up
   my own food
   "Staff don't care about me, nobody cares about me"
   "I'm a miserable bitch"
2. You should hear the way they talk to me- it's not
   fair/it's not right. They can be so rude. It upsets me.
   You don't tell people what to do, you ask them

Behaviour

1. Isolates herself in her room. Disengaged
   from staff and other residents. Refusing to
   take part in any activities
2. Making rude, nasty or derogatory comments
   to care staff being demanding. Refusing to
   comply with personal care interventions

Need & Possible thoughts

1. Needs to feel that people care about her.
   To be valued. Companionship. Inclusion.
   To feel that life still has a purpose.
   Meaningful activity
2. To be respected and valued. Sense of
   control

Mental Health

None until depression recently diagnosed,
scored 18/30 on GDS
Felt bitter about physical problems, and envious
of others, missed family
Wished she was dead but no suicidal ideation

Personality

Likes keeping busy
Describes herself as a perfectionist
Was very caring lady who liked helping others
Very independent – struggles with having to
rely on staff for personal care
Hates being told what to do or given advice
Has to be right, can't contradict/reason with her
Hobbies – Travelling, theatre, reading, sang
in operatic society, listening to 'gentle' music,
dancing, crochet, knitting, icing cakes

Physical Health

Insulin controlled diabetes   Chronic lympoedema
Ischaemic heart disease   Oedematous legs
Ulcerative colitis   Osteoarthritis
Chronic kidney failure   Prone to UTIs
Pressure sore on sacrum   Poor eyesight
Numbness in fingers
Over past 2 months has lost 10kgs

Appearance

1. Sad and depressed
2. Irritable or angry

Fig. 9.1 Ellen's formulation.

- Facilitate transfers of patients to appropriate care settings (from hospital to care facilities and between care facilities).
- Develop links with statutory and regulatory organizations.

Initially, the NCBS team was comprised of a psychologist and a nurse, and was piloted for 2 years. The remit of this team was mainly clinical, but it was quickly recognized that teaching and supervision would play important roles in the work of the team. As the team grew, the NCBS became more involved in conducting action-based research and has numerous publications to its name. Some of these publications have been on controversial topics such as the use of dolls in therapy (James, Mackenzie, & Mukaetova-Ladinska, 2006) and the therapeutic use of lies (James, Wood-Mitchell, Waterworth, Mackenzie, & Cunningham, 2006) with patients with dementia.

Currently, the team is made up of two senior nurses and four mid-grade nurses. It is managed by a psychologist and receives sessional input from a psychiatrist. Over the last decade, 1,000+ people have received interventions using the above approach; currently, the NCBS sees approximately 200 residents per year. Empirical evaluation of the work has demonstrated its efficacy (Wood-Mitchell, Mackenzie, Stephenson, & James, 2007). In recent years, the Newcastle methodology has informed the development of a number of other services in the United Kingdom (e.g. in Northern Ireland, London, Aberdeen, Sheffield, and Southampton). We believe the reason for its success relate to its values and desire to empower all people involved in dealing with "problematic" behaviors (i.e. the resident, staff, family, care home manager). This systemic stance helps to ensure that the formulation-led care plans are initiated and adhered to appropriately.

The formulation framework used by the NCBS draws heavily from Cohen-Mansfield's (2000a, b) model for challenging behavior. This "needs-based" model highlights the fact that challenging behaviors are usually not unpredictable random actions; rather, they are rational activities with a high degree of predictability. Indeed, frequently the behaviors are manifestations of patients' attempts to cope in situations they are misperceiving or are confused by. Cohen-Mansfield's framework involves obtaining two types of information (i) background features (history, premorbid personality, physical health status) and (ii) a comprehensive description of the challenging episodes. The latter are the verbal and non-verbal signs displayed by the person. By putting these two types of information together, one is in a stronger position to accurately identify the person's coping strategy or the need driving the coping response, for example, to be free from pain, respond to an imagined attacker, or defend oneself from perceived molestation during a personal care activity.

The unmet needs perspective illustrated in Cohen-Mansfield's model has influenced other clinicians regarding their philosophies of care, and there is now a tool, the Camberwell Assessment of Needs in Elderly (CANE; Reynolds et al., 2000; Orrell & Hancock, 2004), which seeks to identify people's social, medical, psychological, and environmental needs. This measure covers 24 areas, two of which relate to carers' needs. It has recently been employed by NCBS, although it not a tool used in the current case study.

Protocol of the Newcastle approach

There are a number of stages to consider when using the Newcastle service's 14-week approach; these are outlined in Table 9.1. As one can see, it is a "front loaded" method of working, with most of the intensive work taking place in the first few weeks of the case. In the later stages, the therapist tends to be monitoring and tweaking both the formulation and interventions as a consequence of staff feedback. The guiding ethos when using the approach in care settings is that it is paramount for the staff to feel they are involved in the various stages of the work, from initial assessment to the delivery of the intervention. The methodology used in the Newcastle approach is described in more detail below; specific mechanisms of change employed with Ellen are also reviewed.

Table 9.1 Stages engaged in by NCBS therapist

Week 1: Having received the referral and been allocated the case, the therapist commences the "fact finding" process. An important step is to make sure that all the physical checks have been completed by the medical practitioner to ensure that the problematic behavior has not arisen from either an acute infection or transient difficulty (e.g. pain resulting from a fall, constipation).

Week 2: By the second week, the therapist will have made contact with the home on a number of occasions and spoken to the relevant people, including the patient. In the conversations with staff, it is made clear what the services' expectations are. To reinforce the latter issue, an information sheet is left with the home describing the service and each others' responsibilities in delivering the package of care. During this week further information is collected from the various sources, and a detailed analysis of the behavior is undertaken via monitoring charts. A pre-treatment measure, the Neuropsychiatric Inventory (Cummings et al., 1994), is undertaken with the patient's key worker.

Week 3: The information collected thus far starts to undergo analysis, and greater clarification and specification of the problems are made. If not done previously, the feedback from the family is added to the growing data set.

Weeks 4 and 5: The main event taking place in this phase is the delivery of the ISS. This is a specific session, attended by staff in the care setting (ideally with all levels of staff represented), lasting approximately an hour. In this session, the information about the person's problematic behavior is presented in the context of his/her background. The idea of the session is to develop an understanding of the behavior in relation to the wider context, allowing staff to speculate on the patient's' "needs"—in other words, what is driving the behavior. This process helps to inform the interventions, which are developed by staff during the ISS. One of the goals of the Newcastle therapist is to ensure that the interventions devised meet the SMART criteria.

The therapist facilitates the meeting using effective questioning techniques, feedback, summarizing, education, challenging strategies, and guided reflection techniques. These methods are designed to get the staff to "step back" from the situation, and look afresh at the behavior within its historical and situational context. Collaboration with staff is particularly important when trying to identify the patient's needs and possible interpretation of the situation.

Thus the goal of the ISS is to assist staff to become more knowledgeable, empowered, and motivated to improve the resident's well-being, through the implementation of appropriate interventions. Within the process, an effective ISS will have used information from many sources to give staff an understanding of what factors are contributing toward the patient's actions. Within this approach, it is vital that the interventions are developed by the staff themselves, so that they have ownership of the treatment process.

Week 6: Following the ISS, it is the therapist's responsibility to take away the details discussed at the meeting, and recorded on the flip chart, to produce an A4 summary sheet of the formulation (see Figure 9.1). Attached to the formulation sheet will be a detailed description of the interventions (i.e. a care plan). A vital feature underpinning the success of the interventions is that they are carried out consistently and uniformly by all staff. To gauge how well the information is disseminated, the home is provided with a sheet on which all staff must sign to indicate that they have read and understood the invention sheet.

Weeks 7–11: The remaining sessions involve follow-up work, visiting the home to ensure the interventions are being carried out consistently. In some cases, the formulation may require changing or the interventions tweaking.

Weeks 12–14: Unless there are exceptional reasons for continuing input, this milestone results in discharge. At this meeting a discharge interview takes place, where the key worker is asked to complete a qualitative and quantitative (NPI) measure of change.

In the following subsections, we will examine the process and structural features of the approach from assessment to outcome in more detail.

Process and structural features of the assessment phase

The function of the assessment is twofold, firstly to collect relevant data to help inform the intervention, and secondly to collect the information in a manner that increases the likelihood that the staff will carry out the interventions. The latter requires therapeutic engagement with the staff: empathizing, collaborating, and asking Socratic questions (see Table 9.2, adapted from Fossey & James, 2008). Indeed, it is by using such processes that the NCBS therapist can encourage staff to become inquisitive to learn more about the patient and the causes of the "target" behavior. Thus, this method can be seen as a repersonalization process. This is the reverse of Kitwood's (1997) notion of depersonalization, whereby residents in care often lose their sense of identities due to staff not knowing, or not having regard, for them and their personal histories. Using the Newcastle approach, repersonalization begins during the information collection phase. The repersonalization process was clearly evident in the case of Ellen, as it became clear that the staff knew little about her. Thus, as one can see, the approach is a "systemic" methodology, with every endeavor being made to make the staff true stakeholders in the treatment strategy.

It is evident from Table 9.2 that it requires good interpersonal skills to work in care settings. Further, it is my belief that the skills of a competent clinician in this area would match the abilities of therapist working in any other area of mental health.

The structural framework in which the information is presented is called the formulation. This framework is outlined in detail below and presented diagrammatically in Fig. 9.2.

Background assessment: Background details concerning the person's life, health status, etc. are collected from staff and family (see section "Formulation").

Assessment of the triggers: Information is obtained to determine the events or people who are likely to elicit the behaviors. The use of diaries and assessment charts are helpful to identify the triggers.

Assessment of the challenging behavior: It is very important to obtain a rich description of the challenging behavior. This, again, can be done through personal observations of staff, the use of diaries, and assessment charts. An example of one of the assessment charts used by the service is presented in Fig. 9.3.

Formal assessment measure: The NCBS routinely use the NPI (Cummings et al., 1994) as a pre-/post-assessment measure; the version used includes the caregiver distress scale (the NPI-D). This informant-rated scale measures both the frequency and severity of problematic behaviors and the emotional/psychological distress of caregivers in relation to 12 neuropsychiatric symptoms. For each of the 12 symptoms, a behavior score is obtained by multiplying the frequency (1–4) by the perceived severity of the behavior (1–3). A total behavior score is achieved by adding the individual behavior scores of each symptom (maximum score = 144). The distress caused to caregivers for each symptom is also scored (0–5), and then totaled (maximum score = 60).

Information sharing session and goal-setting process

In the ISS, all the background information collected is presented and put together with the data from the behavioral charts. Patterns are explored and detected, potential triggers elucidated; the staff are encouraged to relate their experiences of the behavior and then lessons are unpicked from these accounts. In many respects, it is the therapeutic work done in the ISS that most resembles a traditional session of psychotherapy for the therapist. As with therapy, the goal of the session is to arrive at a shared conceptual understanding of the problem and develop a plan to

Table 9.2 Some of the skills required to work with staff in care facilities

Technique	Definition	Example (statements you might hear NCBS member say with respect to theme)
Setting goals of the ISS	Negotiating with the staff about the contents and preferred methods of discussion during ISS.	Today we're going to be discussing Ellen's behavior and some of the reasons for her communicating this way. In your view, what are the three things it's essential that we talk through before finishing the session?
Collaborating	Ensuring the staff feel part of the teaching process, encouraging them to be active participants.	You've had lots of experience of this, so before I discuss this issue further, who can tell us what's the best thing to say to her when she calls you a "bitch."
Gathering information	Fact finding and obtaining information from the staff about the situation, feelings, thoughts, and/or behaviors.	What time does she tend to wake up? What expression did she have on her face after she hit you?
Feedback	Providing specific feedback that aids learning, and asking for feedback to help guide the teaching.	The previous care plan was too vague. The ideas we have discussed today are much clearer and specific, well done!
Summarizing/ clarifying	Chunking information to help clarify links and highlight key features.	Great, now let's see if I understand what you did there. You saw her searching for the toilet, and knew she'd be too embarrassed to ask you, so you asked if she'd like to wash her hands and then guided her to the sink in the toilet.
Supporting and understanding	Providing verbal and non-verbal signs that provide reassurance and encouragement to the staff.	That was difficult, but you seemed to have handled it really, really well.
Informing/ educating	Providing factual information aimed at increasing staffs' knowledge.	Multi-infarct dementia is a type of vascular dementia. It is often very difficult to distinguish multi-infarct from Alzheimer's disease.
Aiding reflection	Working with the staff to get them to think through issues in order to come to an increased understanding of key issues.	Let's stop a second and think through the implications of this. If, indeed, pain is a common cause of challenging behavior, what should we do?
Formulating	Working with the staff to develop a framework that helps to explain residents' behaviors and needs.	Ok, we seem to have gathered quite a lot of information about Ellen now. Let's put it all together and see how it helps explain why she's so depressed.
Self-disclosing	Informing staff about personal experiences that help to illustrate issues or concepts.	I must admit, I wasn't aware that diabetes was a side effect of anti-psychotic use. One of the nurses told me during our training session 2 weeks ago.
Challenging	Getting the staff to rethink their views, often by pointing out inconsistencies in their thinking.	Well, both of you can't be right. One of you is saying she is like this with everyone, while the other thinks she is cooperative when with certain individuals.
Disagreeing	Taking a different viewpoint to the staff, in order to highlight an alternative perspective.	I am going have to disagree with that. She is not just being awkward. Remember she has a dementia and thus can struggle at times to make sense of what is happening to her during her personal care tasks.
Behavioral tasks	Using activity-based tasks (role-play, modeling) to help demonstrate skills.	Now that we have discussed the problems and possible strategies for communicating with Ellen, let's try to demonstrate it via a role-play.

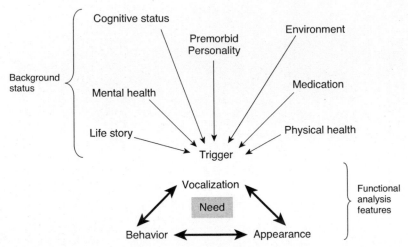

Fig. 9.2 Formulation diagram.
Source: Adapted from James, I.A. (1999). Using a cognitive rationale to conceptualize anxiety in people with dementia. *Behavioural and Cognitive Psychotherapy*, *27*(4), 345–351.

deal with it. In terms of the Newcastle model, the problematic behavior is perceived as an expression of an unmet need on the part of the resident (Cohen-Mansfield, 2000a, b). By the end of the ISS, a set of interventions and approaches will have been developed in collaboration with the staff. It is relevant to note that the therapist plays a major role in ensuring that the goals are realistic and feasible. Indeed, for each intervention the therapist is routinely instructed to employ the SMART (specific, measurable, achieveable, relevant, timely) criteria with respect to the goal setting (Fossey & James, 2008). Further discussion about the goals is presented in the section on interventions.

Formulation

Following the ISS, a formulation is produced (see Fig. 9.1). Much of the information mentioned in Fig. 9.1 will already have been presented to the staff in the ISS via a flip chart. This flip chart information will have helped generate discussion and assisted the staff to achieve a greater level of understanding regarding Ellen's behavior. However, at this stage the information is condensed and written-up in the form of a single A4 sheet of paper. The experience of the Newcastle team suggests that supplying the staff with an overly comprehensive formulation presented on multiple sheets is both off-putting and less likely to be read. In contrast, it has been found that a single formulation sheet with a brief care plan attached provides the most effective treatment strategy. The following section discusses the components presented in Figs. 9.1 and 9.2; both the background features and the features associated with the analyses of the problematic behaviors.

Background

Physical health

Many older people experience declining physical health (e.g. visual and auditory problems) and age-related illness (e.g. arthritis, backache, cancer, toothache, constipation, and chiropody ailments). It is important to note that many challenging behaviors are related to pain and physical discomfort, which are often made worse during staff/resident interactions (such as toileting, transfers, and washing).

Behavioral Chart for …………………………..

Target behavior ………………………………………..
Please record any episodes of the above behavior (day/night).
Aim – to record frequency and circumstances of incidents.

Date and Time	What was the person doing just before the incident? (**A-antecedent**[†])
Where the incident occurred	
	What did you see happen? (**B-actual behavior**[†])
Which staff were involved (initials)	
What did the person say at the time of the incident?	
How did the person appear at the time of the incident? (may be more than one tick)	

Angry	Frustrated
Anxious	Happy
Bored	Irritable
Content	Physically unwell
Depressed	Restless
Despairing	Sad
Frightened	Worried

How was the situation resolved? (**C-consequences**[†])

Fig. 9.3 Example of an assessment chart incorporating an ABC analysis together with elements of the Newcastle approach.

[†] **A**—antecedents are the features happening just prior to the emergence of the behavior that may have served to trigger or reinforce it; **B**—behaviors are simply the factual acts witnessed by the staff. The staff are taught not to interpret the behavior, rather provide factual details; **C**—consequences are the responses of others to the behavioral disturbance. An analysis of this aspect helps to determine what the person might be achieving by acting this way. Also by examining the consequences, one can check the behavior is not being inadvertently reinforced.

Personality

It is important to recognize that a person's personality endures through the course of dementia; his/her individuality will be apparent in many ways and at various stages of the illness. People with severe dementia may still wish to express lifestyle preferences (e.g. relating to accommodation, religious practices, food, and sexual orientation). Although some personality changes are related to changes in brain pathology, others are associated with psychological factors, for example, someone with dementia may feel he/she is vulnerable, becomes more emotional, and seeks out more physical attention. Finding out how the person coped with difficulties in the past can be revealing. Current problems may be explained by someone being unable to use familiar methods of coping such as managing stress by going out for a walk.

Mental health

Mental health problems are common and it is important to acknowledge their potential influence. Past difficulties may interact with current problems; for example, a person with long-standing social phobic tendencies who develops dementia and moves into residential care may feel very anxious in busy communal rooms (James & Sabin, 2002). Changes in brain pathology may result in psychotic symptoms such as visual hallucinations or delusions of theft.

Life story

Gathering information about the person's life, relationships, roles, and losses is critically important in order to put his/her behavior in context. In many types of dementia, the person's long-term and procedural memory (e.g. memory for performing familiar roles, actions, music, and dance) often remains relatively preserved. Such information can be used to engage the person in meaningful activities. For example, providing an ex-cleaner with cleaning materials and an area of the home to brush and polish can provide a meaningful activity for that person. Knowledge of the person's life story is therefore crucial both in understanding his/her behavior and what he/she is communicating as well as in establishing a good therapeutic relationship. Important parts of the person's life story (losses, traumas) may also re-emerge during the development of the dementia.

Social

Environmental factors are important influences on the well-being of older people owing to their levels of dependency. This is particularly the case for people with dementia who have particular difficulties with memory, problem solving, and orientation. We need to recognize the link between people's level of well-being and the opportunities they have to engage in fulfiling personal relationships. It is also worth checking whether a person's "challenging behavior" is triggered by his/her being too hot, too cold, hungry, or exposed to excessive stimulation such as a loud television or radio.

Cognitive status

The way in which a person experiences an event will be affected by his/her ability to process information. All cognitive impairments must be taken into account. Deficits in memory or problem-solving ability may lead to distress, particularly when a person has insight into his/her difficulties. Mental health problems such as anxiety and depression may add to cognitive difficulties, decreasing concentration, and having a negative effect on memory and problem-solving skills. Different forms of dementia affect different abilities and they progress at different rates.

Medication

The framework also considers the effect of medication. Medication is a possible point of intervention: a reduction, increase, or change may be helpful. Medication for the treatment of various conditions may affect the person's cognitive abilities. By considering physical health and medication as important, the framework acknowledges biological factors as well as social and psychological factors. The team often tries to minimize the use of anti-psychotic drugs, but frequently encourages the use of pain relief and antidepressant medications. However, where medication is required, it is tailored to the needs of the individual and is always in keeping with the information obtained from the formulation as per current guidelines (Howard et al., 2001; Sink, Holden, & Yaffe, 2005).

Information on all the background factors listed above is normally obtained by examining case files, speaking to carers and relatives, and by communicating with the person with dementia where possible. Specific forms have been devised by the NCBS to aid data collection, such as the personal profile questionnaires. These are questionnaires given to family that ask about the person's past, his/her likes and dislikes, as well as usual coping styles, favorite pastimes, foods, music, and so forth.

Observing and understanding the behavior

Figure 9.2 shows a triangle comprising three themes: vocalization, appearance, and behavior. The framework uses this triad to understand the person's experience of the episode of challenging behavior. One way of finding out what a person is experiencing is to talk to them; however, the person with dementia may not always be able to tell you what is driving his/her behavior. Valuable information can be gained simply by observing the person. There are three key features to pay attention to:

◆ The person's behavior

◆ What he/she says and/or vocalizes (whether coherent or not)

◆ How he/she appears to be feeling.

These observations can give us important clues to what patients are thinking and toward a better understanding of their needs. It is relevant to note that if there is more than one challenging behavior present, there will be more than one trigger and triad.

Triggers

The box labeled "triggers" is situated between the background details and the triad. This box simply highlights the circumstances in which the problematic behaviors are observed.

Behavior

Part of the assessment involves gathering details of what exactly happens during an episode of challenging behavior, or, in other words, a functional analysis. General labels such as "aggression" or "wandering" tell us little about what a person is actually doing, and even less about why he/she is doing it. As we are assuming that the behavior is a strategy being employed to enable the person to fulfill a need, careful analysis of the behavior helps to determine what the person is trying to achieve via this behavior. This analysis will need to consider antecedents and consequences, and where and with whom the behavior does and does not occur.

Conversations or vocalizations

It is helpful to gather information about the patient's difficulties by asking him/her directly. Most of this information will come from conversations and listening to the person. The verbal communications of people with severe dementia are not always coherent. However, it is important to take into account the type of vocalization (shouting, type of screaming—pain related, calling for help), when it occurs, and its content (the words used).

Appearance

It is important to observe the patient's appearance. Does he/she look anxious, depressed, or angry? Observing how the person appears is key to understanding his/her experience. The three most common forms of emotional distress are anxiety, anger, and depression. Empirical research informs us that each of these has a characteristic theme associated with it (Beck, 1976; James, 2001). These themes are outlined in Table 9.3.

As outlined above, when people feel anxious, they often see themselves as vulnerable and unable to cope with the demands of the situation. When people appear depressed, they often see

Table 9.3 Cognitive themes and their relationships to emotional appearance

Appearance	Cognitive themes
Depressed	The person has a self-perception of being worthless or inadequate, perceiving the world as hostile or uncaring, and viewing the future as being hopeless.
Anxious	The person has a self-perception of being vulnerable, perceiving her environment to be chaotic, and the future as unpredictable.
Angry	The person perceives that someone is acting unjustly toward her, and her rights are being infringed. Also there is a perception of the environment as being hostile, and a need to act immediately to protect her self-esteem from future harm.

themselves as inadequate, worthless, and the situation as being hopeless. Finally, when people are angry, they tend to see themselves as having been badly treated or misused in some way. Understanding these signs helps to inform us what people's needs might be. The anxious person may be fearful for his/her safety, needing to be helped to feel less vulnerable. The depressed person will probably need to be given a greater sense of worth, while the angry resident will need to feel that his/her rights are not being infringed.

Need and possible thoughts

The behavior, vocalization, and appearance observed during an episode of challenging behavior, when combined with the background information, can be used to try to understand what is causing the problem. Part of our role is to try to get the staff to empathize with the person's situation, to reflect on what he/she might be thinking in that situation, and to try to understand the reasons behind the challenging behavior. In other words, the aim is for staff to develop a "theory of mind" perspective with respect to the person with dementia. Table 9.4 summarizes how the information obtained above can be used in devising appropriate interventions.

Treatment and outcome

As stated above, the interventions are based on staff suggestions and are developed and refined at the end of the ISS with the therapist's help. After the group meeting, it is the therapist's task to take away the suggestions and put them together into a coherent treatment programme. As a result, a new care plan is produced based around the problematic behavior. The care plans are honed down to the bare essentials because once again it is common that overly complex treatment goals are not adhered to and often not read. It is relevant to note that psychological approaches are usually the first-line intervention used by the Newcastle Team. In order to illustrate the nature of the interventions further, let us return to the list of approaches suggested for Ellen.

1. Improving her self-esteem and morale by giving her a greater sense of control and a feeling that she was wanted, for example, by asking her if she wanted to go on trips out. The staff were encouraged to say things like—"it would be really nice if you would come—we'd appreciate your company."

2. Encouraging Ellen to help out around the home in order to provide her with a sense of self-worth. She could engage in small, achievable tasks, for example, folding napkins or towels.

3. Specific scripts were outlined to encourage Ellen to join in with the group activities or to socialize with other residents—"it's always nice when you join in." The staff were asked to spend some quality time with Ellen, saying "I've got 20 minutes to spare and thought it would be nice to spend some time with you. What would you like to do?"

Table 9.4 Illustration of how the emotional presentation of the person can help identify need and develop the intervention

Emotional appearance	Theme	Behavior associated with theme	Need	Possible action to deal with theme
Angry when carer removes her dinner plate without asking whether she had finished.	She thinks she is not being shown enough respect.	Swearing at staff: You filthy bitches.	To be respected.	Prior to touching her plate, ask Ellen whether she enjoyed the meal and then whether she's finished.
Depressed and lonely when sees other resident has a visitor	Thinks no one wants her.	Sits by herself, refusing to eat.	To feel valued by others.	At visiting times assign a member of staff to spend some 1:1 time with her.
Shame followed by *Anger* when member of staff points out to Ellen that she has been incontinent.	Initial theme is to do with a sense of embarrassment, but due to her reduced range of coping strategies to deal with the situation, she goes on the offensive.	Threw cup of water on floor and told staff member to f*ck off. Swore again when staff tried to change her.	To have her dignity maintained, while requiring her to change her wet clothes for hygiene/skin integrity reasons.	Use of a therapeutic lie (James et al., 2006), informing her that she must've spilled some water over herself. Hence, would she like some assistance to get changed.

4. Purchasing a mattress variator to help Ellen mobilize independently. Ellen did not want to go to bed simply because she (a) couldn't get up unaided and (b) found it difficult to change her position.

5. Improving communication in situations that had previously been confrontational (i.e. avoiding direct confrontation). The staff were encouraged to be more pleasant and respectful. They were encouraged to see that it is very difficult for someone to maintain his/her anger when the person he/she is venting the anger on is being pleasant and helpful.

6. Getting all the staff to use a standard protocol when responding to Ellen's hurtful and unpleasant comments. (A protocol helps provide consistency and enables the staff to have a greater sense of control of situations.)

In addition to the above, owing to the fact that Ellen was depressed, it was also felt appropriate to change the current prescription of fluoxetine to mirtazapine. It was hoped that mirtazapine, in addition to improving her mood, might improve her appetite.

After a week of using the interventions, the staff reported feeling better equipped to support Ellen. She was much more amenable to their care interventions. They also reported that they were enjoying spending time with Ellen—seeing her in a more positive light. They also described Ellen as being "approachable." Ellen was enjoying the time staff spent with her. She said "the staff are different now—most are pleasant and helpful." Furthermore, Ellen had stopped putting herself on the floor; she had started to interact with the other residents, and enjoyed participating in group activities. She was also helping out around the home. A mattress variator helped with her sleep, and she was going to bed at night without complaint. In addition, as a result of her going to bed, and her legs being in a horizontal position at night, they were not so edematous. The above observation were reflected in changes in the NPI scores with a pre score of 20 reducing to 8, and the "caregiver distress" score reducing from 8 to 2.

Discussion

This case illustrates some of the complexities inherent in treating challenging behavior in care facilities. It highlights the importance of devising inputs at the level of the individual both in terms of the person with dementia and the specific needs of each care home. Of note, I usually refrain from using the term person-centered to describe our work, as this has been so overused and misused that it has lost its currency (James & Fraser, 2009). The members of the NCBS prefer the phrase "Staff-centered, person-focused" as this illustrates the systemic nature of our approach. I think the latter term also stresses the key role that process issues play in delivering good care, which is an important point to highlight as too many of the U.K.'s national guidelines fail to deal adequately with "change processes." Often they merely state we should be using evidence-based psychological treatments, or comprehensive person-centered assessments, but they fail to inform us about how to implement them. I hope the above case study has not committed this error, and that the reader is clear about the mechanism of change we endeavor to use in our work. I believe that when more clinicians clarify not only "what they do well" but "how they do it," our therapeutic skills will improve considerably.

In the near future, I think certified courses will be established in this clinical area. Further, I believe that such courses should be equivalent in breadth and quality to the gold-standard 9-month courses seen in the training of cognitive behavior therapists. Unless such bold moves are implemented, I think many clinicians will continue to struggle against the continued overreliance on psychotropic medication. Interestingly, a number of studies have now shown that psychiatrists would prefer to employ specialist teams in the treatment of challenging behavior (Wood-Mitchell, James, Wateworth, & Swann, 2008; Bishara, Taylor, Howard, & Abdel-Tawab, 2009).

According to Bishara et al. (2009), "From our survey, it appears that the use of pharmacological agents for the management of BPSD (behavioral and psychological symptoms of dementia) does not appear to be favored by the experts. They remarked that they would rather have effective and adequate nursing input and use non-pharmacological options, where possible, but the scarce availability of these options is a major limiting factor for their use" (p. 952). Thus, it behooves us to provide our medical colleagues with credible alternatives to medication. Although the traditional psychotherapies (e.g. reminiscence, reality orientation, validation, music therapy) have their place, it is important to recognize that they are not designed to treat a highly problematic behavior during the acute phase. As such, it is my experience that the only effective alternative to the use of tranquilizers is the quick input of a specialist team, one that is able to work with both the resident and the staff who are experiencing the difficulties.

The present case has described one possible strategy; however, clearly it is not the only psychological framework that can be used with this group of people. For example, Cohen-Mansfield (2000b) has produced a helpful "structured decision tree" protocol to guide individualized interventions (the TREA—treatment routes for exploring agitation). Another approach has been described by Bird, Llewellyn-Jones, Korten, and Smithers (2007), which includes psychotherapeutic methods for working closely with the staff and family members.

The development and modus operandi of the NCBS is consistent with the guidelines of the Dementia Strategy for England (2009), National Service Framework for Older People (Standard 7.54-6; Department of Health, 2001), and Audit Commission (2002, "Forget me not"), concerning the input of a specialist multidisciplinary outreach team into care home settings. It is relevant to note that in the United Kingdom, despite the above guidelines, there is limited evaluation of the impact of the work of community teams into care homes, with relatively few exceptions (Moniz-Cook et al., 1998; Proctor et al., 1999; Fossey et al., 2006; Stevenson, Ewing, Herschell, & Keith, 2006; Wood-Mitchell et al., 2007; Orrell et al., 2007). In the international arena, a handful of researchers have conducted important controlled trials in this area (Rovner, Steele, Shmuley, & Folstein, 1996; Cohen-Mansfield et al., 2007; Bird et al., 2009). Related work has also been undertaken with people living in their own homes, with key studies undertaken by Teri et al. (2005), Mittelman, Roth, Clay, and Haley (2007), and Marriott, Donaldson, Tarrier, and Burns (2000). It may be wishful thinking, but it seems evident by the dates of the above publications that there has been a surge in interest in providing better services for people with dementia over recent years. In support of this view, Esme Moniz-Cook (Hull, UK) has now received a large grant from National Institute for Health Research, UK to undertake two major randomized controlled trials (RCTs): one focused on challenging behavior in care facilities and the other for "people living at home." Further, the Australian Government has funded teams across Australia to use individual-ized psychological approaches in the treatment of challenging behaviors (Australian Government, 2007). It is hoped that with this higher level of interest from researchers and governments that we can start to establish a better evidence-base for our work, and be able to train our therapists to be competent in skills that have been shown to be effective.

Conclusion

The various forms of behavior that constitute the label "challenging behavior" are not diagnostic categories, although they are sometimes treated as such particularly by the medical profession when using psychotropics. These behaviors are usually elicited by residents when they are distressed, confused, disinhibited, misinterpreting situations, deluded, or hallucinating. The behaviors are often transient, but need to be dealt with when they place the resident or others at risk of physical, emotional, or psychological harm. Often the causes are multifactorial, although some can be directly linked to physical problems (delirium, infection, and pain). Owing to the complex nature of many of these behaviors, a comprehensive assessment of the potential causes should be under-taken. This should be done prior to the administration of medication. Once the causes have been identified, individualized approaches aimed at reducing the relevant distress (e.g. improved com-munication, use of aromatherapy, music, etc.) or confusion (use of memory aids, signage, environ-mental changes) have been shown to be helpful. However, such strategies need to take account of the needs of the individual with dementia, the staff, and the resources within the care setting. The present case illustrates an approach used by a clinical team that fulfills the above requirements, and the processes by which successful outcomes can be achieved have been illustrated.

References

Audit Commission (2002). Forget me not. Available at www.audit-commission.gov.uk

Australian Government (2007). *Dementia management advisory service: Operational guidelines*. Canberra: Department of Health and Ageing.

Ballard, C., Waite, J., & Birks, J. ((2006). Atypical antipsychotics for aggression and psychosis in Alzheimer's disease. *Cochrane Database of Systematic Reviews*, Issue 1, Article no. CD003476.

Beck, A.T. (1976). *Cognitive therapy and the emotional disorders*. New York, NY: International University Press.

Bird, M., Llewellyn-Jones, R.H., Korten, A., & Smithers, H. (2007). A controlled trial of a predominantly psychosocial approach to BPSD: Treating causality. *International Psychogeriatrics*, 19(5), 874–891.

Bird, M., Llewellyn-Jones, R.H., & Korten, A. (2009). An evaluation of the effectiveness of a case-specific approach to challenging behaviour associate with dementia. *Aging and Mental Health*, 13(1), 73–83.

Bishara, D., Taylor, D., Howard, R., & Abdel-Tawab, R. (2009). Expert opinion on the management of behavioural and psychological symptoms of dementia (BPSD) and investigation into prescribing practices in the UK. *International Journal of Geriatric Psychiatry, 24*, 944–954.

Cohen-Mansfield, J. (2000a). Use of patient characteristics to determine nonpharmacologic interventions for behavioural and psychological symptoms of dementia. *International Psychogeriatrics, 12*(1), 373–386.

Cohen-Mansfield, J. (2000b). Nonpharmalogical management of behavioural problems in persons with dementia: The TREA model. *Alzheimer Care Quarterly, 1*, 22–34.

Cohen-Mansfield, J., Libin, A., & Marx, M. (2007). Nonpharcalogical treatment of agitation: A controlled trial of systematic individualized intervention. *Journal of Gerontology: Medical Science, 62A*(8), 906–918.

Cummings, J.L., Mega, M., Gray, K., Rosenberg-Thompson, S., Carusi, D., & Gornbein, J. (1994). The Neuropsychiatric Inventory: Comprehensive assessment of psychopathology in dementia. *Neurology, 44*, 2308–2314.

Dementia Strategy for England, Department of Health (2009). Living well with dementia: A National Dementia Strategy. Available at: www.dh.gov.uk/en/socialcare/deliveringadultsocialcare/olderpeople/nationaldementiastrategy/index.htm.

Dempsey, O., & Moore, H. (2005). Psychotropic prescribing for older people in residential care in the UK, are guidelines being followed? *Primary Care Community, 10*, 13–18.

Department of Health (2001). National Service Framework for Older People. DOH, PO Box 777, London SE1 6XH. Fax: 0623 724524.

Fossey, J., & James, I.A. (2008). *Evidence-based approaches for improving dementia care in care homes.* London: Alzheimer's Society.

Fossey, J., Ballard, C., Juszczak, E., James, I., Alder, N., Jacoby, R., et al. (2006). Effect of enhanced psychosocial care on antipsychotic use in nursing home residents with severe dementia: Cluster randomized trial. *British Medical Journal, 332*, 756–758.

Kitwood, T. (1997. *Dementia reconsidered.* Buckingham: Open University Press.

Hancock, G., Woods, B., Challis, D., & Orrell, M. (2006). The needs of older people with dementia in residential care. *International Journal of Geriatric Psychiatry, 21*, 43–49.

Howard, R., Ballard, C., O'Brien, J., & Burns, A. (2001). Guidelines for the management of agitation in dementia. *International Journal of Geriatric Psychiatry, 16*, 714–717.

James, I.A. (1999). Using a cognitive rationale to conceptualise anxiety in people with dementia. *Behavioural and Cognitive Psychotherapy, 27*(4), 345–351.

James, I.A. (2001). The anger triad and its use with people with severe dementia. *Psychology Special Interest Group for Older People (PSIGE) Newsletter, British Psychological Society, 76*, 45–47.

James, I.A., & Sabin, N. (2002). Safety seeking behaviours: Conceptualising a person's reaction to the experience of cognitive confusion. *Dementia: The International Journal of Social Research and Practice, 1*(1), 37–46.

James, I.A., & Fraser, F. (2009). Person-centred care: A conceptual overhaul. *Signpost, 13*(3).

James, I.A., Powell, I., & Kendell, K. (2001). Cognitive therapy for carers: Distinguishing fact from fiction. *Journal of Dementia Care, 9*(6), 24–26.

James, I.A., Mackenzie, L., & Mukaetova-Ladinska, E. (2006). Doll use in care homes for people with dementia. *International Journal of Geriatric Psychiatry, 21*(11), 1044–1051.

James, I.A., Mackenzie, L., Stephenson, M., & Roe, T. (2006). Dealing with challenging behaviour through an analysis of need: The Colombo approach. In M. Marshall & K. Allan (Eds.), *Dementia: Walking not wandering* (pp. 21–27). London: Hawker Press.

James, I.A., Wood-Mitchell, A., Waterworth, A.M., Mackenzie, L., & Cunningham, J. (2006). Lying to people with dementia: Developing ethical guidelines for care settings. *International Journal of Geriatric Psychiatry, 21*, 800–801.

Marriott, A., Donaldson, C., Tarrier, N., & Burns, A. (2000). Effectiveness of cognitive-behavioural family intervention in reducing the burden of care in carers of patients with Alzheimer's disease. *British Journal of Psychiatry, 176*, 557–562.

Mittelman, M.S., Roth, D.L., Clay, O.J., & Haley, W.E. (2007). Preserving the health of Alzheimer's caregivers: Impact of a spouse caregiver intervention. *American Journal of Geriatric Psychiatry*, *15*(9), 780–789.

Moniz-Cook, E., Agar, S., Silver, M., Woods, R., Wang, M., Elston, C., et al. (1998). Can staff training reduce carer stress and behavioural disturbance in the elderly mentally ill? *International Journal of Geriatric Psychiatry*, *13*, 149–158.

NICE (2007). *Dementia: The NICE-SCIE guideline on supporting people with dementia and their carers in health and social care*. National Clinical Practice Guideline 42. London: British Psychological Society and Gaskell.

Orrell, M., & Hancock, G. (2004). *CANE: Camberwell Assessment of Need for the Elderly*. London: Gaskell.

Orrell, M., Hancock, G., Hoe, J., Woods, B., Livingston, G., & Challis, D. (2007). A cluster randomized controlled trial to reduce unmet needs of people with dementia living in residential care. *International Journal of Geriatric Psychiatry*, *21*, 1127–1134.

Proctor, R., Burns, A., Stratton Powell, H., Tarrier, N., Faragher, B., Richardson, G., et al. (1999). Behavioural management in nursing and residential homes: A randomized controlled trial. *Lancet*, *354*, 26–29.

Reynolds, T., Thornicroft, G., Abas, M., Woods, B., Hoe, J., Leese, M., et al. (2000). Camberwell Assessment of Need for the Elderly (CANE); developmemt, validity and reliability. *British Journal of Psychiatry*, *176*, 444–452.

Rovner, B., Steele, C., Shmuley, Y., & Folstein, N. (1996). A randomized trial of dementia care in nursing homes. *American Geriatric Society*, *44*, 7–13.

Sink, K.M., Holden, F.H., & Yaffe, K. (2005). Pharmacological treatment of neuropsychiatric symptoms of dementia: A review of the evidence. *Journal of the American Medical Association*, *293*(5), 596–608.

Stevenson, G.S., Ewing, H., Herschell, J., & Keith, D. (2006). An enhanced assessment and support team (EAST) for dementing elders: Review of a Scottish regional initiative. *Journal of Mental Health*, *15*(2), 251–258.

Teri, L., Logsdon, R., Whall, A., Weiner, M., Trimmer, C., Peskind, E., et al. (2005). Training community consultants to help family members improve dementia care: A randomised controlled trial. *Gerontologist*, *45*, 802–811.

Wood-Mitchell, A., Mackenzie, L., Stephenson, M., & James, I.A. (2007). Treating challenging behaviour in care settings: Audit of a community service using the Neuropsychiatric Inventory. *Psychology Special Interest Group for Older People (PSIGE) Newsletter, British Psychological Society*, *101*, 19–23.

Wood-Mitchell, A., James, I., Waterworth, A., & Swann, A. (2008). Factors influencing the prescribing of medications by old age psychiatrists for behavioural and psychological symptoms of dementia: A qualitative study. *Age and Ageing*, *37*(5), 547–552.

Chapter 10

The importance of feedback and communication strategies with older adults: therapeutic and ethical considerations

Nancy A. Pachana, Natasha S. Squelch, and Helen Paton

Introduction

The aging of the population, well established in developed countries and beginning to be felt now in the developing world, is a well-recognized phenomenon (UN Department of Economic and Social Affairs Population Division, 2007). The practice implications for health professionals interacting with older clients are starting to be more widely discussed (Laidlaw & Pachana, 2009). Older adults themselves are increasingly aware of the effects of aging on their health. In particular, health professionals and older adults are increasingly cognizant of the possibility that memory or other cognitive and behavioral changes may signal the presence of a health concern which warrants investigation. Part of this investigation may include referral to a neuropsychologist.

Neuropsychologists are called upon to evaluate older adults in a wide range of settings. The client himself or herself, a family member, other health professionals, legal professionals, health care, and residential care agencies all may wish to avail themselves of neuropsychological testing. Some common referrals for neuropsychological testing might include establishing a differential diagnosis between dementia and another psychiatric condition such as anxiety, evaluation of financial or health decision-making capacity, or ascertainment of service needs within a rehabilitation or long-term care setting. In nearly all cases, these individuals would expect to get some sort of feedback about the performance of the individual, an interpretation of the data in terms of diagnosis or intervention strategies, as well as the possibility that further referrals are warranted.

It would seem obvious that the neuropsychologist should understand how to give feedback, particularly to older clients who may have some anxieties about having their cognition evaluated. Just as psychotherapy interventions should be guided by empirical research, so too therapeutic and ethical aspects of giving neuropsychological feedback have a small but growing literature. In this chapter, we aim to introduce concepts guiding therapeutic, collaborative, and ethical feedback and recommendations to individuals, families, and organizations.

Clinical neuropsychological feedback

In a more traditional information-gathering approach to neuropsychological assessment, tests are viewed as a method of providing the clinician with standardized samples of the client's behavior, which allow nomothetic comparisons and predictions of such behavior in everyday life.

The value of a test is demonstrated through its psychometric properties and predictive usefulness, with a focus on the test scores and their interpretation and the sequelae of the assessment results. The role of the person being evaluated to be an active participant in the testing is somewhat constrained and passive. Operating solely within such an information-gathering model may subtly or overtly serve to limit the amount of interaction with the client with respect to his or her own personal concerns about the testing process, about questions their family might have about the process of diagnosis or its ramifications, and about their hopes and concerns about the utility of the assessment process (Finn & Tonsager, 1997).

More recently, models of neuropsychological assessment have been developed which emphasize the client's subjective experience and collaboration in the entire assessment process. Such models offer specific collaborative and therapeutic approaches to feedback of neuropsychological test results. Neuropsychological assessment feedback (NAF) refers to the communication of neuropsychological assessment results and implications flowing from these results, such as referrals, rehabilitation recommendations, and potential legal actions such as guardianship orders. NAF has received relatively little focus in the literature (Gass & Brown, 1992; Gorske & Smith, 2008), despite the purported importance of feedback provision in clinical practice (Smith, Wiggins, & Gorske, 2007). Approaches to NAF delivery, and the effects of such feedback on patients and their families, remain relatively unexplored across age groups but particularly so in older adults.

Feedback from a neuropsychological assessment is considered a fundamental component of the process (Gorsky & Smith, 2008). According to Gass and Brown (1992), the provision of NAF is important for a variety of reasons outlined in Table 10.1. In particular, the ethical obligations of the psychologist to the client are widely acknowledged (e.g. Allen, Montgomery, Tubman, Frazier, & Escovar, 2003; Gorske & Smith, 2008; Green, 2006; Ward, 2008). Feedback can help point out strengths or areas of intact functioning, which families can use to facilitate optimal functioning.

In instances where impairment is severe, feedback allows the clinician to share information that may be crucial to the client's self-understanding and future life planning (Smith, Wiggins, et al., 2007). Given that persons experiencing cognitive change are at risk of viewing themselves negatively, feedback can assist with reframing their self-concept by explaining that changes are due to an identifiable disorder rather than personal failings or undesirable personality traits (Green, 2006).

Table 10.1 Obligations of the neuropsychologist regarding feedback to clients

1. There is an ethical and professional responsibility owed to patients and/or their families as they retain the right to be informed of assessment results and implications.
2. Objective guidance to facilitate informed decision-making should be provided to the client. Feedback describing the client's abilities and functional status can assist with a host of decisions relating to competency, independence, and rehabilitation.
3. Feedback assists treatment planning and outcome monitoring. Moreover, feedback offers a rationale for treatment, serves as a basis to select effective interventions, and can act to support the measurement of efficacy and progress in treatment.
4. Informational support provided to carers fosters greater understanding of the client and facilitates effective ways forward for all concerned. Such information can counteract any exaggeration or minimization of client deficits by families; can help to explain difficult behavior that families may find confusing, uncomfortable, or upsetting; and can offer improved coping strategies

Source: Adapted from Gass, C.S., & Brown, M.C. (1992). Neuropsychological test feedback to patients with brain dysfunction. *Psychological Assessment, 4*(3), 272–277.

Although the majority of clients who have untaken psychological and neuropsychological assessments anticipate that they will receive feedback, not all do. For example, a recent Internet survey of the feedback practices of psychologists conducting personality and neuropsychological assessments found that 71% of psychologists *usually* or *almost always* provided in-person assessment feedback to their clients and/or their families, with most respondents (43%) spending 50–60 minutes providing feedback (Smith, Wiggins, et al., 2007). The authors found that only two-thirds (63.6%) of psychologists *usually* or *almost always* provide understandable reports to their clients. Barriers to providing feedback relate to a host of organizational, clinician, and client factors. Feedback delivery may not be covered for payment under health care schemes; the clinician may feel pressured for time due to workload issues; or the organization itself may not support such activities (Green, 2006). There may be an organizational view that neuropsychological test results can be interpreted merely as "normal" or "abnormal," oversimplifying assessment results and implications in terms of outcomes for the client (Green).

When working with older clients and families, feedback may cause the psychologist to experience personal reactions to the client's problems (e.g. heightened concerns about their own future and that of their loved ones) and countertransference (e.g. having unresolved issues regarding placement of a grandparent or parent; Green, 2006; Knight, 1994). Further, psychologists may be exposed to greater client discussion and potential for dispute than is usually encountered with younger adults (e.g. older clients may hold strong spiritual, moral, or biological explanations for their illness; Knight). Having training in providing feedback to clients across the age range is extremely beneficial to the neuropsychologist. Feedback is also important for the clinician. Based on the results of Smith and colleagues' psychological assessment feedback practice survey, psychologists consider the clinical practice of providing feedback a vital part of the assessment process (Smith, Wiggins, et al., 2007). For clinicians, feedback serves as a link between assessment and therapeutic interventions (Groth-Marnet, 1999).

Older clients themselves may present particular barriers to feedback. Feedback may be unfeasible with clients who travel long distances, are frail, are unable to afford the extra cost, or need to lessen appointments due to dependency on others for transportation (Green, 2006). During feedback, a client's ability to attend, learn, and retain the results can be affected by a range of individual factors (e.g. psychological or medical disorders; cognitive deficits; ability to understand and accept results; Crosson, 1994; Mateer & Sira, 2008). Caregivers attending the feedback session can also be affected by such individual factors (Mateer & Sira).

There are several ways NAF can be communicated: face-to-face in a discussion format; in the form of a written report or letter; telephone or video conferencing session, either live or taped. Given the absence of non-verbal reactions during telephone feedback, special attention should be paid to asking questions such as "How are you feeling right now?" as well as ensuring that all parties on the call have a chance to express their reactions and emotions. Irrespective of the format chosen to deliver feedback, when working with older clients, Green recommends that a significant support person, with intact cognition, also attend the session (with the client's permission); preferably this is the same individual that attended the initial interview. The presence of family or friends allows the clinician to assist with differences of opinion, respond to individual questions, and facilitate the patient-family interaction (Green, 2000, 2006).

Several authors advocate for written documentation to supplement the feedback session (Armengol, Moes, Penney, & Sapienza, 2001; Mateer & Sira, 2008; Pope, 1992). Written feedback can assist in overcoming memory constraints encountered during verbal feedback by clients and families, assist clients who have significant verbal comprehension or verbal memory deficits, serve as a concrete reminder for clients and their families of what was said, facilitate understanding of the recommendations, and assist if there is anxiety regarding diagnosis (e.g. Armengol et al., 2001;

Mateer & Sira). With regard to the perceived utility of written test result summaries, Westervelt, Brown, Tremont, Javorsky, and Stern (2007) demonstrated that the majority of participants found the written summary *very much* helpful (71.1%) and *mostly* helpful (19.8%) in explaining their results. In this study, the majority of significant others who attended the feedback session also found the written summary *very much* helpful (83.5%) and *mostly* helpful (10.1%).

Approaches to clinical neuropsychological feedback

Therapeutic neuropsychological assessment

Therapeutic Neuropsychological Assessment (TNA) has been defined as "a clinician's use of neuropsychological test results as a treatment method" (Gorske & Smith, 2008, p. 31). According to Gorske (2008), the specific steps for conducting a TNA feedback session are as follows:

1. *Introduce the purpose of the feedback session.* Clients are given a written report and informed of the purpose of the session: that is, to provide a detailed report of their neuropsychological assessment results, that includes a discussion of strengths and weaknesses, their performance on individual tests, how test findings relate to life situations considered important to the client, and treatment recommendations resulting from the assessment findings. During this step the clinician continues a collaborative and open relationship with the client by eliciting questions and reactions to the information, and by responding with open-ended questions, affirmations, reflective statements, and summarizations (OARS) to enhance understanding;

2. *Develop life implication questions.* To assist personalize and guide the feedback session, clients are requested to think of two to three specific questions that they would like answered by the assessment results.

3. *Provide feedback about strengths and weaknesses.* This step involves an objective description of neuropsychological strengths and weaknesses, and personalizing the information by relating the results to their everyday life. This is achieved by utilizing the Motivational Interviewing method of "Elicit-Provide-Elicit." The clinician first *elicits* the client's view of the skill used in each test, clarifies his/her perception of skills, and then asks the client how he/she may use these skills in day-to-day life. The clinician then requests the client's consent to *provide* information about the cognitive skills assessed by each test, explains these skills in laypersons terms, provides real-life examples of how the skills can be used, and describes the skill as a strength or weakness based on normative data. Following this, the clinician *elicits* reactions to the information, and enhances collaboration by making sure the information is understood and the skills are applied to daily life.

4. *Summarize and provide recommendations.* The clinician summarizes the key topics discussed during the session. In order to individualize treatment planning and engage the client in decision making, the client is then asked how he/she would like to utilize the information. The clinician asks for the client's consent to suggest recommendations based on information gathered throughout the neuropsychological assessment process.

Therapeutic neuropsychological assessment case study

Noeline was 73 years old when she had a bifrontal craniotomy to remove a right frontal tumor. She made rapid improvement following the operation and quickly regained the ability to do many activities of daily living. Six months later a neuropsychological assessment found memory and executive deficits but further improvement was flagged as possible. However after 18 months,

Noeline's husband, Jack, raised concerns regarding her declining memory so she was referred for neuropsychological reassessment. During the feedback session following the reassessment, a discussion began by reflecting on concerns that had been brought up by Noeline and Jack during the assessment interview. Questions were raised by Noeline and Jack which could be addressed by the neuropsychological evaluation.

Do I have Alzheimer's disease even though the tumor's gone? Or have I continued to improve? These were important questions for Noeline. *Might I be doing too much for Noeline?* Jack and Noeline shared this concern around several issues, including making sure Noeline took her medication correctly.

Noeline felt that her memory was improving while Jack felt her memory was deteriorating. The neuropsychologist suggested that comparing the initial baseline assessment with the current assessment could give an objective method of comparison of memory functioning. Regarding memory, Noeline's recall, retention, and recognition of verbal information had improved. Although she was more capable of using effective memory strategies, she was inconsistent in her use of internal cues, self-monitoring, or other tactics. In everyday terms that meant she sometimes repeated herself or failed to keep on task—something more to do with executive functioning *per se* than memory. She showed other improvements such as going back and forth between tasks without difficulty as well as starting to think through ways to solve problems. The remaining deficits meant that she still benefited from routine and structure rather than just being left to her own devices.

Might I be able to get back to driving? Both Noeline and Jack wondered about this, although it was of much greater significance to Noeline. During the testing session, Noeline had confided in the neuropsychologist that she was frustrated at being stuck at home. Jack preferred to stay put and watch subscription television than go out. She found this particularly irritating. A mood questionnaire had found higher than expected stress levels. Not being able to drive was identified as one of her main losses as her previous interests were mainly social ones based outside the home. Yet her mild level of impairment on testing in the context of her life circumstances, suggested that she might be able to resume driving.

Will she ever regain the interests that she once had? How might Noeline do her household chores more quickly? The couple expressed concerns about functional domains more broadly. Noeline often stayed in bed late or appeared at a loose end because she had problems initiating activities. She seemed indecisive because she struggled to come up with or logically think through possible options by herself.

Upon being asked how they felt after discussing the results of the testing and potential implications for their everyday lives, Noeline and Jack expressed great relief. "We were afraid it was too good to be true" and then "Where do we go from here?" The neuropsychologist suggested as a recommendation that Noeline get an on-road driving assessment. Being able to drive to activities would likely reduce stress and frustration as well as help her access enjoyable interests. Routines and partial cues would optimize her chance of success while still boosting independence. For example, a schedule of daily and weekly activities could be set up. Jack or other family members could remind her the evening before of the next day's activities in order to help her start to prepare herself. Pre-sorted medications could be kept close to items used at mealtimes. Having a series of written steps to work through might assist in situations requiring problems to be solved or decisions to be made: *What do you want to happen? What is standing in your way? What do you need to do? Do you need help?* Jack nodded and suggested to Noeline, "How about going out for walks with me in the morning?" They both left the office with a light step and Noeline's recovery took a turn for the better.

Collaborative neuropsychological assessment

Collaborative Neuropsychological Assessment (CNA; Smith, Green, et al., 2007) is similar to TNA, with a collaborative stance emphasized. The three main goals of CNA are to answer questions about functioning from the referral source as well as the client; to assist the client in feeling understood, seen, and listened to by the clinician; and to provide the client with information and understanding to allow improved insight, acceptance, and the ability to move forward with his/her life (Smith, Green, et al.). Working collaboratively with the client and paying attention to his/her needs, wishes, and emotional experiences is expected to lead to an improved client-therapist alliance, more useful assessment findings, and better follow-through on recommendations (Gorske & Smith, 2008; Smith, Green, et al.). The authors acknowledge that the CNA approach may not be appropriate for all clinical settings or populations (e.g. severe dementia or brain injury may distort the client's perception of reality and reduce the ability to fully engage in the process; Smith, Green, et al.).

CNA views the client as the most important informant of all possible informants (Gorske & Smith, 2008; Smith, Green, et al., 2007; Smith, Werner, & Green, 2005). The clinician assumes an open, accepting, interested, and concerned stance, and works to obtain answers to the specific questions proposed by the clients (and their families), and to increase their understanding of their self-concept, cognitive problems, and daily living (Gorske & Smith; Smith, Green, et al.; Smith et al., 2005). CNA acknowledges that client difficulties impact on the client emotionally, producing distress, anger, and depression. The feedback session is recognized as the most powerful intervention during the assessment process, where the client and clinician collaborate to understand the relationship between the assessment results and the client's life troubles (Gorske & Smith; Smith, Green, et al.).

CNA entails a pre-interview questionnaire, an initial interview, an assessment session, a written report, and a feedback session. Before the initial interview, the client completes a questionnaire inquiring into the three reasons for the neuropsychological assessment. This gives the client an opportunity to convey specific questions he/she would like answered by the assessment as well as any concerns he/she may have. The clinician uses these three questions as the focus of the interview and feedback session in order to address the client's concerns (Smith, Green, et al., 2007).

During the initial interview, the clinician seeks to understand the presenting problem from the client's perspective, as well as the client's emotional experience of the problem. Open-ended questioning and eliciting the client's thoughts and feelings about the effect the problem has on the client's subjective experience are important at this stage. Utilizing information gained thus far, the clinician forms an interpretation of a central cognitive-emotional complaint (CCEC; Smith, Green, et al., 2007; Smith et al., 2005). Adapted from the work of Luborsky (1984), the CCEC concisely summarizes the client's main problem and the emotional consequence of that problem. There are three components to the CCEC: (1) a client's wish/desire; (2) a behavioral/cognitive reaction (i.e. the client's statement of his/her main problem); and (3) an emotional response to the problem (Smith, Green, et al.; Smith et al.).

Understanding the client's beliefs about how the evaluation will help requires the clinician to understand what the client desires from the evaluation and to advise if such expectations are realistic or not (Smith, Green, et al., 2007; Smith et al., 2005). Using the client's three questions completed pre-interview, the clinician inquires about the problems listed and the degree of concern each evokes. The client's wishes for the assessment and its outcome are established, allowing any misconceptions to be clarified (Smith, Green, et al.).

Socialization to the assessment process, the final component to the initial interview, endeavors to improve feelings of collaboration by socializing the client and/or family members to the neuropsychological assessment process (Smith, Green, et al., 2007; Smith et al., 2005). The clients are given examples of what to expect such as the types of tests they will be asked to complete, that clients cannot be told how they are doing during the assessment (e.g. whether they got a particular answer correct or not), and that two reports will be completed (one for the referral source and one for themselves) and a feedback session scheduled.

Two reports are completed: a technical report for the referrer and a CNA report for the client (Smith, Green, et al., 2007; Smith et al., 2005). The CNA report is written in layperson's language; presents test results representing strengths and challenges in bar charts compared to normative samples; and outlines the client's (and/or his/her family's) primary concern, other cognitive challenges, and cognitive strengths, in that order. This is followed by achievement and personality assessment results, the interaction between the personality and cognitive findings, general summary of findings in terms of strengths and weaknesses and a diagnosis if appropriate, summary answering the client's three questions, recommendations, and a list of resources (Smith, Green, et al.; Smith et al.). Smith et al. (2005) provide templates of CNA reports for adults and children.

The feedback session is the most important part of CNA (Smith, Green, et al., 2007). The clinician collaborates with the client to understand his/her functioning and current life difficulties, enlisting the client to help with interpretation of test results. The feedback session begins with "Check In," where the clinician inquires into any changes that have occurred since the assessment session; this offers an opportunity to re-establish rapport and modify interpretations if necessary (Smith, Green, et al.; Smith et al., 2005).

The clinician then provides an "Introduction to the Feedback Session," during which the CCEC is restated along with the client's reason for and expectations of the neuropsychological assessment (Smith, Green, et al., 2007, p. 15; Smith et al., 2005). The clinician reminds the client that he or she is a collaborator in the process of understanding the results and implications; and orients the client to the written feedback reports by outlining the differences between the technical report and the CNA report (Smith, Green, et al.; Smith et al.). The client is given a copy of the CNA report, which is referred to throughout the feedback session; a copy of the technical report is issued to the client at the completion of the session (Smith, Green, et al.).

Feedback begins with the clinician summarizing the client's primary concerns. The fact that different tests were used to assess key cognitive domains is discussed. The clinician goes over in detail five key statements considered important for the client to remember about the assessment (see Appendix A). The client's test results relating to his/her primary area of concern are addressed first, followed by cognitive challenges, cognitive strengths, and achievement results if applicable. For each of these sections, the clinician asks the client to recollect the experience with the assessment, and express the perception of how he/she performed on the tests; gives acknowledgment if the client's perception is consistent with the results and clinician's interpretation; and reviews the results in terms of being above or below average, and as relative strengths and weaknesses moving from global to more specific skills. The clinician assesses the client's feelings, agreement, and understanding of the information, using questions such as "How does that sound?" and "How does it feel to see these results?" The client is asked to provide an example of how each strength or weakness is reflected in his/her everyday life, and is given an opportunity to ask questions or for clarification if required. Following this, personality assessment feedback is provided if this sort of testing was completed with the clinician assessing the client's feelings, agreement, and understanding of the information provided (Smith, Green, et al., 2007; Smith et al., 2005).

A general summary is offered, restating the major sections of the report and giving a diagnosis, if appropriate, using non-technical language. If a diagnosis is given, the clinician specifically inquires how the client feels about this diagnosis (Smith, Green, et al., 2007; Smith et al., 2005). Next, the clinician provides answers to each of the client's initial three questions using any relevant assessment information, and checking for client satisfaction with these responses. Prior to presenting recommendations, the client is asked to suggest several of his/her own recommendations. The clinician essentially supports these, and follows on with any remaining recommendations contained in the report providing a rationale for each (Smith, Green, et al.; Smith et al.). Potentially useful resources are reviewed (e.g. names of relevant service providers). During the "Sign Off," the clinician answers any remaining questions, makes himself or herself available to answer any questions in the future, and provides the copy of the technical report (Smith, Green, et al.; Smith et al.). Smith et al. provide scripted examples of how to conduct components of the CNA interview and feedback session.

Collaborative neuropsychological assessment case study

John was a 72-year-old gentleman referred by a geriatrician in order to provide information to assist with the differential diagnosis of dementia and depression. Upon initial telephone contact, John consented to the neuropsychological assessment and to his wife Judy's involvement in the assessment process. Prior to attending the interview session, John and Judy were mailed a neuropsychological assessment information sheet, a questionnaire inquiring into three specific questions they each would like answered by the assessment, and measures of depression and anxiety.

At the interview session an understanding of John's problems from both his and his wife's perspective was obtained, along with their respective emotional experience of John's memory problems. This information provided by John was presented back to the couple using the CCEC. John's wish for himself (W), his behavioral or cognitive reaction (CR), and emotional response (ER) was presented as follows:

> From what you have told me today, it sounds like you want to be able to remember things for yourself (W), but no matter how hard you try you still forget things such as what to buy at the supermarket (CR). And this leaves you feeling frustrated, embarrassed, and depressed at times (ER). Does that sound right?

The information provided by Judy was then presented using the CCEC:

> It sounds like over the past three years John has had worsening memory problems such as forgetting to take a shower each day (CR). You feel like you constantly have to think for him or remind him to do things (ER) but you just want John to be able to remember things for himself (W).

Following this, an understanding of John and Judy's expectations of how the assessment could help was gained using the three questions they each completed prior to the interview (see Appendix B). It was necessary to clarify John and Judy's misconception that the assessment would be able to answer the question of whether John had dementia. The couple was informed that the neuropsychological assessment could only provide information regarding how John's results are similar or dissimilar to those of people with dementia; and it would be the geriatrician who would provide a diagnosis based on a variety of tests ordered, including neuropsychological test results. Before closing the interview, John and Judy were socialized to the neuropsychological assessment session, which John completed 4 days later.

The couple attended a feedback session 2 weeks following John's neuropsychological assessment. With no reported changes since the assessment, John and Judy's CCEC's were restated, along with their reasons for and expectations of the assessment. John and Judy were reminded of the collaborative process of understanding the assessment results, and were oriented to the CNA report.

John's test results relating to his primary area of concern, his memory, were presented first. He was able to recall having completed memory tests such as list-learning, and his perception that he did poorly on most memory tasks was acknowledged as consistent with what his results showed. John and Judy felt that the results reflected his difficulties in daily life, particularly his improved ability to remember things when he is provided with cueing.

John's cognitive challenges were discussed followed by his cognitive strengths. His and Judy's agreement with the findings were discussed, along with whether the challenges and strengths reflected in John's daily life. Both agreed that John's below average psychomotor speed and executive functioning abilities were challenges for him, manifested as requiring more time to complete daily tasks such as showering and dressing, and difficulty sequencing steps required for cooking a meal.

The results of the couple's depression and anxiety measures were presented. John's questionnaire responses indicated the presence of moderate levels of depression and anxiety; and upon further evaluation during the neuropsychological testing session he met clinical criteria for depression with anxiety features. John agreed that he had felt depressed over the past few years, with no identifiable trigger—just a feeling of having no purpose in life since he retired.

Judy's consent to discuss her questionnaire responses in the presence of her husband at the feedback session was obtained prior to the session being scheduled. Her responses indicated levels of mood disturbance that rivaled John's. Judy tearfully conveyed a high level of burden caring for John, leaving no time to attend to her own needs. Judy appeared somewhat comforted by the fact that depression and burden is common in carers and help was available. Judy was strongly encouraged to contact her general practitioner (GP) for a referral for psychological evaluation and treatment to address her symptoms of depression, anxiety, and burden as appropriate.

With the assessment results and depression diagnosis summarized, John and Judy's initial three questions they sought to have answered by the assessment were discussed (see Appendix C). The couple was reminded that the question of whether John had dementia was probably best and most fully answered by the geriatrician in light of all the data gathered by the team. In particular though, a vascular component was acknowledged and discussed, given his computed tomography (CT) head scan results were reported as indicating minor white matter changes, and his cognitive challenges such as psychomotor slowing. However, John's test results were not typical of those seen in people with dementia; his pattern of results were more suggestive of possible depression. John and Judy expressed great relief that dementia was unlikely; and John acknowledged more hope for the future.

John and Judy were asked to suggest any recommendations. Their suggestions were supported, and the remaining recommendations and resources outlined in the CNA report were discussed (see Appendix C for recommendations such as treatment for depression). A copy of the technical report was provided, along with a separate list of carer resources for Judy. The couple was welcomed to discuss any questions at a later date if needed.

Judy telephoned 2 weeks later to express her gratitude regarding the care her husband received from staff members at the hospital, and in particular to say thank you for the opportunity to discuss, and to have someone acknowledge, the impact that her husband's condition was having on her emotional health.

Collaborative therapeutic neuropsychological assessment

Gorske (Gorske & Smith, 2008, p. 31) developed a form of TNA known as the Neuropsychological Assessment Feedback Intervention (NAFI). The NAFI is a brief "treatment entry intervention" that utilizes a semi-structured individualized feedback report in order to boost treatment adherence motivation. Collaborative Therapeutic Neuropsychological Assessment (CTNA) represents a hybrid of Gorske's NAFI and Smith's CNA outlined earlier. More specifically, the initial interview and general approach follows CNA, while the feedback session and report is borrowed from the NAFI. Gorske and Smith provided comprehensive direction and detailed scripted examples of how to conduct feedback, along with a sample CTNA feedback report.

Family issues

Bennett-Levy, Klein-Boonschate, Batchelor, McCarter, and Walton (1994) consider the attendance of relatives at the initial interview and the feedback session helpful for numerous reasons: (a) families can provide information that the client may be unable to remember, and can assist the client to recall the feedback after the session; (b) relatives can offer a different perspective to presenting issues, and can advocate for the client when necessary; (c) family members are also inclined to ask questions about the relationship between test results and daily functioning, and ways to manage presenting problems; and (d) relatives provide emotional support, and can assist in clarifying any misunderstandings the client has about the assessment. Indeed, Bennett-Levy and colleagues in their study showed that having a relative present during the neuropsychological assessment process protected the client against feeling worse or less confident after the assessment.

Knight (1994, p. 142) stresses the importance of a family-oriented approach to feedback, with the client retaining overall control of the process. Knight offers four underlying principles for the feedback session: (1) families respond to feedback as "long-standing homeostatic systems"; (2) client competence is presumed; (3) varying degrees of competency are held by clients with dementia; and (4) persons with dementia possess some level of awareness of deficit. Knight also emphasizes the need for clinicians to preserve older clients' confidentiality and obtain their consent before sharing information with other people.

Approaches to providing feedback to clients suffering from depression and dementia are outlined by Knight (1994). In cases of depression, a family feedback session is recommended that includes psychoeducation (namely suicide prevention, and the role of depression in feeling helpless and hopeless), treatment prognosis, psychotherapeutic treatment options and rationale, recommendation for family therapy if applicable, and engagement of family assistance in aspects of treatment.

For clients with dementia, Knight (1994) recommends a conjoint session with the client and his/her family (with the client's consent) in order to discuss the client's cognitive impairment, diagnosis, and to provide psychoeducation. Discussion about misconceptions, memory-behavior relationships, symptom-specific improvement with disease progression, and legal and financial planning issues (Friss, 1990) could be included. However, the quantity of psychoeducation provided at any one time is to be judged cautiously by the clinician (Knight).

Family case study

Hazel was an 82-year-old woman who had been seen by the psychiatrist at Mental Health Services for Older People following a 3-month history of increasing worry, shakiness, insomnia, and subjectively declining memory. She described to the psychiatrist her fear that she may have "Alzheimer's" although she was unable to say exactly what symptoms led her to this conclusion. She described her experience of people she knew getting older and losing their memory. On the Mini-Mental State Examination (MMSE), she achieved a score of 29 out of 30. The psychiatrist explained that it was unlikely she had dementia. He suggested that she continue to take Dothiepin (25 mg nocte) for sleep.

Fifteen months later, her daughter (who lived out of town) wrote a letter accompanying a new referral from the GP. She was concerned that, in addition to depressed mood and anxiety, memory problems were evident. During a recent stay, she had noticed Hazel repeating herself, not managing her medications, and losing motivation to do household chores as well as to socialize. During the subsequent psychiatric assessment, Hazel's MMSE score was unchanged. She reported no symptoms of depression while her husband, Ernie, reported that she had some symptoms consistent with depression, such as feeling worse in the mornings and better in the evenings. Dothiepin was increased to 50 mg nocte and she was referred for neuropsychological assessment in order to determine whether she did have cognitive impairment or whether her memory was being affected by depressed mood.

Hazel came to the neuropsychological assessment accompanied by Ernie. She consented to him being present during the pre-testing interview. Before gathering any background information, a guided discussion regarding informed consent about undergoing the assessment and disclosure of diagnosis was undertaken. This began with a discussion about the reason she had been referred: did she know why she was there and what did she think of others saying that her memory was poor? From her perspective, she was experiencing normal age-related memory change ("After all I am 82, aren't I?"). She described an incident a few months ago that had caused her some alarm at the time. She had woken up struggling to remember what day it was. In her mind the issue had resolved itself once she recalled the information later in the day. Ernie sat quietly mostly agreeing with what she said.

The guided discussion continued with examining the purpose of assessment. Although the cause of her reported problems was unknown, the assessment aimed to find out whether there was a significant problem and, if so, identify the reason. She continued to assert that her memory difficulties were linked with aging. More specific questions were asked regarding whether she knew someone with serious memory problems, and what her worst fear might be about the cause of her difficulties. Well-known public figures with similar issues were mentioned. During this discussion, the terms "dementia" and "Alzheimer's disease" were specifically used. Although she sometimes shifted uneasily in her chair, both she and Ernie were able to discuss some of their concerns in a reasonably open and frank fashion. She did know about these problems and she would dread the thought of having them. Ernie admitted that he and their children had discussed whether it was possibly Alzheimer's disease among themselves on a couple of occasions.

The frank discussion continued: there were pros and cons of doing the assessment and knowing the diagnosis. Benefits included treating reversible causes, starting medication to slow the progress of disease, and allowing for the possibility to plan for the future. The costs included the stress of knowing that one had an illness that could only be managed rather than cured. Upon further inquiry, Hazel revealed herself to be someone who had always preferred to use a passive avoidant style of coping as compared with an active style of coping. So, after having discussed things, did Hazel want to go ahead with the assessment? After some thoughts of ambivalence, "Yes." And did she want to know the outcome if it looked like it was dementia? There was a diffident verbal "Yes," but her body language said "No." She stated that she would like family members to be informed.

So the assessment went ahead. Although most cognitive domains were found to be intact, on testing several aspects of memory were clinically impaired. However, functionally she remained independent and able to take care of her needs quite well. In an ensuing feedback session, Hazel and her family were informed that she had amnestic mild cognitive impairment (MCI). The implications of this were discussed including the possibility of further cognitive deterioration, which meant that reassessment in 12 months was recommended. She undertook several therapy sessions focussing on anxiety and mood management.

After the 12 months had elapsed, Hazel was invited for a reassessment. According to her children, she was "happier within herself" despite the memory problems having got progressively worse and her becoming increasingly reliant on Ernie now to help her in her day-to-day functioning. Clearly at this point it was likely she had progressed beyond MCI.

Once more she consented to Ernie coming in for the initial interview and a guided discussion ensued. Upon questioning, she had minimal recall of the initial assessment. She reported little change in her memory problems and stated that she did not recall things if they were not "life and death." Ernie gave several examples of worsening memory compared with a year ago. When asked about completing the assessment, Hazel again consented. However, upon being asked if she wanted to know whether she had a dementia diagnosis, her response had changed: "No." Yet she was happy for Ernie and her children to be informed.

Her preferred style of avoidant coping again showed during testing when she used humor to divert attention away from evidence of memory impairment. She also readily gave explanations to rationalize away problems when they occurred. However, as with the family's subjective report of everyday deterioration, testing showed further impairment which had spread to semantic memory, complex processing, and goal-directed behavior. Her mood had improved though and she was much less anxious than she had been previously.

Hazel was invited to the subsequent feedback session both by telephone and letter. If she had decided to come, the assessor planned to ask to spend time with her family separately in which to discuss the diagnosis of Alzheimer's disease. However, Hazel chose to stay away and instead busied herself with activities at home reportedly forgetting all about the session. The results and outcome were discussed with Ernie and their two children along with ways to support the family in the future. They gained an appreciation of how they could help her put into place compensatory strategies (such as using written reminders) without compromising her preferred coping style. Written information was provided too. Finally, a review with the psychiatrist saw her commenced on cholinesterase-inhibiting medication. In an informal catch-up with a family member at a later stage, she was still participating in pleasurable activities and her cognitive problems had stabilized.

Green (2000, 2006) states that it is not uncommon for family system and interpersonal issues to surface during feedback sessions. As such, the clinician should be alert to the thoughts, feelings, and needs of the family in addition to those of the client during feedback (Allen et al., 1986; Gorske & Smith, 2008). Family counseling may be indicated if family conflicts or tensions arise (e.g. when discussing how responsibilities will be shared among members); and those emotionally supported by the client may find himself or herself in need of psychological assistance. The feedback session can offer the primary caregiver the opportunity to discuss his/her feelings about the client's illness and ways to manage these feelings. Assessing the needs and distress level of the primary caregiver in a separate session may be required (Green).

Lastly, the psychologist should reinforce during feedback that the client can take on roles and responsibilities as a family member despite having an illness, particularly if the family propose unnecessary drastic changes (Green, 2000, 2006).

Ethical feedback

Among clinicians a lack of awareness or adequate training in feedback processes exists, and consequently, uncertainty surrounds the propriety of sharing feedback and the presentation of feedback information, especially when results are unfavorable (Butcher, 1992). Clinicians may be reluctant to share negative information with their clients (Knight, 1994) and may be concerned with potential adverse effects and consequences of disclosing critical information (Butcher). Unease can also exist about translating clinical information into layperson terms, and providing inconclusive results to clients expecting clear results (Pope, 1992). Green (2006) acknowledges that psychologists working with older adults in particular may anticipate that families expect a definitive diagnosis, and the inability to provide this may leave clinicians feeling less competent.

Pope (1992) argues strongly that neuropsychologists have an important ethical obligation to inform clients about the results of testing, including diagnostic implications. However, an element of paternalism may creep into feedback, on the part of either the clinician or the family, where complete disclosure of results is not undertaken in order to "protect" the client from unpleasant news. In reality, this robs the person of the opportunity to take stock of his/her life and complete unfinished business, particularly if the diagnosis implies shortened lifespan.

The pill bottle story

Here is the story of one person with dementia, as written by her daughter (who also happens to be a health care professional):

> My Mum has Alzheimer's. She's had the symptoms for years but because of both family's and GP's reluctance to 'say it', she's just recently been diagnosed. They decided to start her on medication and told her the pills were to help her memory. They failed to tell her that she had Alzheimer's.
>
> One day my sister came upon her in the bathroom, crumpled to the floor—sobbing and wailing. She held in her hand the bottle of medication. The label indicated that she had Alzheimer's—something she'd not been told. To find out from a bottle, instead of her family and GP, was almost too much to bear!
>
> Unfortunately my sister didn't know how to manage her anxiety or new knowledge and reassured her by stating: 'It doesn't mean you have Alzheimer's. It's just to help improve your memory'. Mum was temporarily mollified and went on with her day.
>
> Later, while sitting together, Mum told me that she thought she might have Alzheimer's. We talked about how she understood her illness, what she felt she needed to manage it, and how we could be most helpful. She was able to tell us *who* she wanted to manage her finances, what plans she had for long-term care, and her preferences for care.
>
> Early discussions about the disease, while emotionally upsetting, allow us time to manage and plan and prepare.

On the other hand it is also the client's right not to know his/her diagnosis, especially in the case of dementia. Rather than making disclosure a routine practice, it is up to the neuropsychologist to determine beforehand what the client wants and follow-through in view of that. This might entail carrying out pre-assessment counseling to gain informed consent and documenting the outcome within the client record: "Would you like to know how well you have done on the memory tests? And would you like to be told what your diagnosis might be, even if it is not certain?" (Williams, 2004, p. 15). Equally, clients might be given the choice of who delivers the results. For example, they may prefer to be told by their GP with whom they have already established an ongoing relationship. Should clients wish to be told and the diagnosis is that of dementia, they and their carers benefit from a staged feedback process taking place across more than one session. Wald, Fahy, Walker, and Livingston (2003) recommend for "The Rule of Threes" to prevent overload in carers. A similar format would be useful for clients too. The initial session would focus on disclosing the results followed by explaining dementia, associated behavioral and psychiatric problems, and medications. A subsequent session(s) would address other issues such as the course of the illness and planning ahead. Such a supportive feedback approach is most appropriate considering the challenges of a dementia diagnosis.

Skills required for effective neuropsychological assessment feedback

Providing feedback is considered a core skill a neuropsychologist should possess (Kaplan & Moes, 2001). Green (2000, 2006) states that the clinician must combine expertise in neuropsychological assessment with clinical psychotherapeutic skills to ensure a successful feedback session. Further, the usefulness of the assessment is dependent on the extent and quality of feedback, and the manner of feedback delivery.

The neuropsychologist must endeavor to communicate information in layperson's terms, as professional terminology may be unfamiliar or can differ from ordinary usage (Crosson, 1994). This reduces potential misunderstandings and increases the effectiveness of the feedback (Mateer & Sira, 2008). Frequent checking for understanding should be undertaken, particularly when presenting more abstract or complex concepts, and when ascertaining the presence of assumed knowledge (Crosson).

The neuropsychologist should be aware that clients and their families might feel intimidated by clinicians. Such feelings may result in an absence of client questions that clarify misunderstanding, thereby compromising the interactive nature of the session (Crosson, 1994). Further, clients should be made to feel comfortable to agree or disagree with information presented during the feedback session. If the client makes an objection, the clinician should manage this "in an open-minded, collaborative, problem-solving manner" (Armengol et al., 2001, p. 152).

Green (2006) outlines several clinical skills important to the success of the feedback session. The clinician should: (1) encourage interaction, such that clients and supportive others feel at ease posing questions, voicing concerns, and replying to the clinician; (2) maintain rapport with the client and develop rapport with attendees; (3) listen, check, and attend to verbal and non-verbal cues, to ensure information is understood; and (4) be sensitive to the type and amount of information the participants are ready to receive and to their reactions. Green also states that the clinician should not impart feedback in a way that leaves attendees feeling "overwhelmed," "hopeless," or "powerless" (p. 233).

Green (2000, 2006) outlines several specific objectives of feedback sessions with older adults (see Table 10.2). In addition, Green also recommends addressing the implications of the neuropsychological assessment results on the client's daily functioning and competence to maintain certain responsibilities (e.g. driving; managing finances; minding the grandchildren). A discussion regarding the clients' ability to continue living in their current environment may be necessary, along with ways to increase existing support systems and independence for those requiring additional support to remain in their home.

Participant level of acceptance of neuropsychological sequelae can impact on their ability to integrate feedback. Differences of opinion between attendees and the clinician should be clarified, or clearly stated if resolution is not successful (Crosson, 1994). The client's level of acceptance may also guide the amount of feedback given pertaining to weaknesses. Crosson advocates for a balanced approach to feedback, focusing as much on strengths as on weaknesses, as this may decrease the likelihood of denial.

Results from a study by Bennett-Levy et al. (1994) suggest several clinical practices that may enhance client experiences of the neuropsychological assessment process: (1) prepare the client adequately for the assessment. This includes clinicians either educating referrers to provide improved information, or assuming responsibility for preparing the client and sending an information sheet; (2) offer a reasonable rationale for the tests, so that clients understand the relationship between the tests and everyday life; (3) provide memorable, understandable, and useful feedback, that focuses on strengths and weaknesses, on how the results may impact on daily life,

Table 10.2 Neuropsychological feedback points for older clients

1. Discuss neuropsychological strengths and weaknesses compared to normative data and to expectations of pre-morbid functioning.

2. Provide an explanation of how these strengths and weaknesses contribute to observed real-life changes (e.g. unreliable medication management or the repetition of questions may be explained in terms of the client's significant memory impairment). Rather than stating, for example, that "memory" is "impaired," the nature and severity of dysfunction within a domain should be described. Similarly, explaining the difference between short- and long-term memory, and between other memory processes (e.g. storage; retrieval) can also assist in better explaining the client's behavior and rationale for treatment recommendations (e.g. external memory aides).

3. Discuss possible diagnostic explanations for the behavior changes and their respective degrees of certainty. The conclusiveness of results should not be overstated; it is important to stress that results offer possible explanations for cognitive dysfunction rather than a definitive diagnosis. Client consultation with specialist practitioners (e.g. neurologist; psychiatrist) skilled in interpreting supplementary tests (e.g. brain imaging) is required for definitive diagnostic statements.

4. Identify steps toward finalizing the diagnosis, such as follow-up evaluations (e.g. brain imaging; relevant blood tests)

5. Describe effective treatments for the disorder (e.g. Alzheimer's disease medications)

6. Determine if other treatments (e.g. cognitive therapy; behavioral management; psychotherapy) are appropriate.

7. Identify psychological issues affecting the client and family members in relation to the disorder, and plan associated interventions.

Source: Adapted from Green, J. (2000). *Neuropsychological evaluation of the older adult: A clinician's guidebook.* San Diego, CA: Academic Press; Green, J. (2006). Feedback. In D.K. Affix & K.A. Welch-Bohmer (Eds.), *Geriatric neuropsychology: Assessment and intervention* (pp. 223–236). New York, NY: Guilford Press.

and on the management of problem areas; (4) encourage the client to have a relative present during the process by stating the potential benefits of this; and (5) be mindfully sensitive to clients who exhibit anxiety, as the assessment process can have positive and negative influences on self-confidence. Other non-significant factors in Bennett-Levy et al.'s study that may enhance quality of service include making the client comfortable by ensuring adequate breaks and refreshments, giving the client the choice between completing the assessment in one session or splitting the session, and providing feedback in writing or by audio recording.

Bennett-Levy et al. (1994) consider neuropsychological assessment preparation particularly important for three reasons: (1) it may reduce pre-assessment anxiety as shown in previous intervention studies (Deane, Spicer, & Leathem, 1992; Wallace, 1986); (2) clients can consider what questions they would like answered by the evaluation, allowing for a more satisfying experience; and (3) it may prompt clients and their families to reflect on recent experiences, thereby providing the clinician with more complete historical information (Connell, 1992). Bennett-Levy et al. provide a copy of the neuropsychological assessment information sheet, developed by Connelly, Bennett-Levy, and Klein-Boonschate, to be sent to clients awaiting neuropsychological assessment. Webster (1992) found that sending mental health center clients an information sheet explaining the nature of initial assessment sessions significantly increased client satisfaction overall, possibly due to the perception of increased levels of personal attention.

In an Internet survey, Smith, Wiggins, et al. (2007) were the first to explore psychologist perceptions of the psychological and neuropsychological feedback experience of their clients and families. The majority of psychologists reported that feedback information facilitated discussions with patients and assisted patients in understanding their cognitive and functional issues better. However, psychologists were in less agreement about whether such feedback increased motivation to follow treatment recommendations.

Several authors have observed that following feedback clients feel greatly relieved at having their experiences explained through the course of feedback. Newman and Greenway (1997) offer the view that clients feel better because they are provided with a new vocabulary with which to discuss their issues. Naming and understanding the nature of the illness appears particularly relevant to older adults presenting with cognitive complaints. Because older clients and their families begin the assessment process with a host of changes, and concerns about what such changes may indicate, being given a diagnosis may provide some relief in terms of having a name and some explanation for their cognitive changes (Knight, 1994).

As this final short case study suggests, individually tailored feedback, provided in a timely and sensitive fashion, may have effects that the clinician and client may find difficult to predict in full.

The thank you

Faith was an 81-year-old woman referred for neuropsychological assessment due to cognitive changes and episodes of confusion. Years before, her father had developed behavioral problems of dementia such as wandering. She reported that she was very anxious about the possibility of facing similar issues. Partway through testing she complained of being mentally fatigued. On further discussion, it was evident that she was becoming upset about the possible implications of performing poorly. She said that if it was confirmed that she did have a problem with dementia, she would become very down and would not wish to continue with life, although she stated that she would not become actively suicidal. A break was taken from testing and the opportunity was taken to discuss her concerns in depth for returning to the assessment.

It was eventually concluded that she most probably did have dementia. The results and diagnosis were discussed with her in a joint session (psychiatrist and neuropsychologist) in her own home with family members present. A while later the neuropsychologist received a letter which read as follows:

> Thank you—the material you promised me came in the mail as promised [sic] and I sat down and read it through while [news about the diagnosis] was fresh in my head. I couldn't be getting better care and attention though I wish I didn't need it. The family check on me to make sure I'm doing what I'm supposed to do which is just as well as I forget a lot. The medicine arrived yesterday and was delivered at the house. With the family helping, I am managing fine and it is surprising how many people (like the supermarket assistant) who say 'Look, I've heard you've got Alzheimer's—can I help?' Am taking my 'dope' regularly. Thanks for your help. Faith.

The reader might wish to think about these issues in relation to the exploration of a more collaborative therapeutic approach with his/her own assessment practices:

1. In the context these cases, what do you see as the main similarities and differences with your own current practice? What steps might you wish to take to augment or change your own approach to be more therapeutic in focus?

2. How might various mental health settings with which you are familiar constrain use of these feedback techniques? What sorts of settings might actually facilitate their use?

3. In reflecting about the specific older patients that you see, which might benefit most from adopting such an approach to testing? Which might benefit least?

4. To what degree do you believe other health professionals, including other neuropsychologists, might need to be educated about the processes as well as the pros and cons of the assessment approaches described in this chapter?

References

Allen, J.G., Lewis, L., Blum, S., Voorhees, S., Jernigan, S., & Peebles, M.J. (1986). Informing psychiatric patients and their families about neuropsychological assessment findings. *Bulletin of the Menninger Clinic, 50*, 64–74.

Allen, A., Montgomery, M., Tubman, J., Frazier, L., & Escovar, L. (2003). The effects of assessment feedback on rapport-building and self-enhancement processes. *Journal of Mental Health Counselling, 25*(3), 165–182.

Armengol, C.G., Moes, E.J., Penney, D.L., & Sapienza, M.M. (2001). Writing client-centred recommendations. In C.G. Armengol, E. Kaplan, & E.J. Moes (Eds.), *The consumer-oriented neuropsychological report* (pp. 141–159). Lutz, FL: Psychological Assessment Resources.

Bennett-Levy, J., Klein-Boonschate, M.A., Batchelor, J., McCarter, R., & Walton, N. (1994). Encounters with Anna Thompson: The consumer's experience of neuropsychological assessment. *Clinical Neuropsychologist, 8*(2), 219–238.

Butcher, J.N. (1992). Introduction to the special section: Providing psychological test feedback to clients. *Psychological Assessment, 4*(3), 267.

Connell, T. (1992). Neuropsychological assessment: A guide for families. *Think Magazine, 2*(4), 20–23.

Crosson, B. (1994). Application of neuropsychological assessment results. In R.D. Vanderplog (Ed.), *Clinician's guide to neuropsychological assessment* (pp. 113–163). Hillsdale, NJ: Lawrence Erlbaum Associates.

Deane, F.P., Spicer, J., & Leathem, J. (1992). Effects of videotaped preparatory information on expectations, anxiety, and psychotherapy outcome. *Journal of Consulting and Clinical Psychology, 60*(6), 980–984.

Finn, S.E., & Tonsager, M.E. (1997). Information-gathering and therapeutic models of assessment: Complementary paradigms. *Psychological Assessment, 9*(4), 374–385.

Friss, L. (1990). A model state-level approach to family survival for caregivers of brain injured adults. *Gerontologist, 30*, 121–125.

Gass, C.S., & Brown, M.C. (1992). Neuropsychological test feedback to patients with brain dysfunction. *Psychological Assessment, 4*(3), 272–277.

Gorske, T.T. (2008). Therapeutic neuropsychological assessment: A humanistic model and case example. *Journal of Humanistic Psychology, 48*(3), 320–339.

Gorske, T.T., & Smith, S.R. (2008). *Collaborative therapeutic neuropsychological assessment*. New York, NY: Springer.

Green, J. (2000). *Neuropsychological evaluation of the older adult: A clinician's guidebook*. San Diego, CA: Academic Press.

Green, J. (2006). Feedback. In D.K. Affix & K.A. Welch-Bohmer (Eds.), *Geriatric neuropsychology: Assessment and intervention* (pp. 223–236). New York, NY: Guilford Press.

Groth-Marnet, G. (1999). Financial efficacy of clinical assessment: Rational guidelines and issues for future research. *Journal of Clinical Psychology, 55*(7), 813–824.

Kaplan, E., & Moes, E.J. (2001). Who is a neuropsychologist? In C.G. Armengol, E. Kaplan, & E.J. Moes (Eds.), *The consumer-oriented neuropsychological report* (pp. 1–12). Lutz, FL: Psychological Assessment Resources.

Knight, B.G. (1994). Providing clinical interpretations to older clients and their families. In M. Storandt & G.R. VandenBos (Eds.), *Neuropsychological assessment of dementia and depression in older adults: A clinician's guide* (pp. 141–154). Washington, DC: American Psychological Association.

Laidlaw, K., & Pachana, N.A. (2009). Demographics in older adults. *Professional Psychology: Research and Practice, 40*(6), 601–608.

Luborsky, L. (1984). *Principles of psychoanalytic psychotherapy: A manual for supportive-expressive (SE) treatment*. New York, NY: Basic Books.

Mateer, C.A., & Sira, C.S. (2008). Practical rehabilitation strategies in the context of clinical neuropsychology feedback. In J.E. Morgan & J.H. Ricker (Eds.), *Textbook of clinical neuropsychology* (pp. 996–1007). New York, NY: Taylor & Francis.

Newman, M.L., & Greenway, P. (1997). Therapeutic effects of providing MMPI-2 test feedback to clients at a university counselling service: A collaborative approach. *Psychological Assessment, 9*(2), 122–131.

Pope, K.S. (1992). Responsibilities in providing psychological test feedback to clients. *Psychological Assessment, 4*(3), 268–271.

Smith, S.R., Werner, G.A., & Green, J.G. (2006). Collaborative neuropsychological assessment. Paper presented to the annual meeting of the National Academy of Neuropsychology. San Antonio, TX.

Smith, S.R., Wiggins, C.M., & Gorske, T.T. (2007). A survey of psychological assessment feedback practices. *Assessment, 14*(3), 310–319.

UN Department of Economic and Social Affairs Population Division (2007). World population prospects: The 2006 revision, highlights (Working Paper No. ESA/P/WP/WP.202).

Wald, C., Fahy, M., Walker, Z., & Livingston, G. (2003). What to tell dementia caregivers—the rule of threes. *International Journal of Geriatric Psychiatry, 18*, 313–317.

Wallace, L.M. (1986). Communication variables in the design of presurgical preparatory information. *British Journal of Clinical Psychology, 25*, 111–118.

Ward, R.M. (2008). Assessee and assessor experiences of significant events in psychological assessment feedback. *Journal of Personality Assessment, 90*(4), 307–322.

Webster, A. (1992). The effect of pre-assessment information on clients' satisfaction, expectations and attendance at mental health day centre. *British Journal of Medical Psychology, 65*, 89–93.

Westervelt, H.J., Brown, L.B., Tremont, G., Javorsky, D.J., & Stern, R.A. (2007). Patient and family perceptions of the neuropsychological evaluation: How are we doing? *The Clinical Neuropsychologist, 21*, 263–273.

Williams, C.M. (2004). Pre-diagnostic counselling with people with memory problems: What can we learn from HIV/GUM services? *Psychology Special Interest Group for Older People (PSIGE) Newsletter, 87*, 11–16.

Appendices

Appendix A

Collaborative neuropsychological assessment report—key statements

Things to remember about a neuropsychological evaluation:

1. Everyone has personal strengths and weaknesses (these strengths and weaknesses will be outlined in the following pages). Just because you have a personal weakness may not mean that this is a weakness in comparison to other people.

2. A neuropsychological assessment is like a photograph, not a movie. That is, this is a picture of your functioning at the time of the assessment; things change over time and circumstances differ.

3. You are the expert on you and neuropsychological tests are tools to help you better understand your mental life.

4. All of us have personal strengths and we are more successful when we focus on these strengths. The following pages will help you identify these strengths and the ways you can use them to your greatest advantage.

5. This report is designed to help you discuss the test results with your clinician; you are encouraged to discuss, disagree, or share any reactions you might have (Smith et al., 2005).

Appendix B

Collaborative neuropsychological assessment—example from pre-interview questionnaire

John's questions and concerns:

Question 1:

Do I have dementia?

- *Specifics:* I have a lot of trouble with my memory. When I go to the supermarket I can't remember what to buy. When I walk into a room I can't remember what I went in there for.
- *Effects:* I feel frustrated and embarrassed when I can't remember things. I have to rely on my wife to remind me to do things. I feel depressed sometimes because of my memory problems.

Question 2:

If I have dementia, can it be cured?

- *Specifics:* I have been told that dementia can't be cured.
- *Effects:* I feel concerned about what will happen to me in the future if I have dementia.

Question 3:

Is there a medication that can help with dementia?

- *Specifics:* I have been told there are medications I can take to help with my memory problems.
- *Effects:* Medication gives me some hope that my memory problems will improve.

Your wife Judy's questions and concerns:

Question 1:

Does John have the beginnings of dementia?

- *Specifics:* John asks the same question over and over. He has trouble remembering to have a shower.
- *Effects:* I feel I have to think for John all the time and remind him to do things during the day so that he remembers.

Question 2:

If John has started to develop dementia, what is the treatment you would advise?

- *Specifics:* I have heard that medication and keeping your brain active can help dementia.
- *Effects:* I feel helpless because I don't know what to do to make his memory problems better.

Question 3:

Is there anything I can do to help with John's memory problems?

- *Specifics:* I have been told that I could play cards with John to keep his mind active.
- *Effects:* I feel good when I'm doing something that helps John with his problems.

Collaborative neuropsychological assessment report—responses to example pre-interview questionnaire and recommendations

Summary of your questions and concerns:

Question 1:

Do I have dementia?

- *Assessment results:* You said that you have trouble with your memory. The test results did not indicate that you have trouble learning new things compared to other people most similar to you. However, your memory appears to improve when you are given assistance, such as being given the beginning letter of the word you are trying to think of. This suggests that you have difficulties retrieving information from your memory. This could be related to depression or vascular problems.

Question 2:

If I have dementia, can it be cured?

- *Assessment results:* Your test results don't suggest that you have dementia. Unfortunately, there is no current cure for dementia. Things you can do to reduce your risk of getting dementia include keeping your mind and body active, and eating a healthy diet low in fat and salt.

Question 3:

Is there a medication that can help with dementia?

- *Assessment results:* There are medications that can help with dementia. They do not cure dementia but may slow down the progression of the disease. There are also medications that can help improve depression. In a lot of cases people find that when their depression improves, their ability to remember things also improves.

Summary of your wife Judy's questions and concerns:

Question 1:

Does John have the starting of dementia?

- *Assessment results:* You said that John asks the same question over and over, and forgets to take a shower. The test results did not indicate that John has trouble learning new things compared to other people most similar to him. However, his memory appears to improve when he is given assistance, such as giving him the beginning letter of the word he is trying to think of. This suggests he has difficulties retrieving information from his memory. This could be related to depression or vascular problems.

Question 2:

If John has the beginning of dementia, what is the treatment you would advise?

- *Assessment results:* John's test results don't suggest that he has dementia. Unfortunately, there is no current cure for dementia. Things people can do to reduce the risk of getting dementia include keeping the mind and body active, and eating a healthy diet low in fat and salt.

Question 3:

Is there anything I can do to help with John's memory problems?

- *Assessment results:* John has trouble retrieving information from his memory. John could use retrieval memory strategies, such as going through the alphabet to help him remember a friend's name. If this does not help at the time, you could provide John with a prompt such as "His name starts with Bru."

Based on your test results, we can make these recommendations:

1. To help with your depression, you may wish to ask your doctor about treatment options for depression. Common treatments for depression include medication, and psychological treatment such as cognitive behavior therapy.

2. Your doctor may wish to consider a magnetic resonance imaging (MRI) head scan to further explore the extent of vascular changes that were reported on your CT head scan. MRI head scans are more sensitive to showing vascular changes in the brain than CT head scans.

3. I will provide you with some retrieval memory strategies that may assist you to better access information from your memory. Your wife can also use these strategies to help you to remember things.

Chapter 11

Treating late-life insomnia: a case study

Simon S. Smith

Introduction

Insomnia is broadly defined as difficulty initiating sleep, difficulty maintaining sleep, waking up too early, or sleep that is chronically non-restorative or poor in quality. Insomnia is associated with impaired work performance and reduced quality of life, and has high associated direct and indirect health care costs (Walsh, 2004). Although almost everybody experiences occasional nights of poor sleep, a very wide range of prevalence has been reported for complaints of persistent insomnia or poor quality sleep. Older estimates of population prevalence rates varied from around 12% (Broman, Lundh, & Hetta, 1996) to over 40% (Bixler, Kales, Soldatos, Kales, & Healey, 1979). This wide variation reflects historical difficulties in the definition and measurement of insomnia, with inconsistent definition of clinically significant insomnia. The most robust international estimates of prevalence (Ohayon, 2002) suggest that at least 30% of the general population report symptoms of insomnia, and perhaps 6–9% would meet conservative criteria for a clinical diagnosis.

The frequency of sleep disturbance is likely to be higher in selected populations. For example, persistent insomnia often appears concomitant with disorders such as chronic pain, depression and anxiety, heart disease, and diabetes (Katz & McHorney, 1998; Smith, Perlis, Smith, Giles, & Carmody, 2000; Foley, Ancoli-Israel, Britz, & Walsh, 2004). Prevalence of insomnia in the range of 25–70% has been reported in general medical and in-patient populations (Shochat, Umphress, Israel, & Ancoli-Israel, 1999; Wittchen et al., 2001). The annual incidence rate may be about 5% for adults over the age of 65 (Foley, Monjan, Simonsick, Wallace, & Blazer, 1999), although other epidemiological parameters are not well described.

The prevalence of insomnia is often reported to increase with age; however, most estimates of insomnia prevalence in community dwelling older adults (Ohayon, 2002) are within the same range as for the general population. Specific issues impacting sleep quality in older adults include the potential for normal changes in sleep architecture (Van Cauter, Leproult, & Plat, 2000), medical or psychiatric co-morbidities, potentially increased social isolation (Cacioppo & Hawkley 2003), and potential changes to circadian rhythm dynamics leading to increased susceptibility to circadian phase misalignment (Dijk, Duffy, Riel, Shanahan, & Czeisler, 1999; Zhou, Liu, van Heerikhuize, Hofman, & Swaab, 2003). However, in common with other putative age-related changes, concomitant factors including inactivity, dissatisfaction with social life, and the presence of other disorders have been found to be stronger determinants of insomnia than age *per se* (Lichstein, Durrence, Bayen, & Riedel, 2001; Ohayon, Zulley, Guilleminault, Smirne, & Priest, 2001; Nau, McCrae, Cook, & Lichstein, 2005).

The primary determinants of when, and how, good sleep can be achieved are strongly biological. General models of sleep propensity are consistent with an interaction between sleep drive (a homeostatic process) and the circadian pacemaker (Pace-Schott & Hobson, 2002; Cajochen Münch, Knoblauch, Blatter, & Wirz-Justice, 2006). There are zones within the circadian cycle during which sleep is strongly promoted (and relatively easy to attain), and other periods during which sleep is very difficult to achieve (Strogatz, Kronauer, & Czeisler, 1987). Variations in either of these two processes can make it very difficult to sleep at the desired time of day, irrespective of other barriers to sleep. This is seen most obviously with "jet lag" after transmeridian travel. Despite this strong biological drive to sleep, we have a clear capacity to wilfully delay and inter-rupt our sleep. This capacity has potential ecological benefits, such as the capacity to respond to environmental threats. In common with anxiety and other disorders, we can easily substitute subjective negative cognitions for objective environmental threats, both leading to increased autonomic arousal and emotional distress incompatible with sleep onset and maintenance (Harvey, 2002).

The classification and clinical significance of insomnia can be determined by measuring the severity, duration, frequency, and daytime consequences of the complaint. A number of classifi-cation schemes have been devised. The most common of these in use by psychologists in the field of behavioral sleep medicine are the Diagnostic and Statistical Manual of Mental Disorders (DSM; American Psychiatric Association, 2000) and the International Classification of Sleep Disorders (ICSD; American Academy of Sleep Medicine, 2005). The DSM-IV-TR identifies three main groups of sleep disorders. The first of these are the primary sleep disorders, which in turn are comprised of two subgroups. The first is the dysomnias, which are changes in the quality, quantity, or timing of sleep itself. For example, dysomnias include disorders that result in a com-plaint of insomnia, or of excessive daytime sleepiness. The second is the parasomnias, which include behavioral or physiological events occurring during sleep, or at sleep-wake transitions. The second main group contains sleep disorders related to another mental condition and the third contains other sleep disorders (including sleep disorders related to a medical condition and substance-induced sleep disorders). Primary sleep disorders can only be identified in the absence of involvement of disorders from the other two groups (Rothenberg, 1997). The DSM-IV-TR criteria describe a complaint of insomnia as primary only after other mental, medical, substance-induced, or environmental causes have been discounted.

The ICSD-II classification system differs from DSM-IV nosology in that it is non-axial, and is only concerned with sleep disorders. Sleep disorders are divided into eight categories: insomnia, sleep-related breathing disorders, hypersomnia of central origin, circadian rhythm sleep disorders, parasomnias, sleep-related movement disorders, isolated symptoms, and other sleep disorders. Within the insomnia category, there are 11 insomnia subtypes with adequate, although varying, levels of empirical support. The DSM-IV category of "primary insomnia" subsumes a number of insomnia diagnoses in the ICSD, including psychophysiological insomnia, sleep state misperception, idiopathic insomnia, and some cases of inadequate sleep hygiene. According to DSM-IV, the insomnia complaint must satisfy a number of additional criteria. A structured inter-view for sleep disorders according to DSM-III-R had been developed (Schamm et al., 1993). Although good reliability and validity properties were reported for this instrument, no such structured interview has been published for the DSM-IV, while the primary care version of the DSM-IV, the DSM-IV-PC (Pincus et al., 1995) provides a sleep disturbance algorithm to aid in the diagnosis of primary insomnia. Only partial empirical support has been found for either DSM-IV- or ICSD-specific diagnostic categories, based on a cluster analysis of data from questionnaires and polysomnography (PSG) monitoring (Edinger et al., 1996). For this reason, caution should be used in assigning specific subtypes to a complaint of insomnia; however, the

DSM-IV categorizations are probably the most robust schema for classification of insomnia for most practitioners.

In the past, the relationship between insomnia and other disorders has resulted in insomnia being often viewed as a symptom, or at least secondary to the other disorder (Harvey, 2001). More recently, this view has changed so that insomnia is now more properly seen as a co-morbid condition where it appears with another disorder (National Institutes of Health, 2005). This change has important treatment implications, particularly in medical environments. The consensus view is now that clinically significant insomnia warrants treatment in its own right, and is likely to improve total health in patients with co-morbid conditions (Smith, Huang, & Manber, 2005). Further, meta-analyses suggest that primary insomnia is a predictor or precursor of late-life depression (Riemann & Voderholzer, 2003), raising the potential for early intervention into mood disorders.

These findings provide a good rationale for early and effortful intervention to improve sleep quality in older adults, especially in the context of co-morbid health concerns. The importance of adequate sleep is further reinforced by relatively new understanding of the critical role of sleep in health, with strong interactions between sleep and metabolic health (Spiegel, Leproult, & Van Cauter, 1999) and sleep and cognitive functioning (Walker & Stickgold, 2004). Our management philosophy begins with the understanding that sleep, together with diet and exercise, forms the "triumvirate of good health" (after Professor William Dement of Stanford University). This approach helps to reframe sleep as positive health behavior.

Behavioral or cognitive behavioral treatment (CBT) is highly effective for treatment of insomnia. CBT for insomnia (CBTi) is recommended as the first-line therapy in the 2008 American Academy of Sleep Medicine Clinical Guidelines for the Evaluation and Management of Chronic Insomnia in Adults (Schutte-Rodin, Broch, Buysse, Dorsey, & Sateia, 2008). Three Cochrane Reviews support the clinical use of CBTi, and a major review by the Standards of Practice Committee of the American Academy of Sleep Medicine also strongly supports the efficacy of CBTi (Morgenthaler et al., 2006; Morin et al., 2006). The efficacy of CBTi demonstrated in highly controlled studies also translates to effectiveness in the real-world clinical environment (Espie, Inglis, Tessier, & Harvey, 2001), including cases where insomnia is associated with co-morbid medical conditions (such as cancer, pain, and alcohol abuse; Morin et al.). The cost per quality-adjusted life-year for CBTi is regarded as "good value for money" (e.g. by the National Health Services [NHS] in the United Kingdom; Morgan, Mathers, Thompson, & Tomeny, 2003). Thus, CBTi provides an efficacious intervention for insomnia, even when it is co-morbid with another medical condition (Ozminkowski, Wang, & Walsh, 2007). The term CBTi generally refers to a package of strategies that are delivered together (Harvey, Inglis, & Espie, 2002); this typically includes components of stimulus control (Bootzin, Epstein, & Wood, 1991; Harvey et al., 2002), sleep restriction (Spielman, Caruso, & Glovinsky, 1987), and cognitive therapy (Morin, Kowatch, Barry, & Walton, 1993) and may also include additional components common in psychological practice such as relaxation therapy (Means, Lichstein, Epperson, & Johnson, 2000) and other strategies. Meta-analysis of randomized controlled trial studies (Wang, Wang, & Tsai, 2005) demonstrated that this type of CBT package is superior to any of the single component treatments delivered alone.

A major meta-analysis of the benefits of CBTi versus pharmacological interventions for insomnia (Smith et al., 2002) found that there was no benefit for drug treatment for most measures of sleep quality, and that CBTi actually produced a greater reduction in sleep-onset latency. More recent trial data suggest that combination treatments (i.e. hypnotic medication plus CBTi), followed by CBTi alone, may provide the best outcomes (Morin et al., 2009), although the application of such a strategy to patients with longer-term sleep complaints is uncertain.

There may be particular reasons for not instituting treatment with sedative-hypnotic medication in older patients. These reasons could include an increased risk of falls (Berdot et al., 2009), increased risk of road crash (Verster, Monique, Pandi-Perumal, Ramaekers, & Gier, 2008), and potential contraindication for use with other medications. Despite the evidence of benefit of CBTi, pharmacological treatment prescribed by a general practitioner (GP), or over-the-counter and complementary medicines obtained from a pharmacy (Prakash et al., 2007) is still the primary treatment modality for insomnia in Australia.

Treatment setting

Our patients are seen in an insomnia clinic provided as a service in a tertiary Sleep Disorders Center sited in a public hospital. The center primarily provides assessment and treatment for patients with suspected obstructive sleep apnea (OSA); however, patients with a wide range of other sleep disorders are also referred for investigation. The nature of this setting means that most patients referred to the insomnia clinic have had a thorough medical review, and in many cases have undergone an overnight sleep study (PSG) in the laboratory. The service focuses on the insomnia complaint only, with referral if needed for other untreated medical or psychological complaints. The patient population seen in this tertiary environment is therefore unlike most seen in community practice. They frequently have very long-term or severe complaints about their sleep quality, and have frequently attempted a range of treatment modalities previously. Co-morbid disorders are typically addressed by other health professionals. Patients are assessed to specific ICSD-II (American Academy of Sleep Medicine, 2005) criteria as part of long-term clinical research program. Patients are typically only seen for two or three sessions, each an hour in length, with follow-up provided by their GP. Limited treatment duration data suggest that effective treatment can be provided within two sessions, although four to six sessions may be optimal (Edinger, Wohlgemuth, Radtke, Coffman, & Carney, 2007). To make the best use of this short time with the patients, they are sent a questionnaire pack, together with a 2-week sleep diary, to be completed before the initial session. Current assessment guidelines for insomnia research (Edinger et al., 2004) and clinical practice (Lichstein, Durrence, Taylor, Bush, & Riedel, 2003) focus on self-report measures. In most cases an overnight sleep study is not recommended, unless there are clinical suggestions of another sleep disorder. The questionnaire pack contains brief standardized measures to quantify the sleep complaint; the Insomnia Severity Index (ISI; Bastien, Vallieres, & Morin, 2001; Smith & Trinder, 2001), the Dysfunctional Beliefs and Attitudes About Sleep Scale (DBAS; Smith & Trinder; Morin, Vallières, & Ivers, 2007), and the Depression, Anxiety, and Stress Scale (DASS-21; Lovibond & Lovibond, 1995).

The sleep diary (Åkerstedt, Hume, Minors, & Waterhouse, 1994; Monk et al., 1994) provides a prospective self-report of daily sleep and wake behaviors. The diary enables a number of assessment and outcome parameters to be calculated. These include the timing of bedtime (i.e. the first attempt to sleep), sleep-onset latency (sleep time-bedtime), wake after sleep onset, early morning wake, out-of-bed time, and secondary parameters such as sleep efficiency (sleep time/time in bed) and can also provide a robust estimate of circadian phase position, at least in young adults (Martin & Eastman, 2002). The diary can serve a psychoeducational purpose, in some cases providing the patients with a more realistic self-assessment of the frequency of their sleep complaints. The diary is also used as a treatment platform, both for determining new sleep schedules, and for assessing adherence to the intervention at follow-up.

Our patients are explicitly informed that their first appointment will involve an assessment of their current sleep habits, and that the subsequent sessions will focus on changing their sleep patterns, improving their sleep habits, reducing intrusive and anxiety-provoking thoughts at bedtime, and sleep education.

Case study

Session 1

Mr. Albert was a 74-year-old man, referred to the insomnia service by a consultant respiratory and sleep physician. His medical history included a diagnostic sleep study with a subsequent diagnosis of mild OSA, a very long-term (30-year) complaint of insomnia, and current treatment for depression by his GP. Mr. Albert attended the insomnia clinic with his wife, for assessment and further management of his sleep complaint. The initial session included a structured clinical interview designed to assess more specific information about his current sleep-wake schedule, sleeping problem history (e.g. chronicity, precipitants), functional analysis (e.g. cues to treatment seeking action, any indicators of negative associations between the bed environment and insomnia), symptoms of other sleep disorders, recent medical history, brief clinical assessment of psychopathology, use of sleep medications (including over-the-counter and complementary and alternative medicines), and information about his current diet, exercise, and substance use habits. A similarly comprehensive interview schedule is provided by Morin (1993) and Morin and Espie (2003).

Mr. Albert did not identify any clear precipitating event that led to his current sleep problems. A precipitating event (such as an acute stressor) is a component of the classic Spielman model that describes the process whereby the type of ordinary transient sleep disturbance encountered by almost everyone at some point in the their lives leads to chronic persistent insomnia is others (Spielman et al., 1987). Mr. Albert did feel that he had slept very well as a young man, and did feel that he now slept much worse than his peers.

Dated clinical stereotyping once held that insomnia patients should be "sleepless" and OSA patients should be "sleepy." In contrast, our group has reported that the prevalence of clinically significant insomnia in "typical" Australian OSA patients is as high as 39% (Smith, Sullivan, Hopkins, & Douglas, 2004). Several international studies support this finding, with co-morbid insomnia in 17–50% of OSA patients (Krakow et al., 2001; Chung, Krakow, Melendrez, Warner, & Sisley, 2003; Scharf, Tubman, & Smale, 2005; Rebbapragada et al., 2006). Conversely, there is a growing understanding of the potential presence of clinically significant OSA in patients presenting with an insomnia complaint (Lichstein, Riedel, Lester, & Aguillard, 1999), and it is possible that home monitoring with oximetry of other screening devices may be useful in some practice settings.

Mr. Albert did not find medical treatment of OSA with continuous positive airway pressure therapy (CPAP) useful, and he had discontinued treatment shortly after it had been prescribed. Poor adherence to CPAP is currently a major issue in sleep medicine. The treatment requires nightly use of a face mask and pressure pump for a lifetime. There has been recent commentary on the impact of untreated insomnia on subsequent acceptance and adherence to CPAP treatment in patients with co-morbid OSA (Lavie, 2007). Poor adherence to CPAP may reflect a complex relationship between insomnia, OSA, and perceived treatment benefit in many patients (Olsen, Smith, & Oei, 2008), but the potential benefit of treating insomnia in such patients hasn't yet been tested in a controlled trial. In this case, Mr. Albert felt that his major sleep problem was insomnia, and this was the indication for assessment and treatment. His wife was also a patient of the sleep clinic, with severe OSA effectively treated with CPAP. Although there are reports on the impact of untreated OSA on bed-partners, Mr. Albert did not find his wife's CPAP treatment to be a problem for his own sleep (the pump makes a low hum throughout the night), and was very supportive of her treatment.

Assessment

Mr. Albert's responses to the ISI (Bastien et al., 2001) indicated clinically significant insomnia, with very severe difficulty falling asleep. He did not report difficulty staying asleep, nor with waking up too early in the morning. Mr. Albert reported that poor sleep interfered "very much" with his ability to function during the day. Specific problems that he attributed to his poor sleep included daytime fatigue, problems with memory and concentration, increased irritability and tension, muscle aches, and heartburn. He believed that his sleep problems were primarily due to "racing thoughts" or worries at night, and also partly due to bad sleeping habits. He had been provided with "sleep hygiene" advice by his GP, and had read other patient education materials during his route through the tertiary referral process. It has been reported that patients prefer sleep hygiene education over more active interventions (Vincent & Lionberg, 2001), but it is now regarded as a largely ineffective strategy (Harvey et al., 2002). Mr. Albert did not believe physical symptoms (such as pain or another medical condition) or natural aging processes contributed to his poor sleep.

Mr. Albert's responses to the DBAS (Morin et al., 2007) suggested strong concerns regarding possible immediate and long-term negative effects of insomnia, and he also expressed a strong perceived need for control over his sleep. A typical misapprehension about sleep reported by Mr. Albert was that he believed that 8 hours of uninterrupted sleep was an absolute societal norm. In fact, sleep need varies widely among individuals. A potential issue for some patients is a discrepancy between their actual sleep need (i.e. the amount of sleep required for optimum daytime functioning) and its perceived norm. One consequence of this discrepancy can be spending too much time in bed in an attempt to achieve this sleep duration goal. Mr. Albert reported a strong reluctance to get out of bed, driven by this rationale. Mr. Albert also commented that "just the anticipation of being awake makes me tense," consistent with negative cognitions around sleep itself.

Mr. Albert indicated in his sleep diary that both his bedtime (9:00–11:00 pm) and wake times (5:30–8:00 am) varied considerably from day to day across the 2 weeks. Importantly, his sleep-onset latency (the time between going to bed and falling asleep) was up to 2 hours, and he sometimes did not fall asleep until 1:00 am. His habitual sleep duration therefore varied from 4 to 9 hours, resulting in poor "sleep efficiency" (the ratio between time in bed and time asleep; Monk, Buysse, Rose, Hall, & Kupfer, 2000).

Mr. Albert's responses to the DASS-21 (Lovibond & Lovibond, 1995) suggested at least moderate symptom levels of depression, normal symptom levels of anxiety, and moderate symptom levels of stress. He had received pharmacological treatment for depression intermittently over two decades. He believed that his insomnia was a more persistent problem than was his mood, despite episodes of severe depression. Retrospection can be unreliable but he was confident that symptoms of insomnia did not always co-occur with other symptoms of depressed mood.

Mr. Albert reported his average alcohol intake to be approximately 140 g/week, predominantly "nips" of spirits. Although a relationship between self-medication with alcohol leading to further disrupted sleep has been described (Roehrs & Roth, 2001), this level of intake is regarded as "low risk" by Australian guidelines published by the National Health and Medical Research Council (NHMRC). Alcohol in the evening can be a problem for patients with OSA, increasing the frequency and severity of upper airway obstruction (Scrima, Broudy, Nay, & Cohn, 1982), and this had been explained to Mr. Albert previously. His self-reported caffeine intake of approximately 165 mg/day (three cups of tea) was also within recommended limits of 220 mg/day, and was not likely to be a significant problem for sleep. He had never smoked.

Mr. Albert's current medications included lorazepam (a benzodiazepine used as an anxiolytic), amitryptaline (a tricyclic antidepressant and anxiolytic), omeprazole (a proton-pump inhibitor used to treat symptoms of gastroesophageal reflux disease), and ranitidine (a histamine receptor antagonist also used to treat gastroesophageal reflux disease). Sedation has been reported as a "more common" adverse reaction, and sleep disturbance a "less common" adverse reaction, to lorazepam. Disturbed concentration, insomnia, and drowsiness are reported adverse reactions to amitryptaline. Mr. Albert had previously tried alprazolam and zolpidem to improve his sleep. In this setting, a medication review by a hospital pharmacist or by a hospital physician is sometimes possible, but in general this is left to the patient's GP. Polypharmacy is very common in this older adult population and may directly impact on sleep quality (Smith, Dingwall, Jorgenson, & Douglas, 2006).

Mr. Albert held some common beliefs and attitudes regarding the consequences of poor sleep that can perpetuate insomnia. The cognitive aspects of CBTi are the least developed (Harvey & Tang, 2003), and there is limited support for doctrinaire CBT as a single treatment. A number of reports suggest that dysfunctional cognitions around sleep can improve with institution of standard CBTi (Edinger, Wohlgemuth, Radtke, Marsh, & Quillian, 2001a, b; Morin, Blais, & Savard, 2002). Our standard practice is to provide psychoeducation in the form of a patient education manual designed to alter unrealistic expectations about sleep need, misattributions about the consequences of insomnia, and erroneous beliefs about how to improve sleep. This manual has been validated in a major CBTi trial (Edinger et al., used with permission), but there are other excellent patient resources (e.g. Lack et al., 2003). The manual aims to provide factual content about circadian rhythms, sleep quality, and sleep quantity. The education component also reviewed sleep hygiene principles about the effects of diet, exercise, caffeine, alcohol, and other environmental factors on sleep. The purpose of the education is to provide the knowledge necessary for self-management using specific behavioral strategies introduced in the second session. Mr. Albert was asked to return the following week for a second session. This time allows for scoring of the questionnaire package and sleep diary, and the time to generate an individualized program for CBTi.

Formulation

The key features of the assessment were a chronic sleep-onset problem with high night-to-night variability in sleep-onset time and sleep duration, poor sleep efficiency, decreased functioning during the day resulting from the insomnia, together with evidence of sleep-preventing associations. Mr. Albert presented with a complaint of sleeping difficulties consistent with at least minimal diagnostic criteria for psychophysiological insomnia by ICSD-II criteria (American Academy of Sleep Medicine, 2005). His current mood, long-term medication use, and aspects of his sleep habits such as variable sleep and wake time, together with previously demonstrated mild OSA were significant contributors to these problems.

Session 2

During the second session, Mr. Albert's presenting complaints, and his self-report on questionnaires, were confirmed with him. His general understanding of the manual content was also checked. He was then introduced to a structured self-management program, designed to target specific aspects of his sleep problems. The primary behavioral component of this program incorporated sleep restriction therapy (Spielman, 1986; Spielman, Saskin, & Thorpy, 1987) to improve his sleep efficiency. Sleep restriction aims to consolidate sleep by reducing the time spent in bed to something approximating the time actually spent asleep. Practically, this means that an estimate of actual sleep need must be made (e.g. mean sleep duration over a 2-week period). In Mr. Albert's case, his earliest bedtime was set initially at 11:00 pm, with wake time set at 6:30 am. This initial regime was designed to provide him with 7½ hours of sleep opportunity. This reflects his self-reported mean sleep duration of 7 hours, with ½ an hour allowed for normal sleep-onset latency and wake periods during the night. The rationale for this intervention was carefully discussed with him and the decision about where to "place" his sleep times relative to the day were made in the context of his preferred lifestyle and in discussion with his wife. It is common for individual sleep need to vary, and this can sometimes cause some conflict around bedtimes in couples. Mr. Albert's wife typically slept for about 1 hour more than his average sleep duration. This meant practically that they could either go to bed together, or get up together, but not both. They both agreed to wake at 6:30 am, and both thought that this cooperation was likely to help Mr. Albert adhere to sleep restriction protocol. It was also seen by Mrs. Albert as an active way to help her husband.

The standard approach to sleep restriction therapy is to titrate time in bed in light of daytime functioning, but to do this slowly (over weeks) rather than in response to a single night's sleep. Mr. Albert was provided with an additional diary designed to help him to easily calculate any changes to his initial sleep restriction protocols. In general, if he can adhere to the protocol for 2 weeks, and still experiences substantial wake time before falling asleep, then his bedtime will be delayed further. In contrast, if his sleep efficiency has improved, the protocol is maintained. If he finds that he is falling asleep rapidly, has minimal wake after sleep onset, but feels sleepy during the day, then the protocol can be relaxed by advancing his bedtime. These changes are typically made in 15-minute increments, with at least a week between changes. Patients tend to resist the idea of sleep restriction because of the paradox around less time in bed (Vincent & Lionberg, 2001), but it is nonetheless probably the most effective CBTi component (Harvey et al., 2002).

The stimulus control procedures, designed to reduce negative associations with his sleeping environment, were also introduced. The stimulus control for insomnia provides very specific instructions designed to strengthen the bed and bedroom as cues for sleep (Bootzin et al., 1991). In short, patients are to get out of bed if they are not asleep, and get into bed when they are sleepy. The requirement to get up is seen by many patients as counterintuitive, requiring significant discussion directed at overcoming barriers to this behavior change. The stimulus control and sleep restriction protocols together meant that Mr. Albert was instructed not to go to bed before 11:00 pm, and not to go to bed after that time unless he felt sleepy. If he could not then fall asleep within about 30 minutes, he was to get back out of bed and engage in a non-stimulating activity until he again felt sleepy. This was to be repeated until sleep was achieved. Mr. Albert reported occasionally falling asleep in front of the television at night, but then feeling aroused and unable to sleep when retiring to bed. This is an archetypal report consistent with the need for stimulus control. Mr. Albert found the stimulus control explanation for his own experience convincing, and chose to read quietly in another room during the "awake" times of the protocol. The combined behavioral strategies can cause partial sleep deprivation initially, and this may lead to an increase in daytime sleepiness. This reinforces the behavioral strategy by increasing homeostatic drive to sleep on subsequent nights. This potential side effect of the therapy was explained to Mr. Albert, and he agreed to specifically avoid driving when sleepy.

Mr. Albert was encouraged to increase his level of daily exercise (aiming initially for 30 minutes of brisk walking), in combination with early morning light exposure (up to 1 hour of sunlight, wearing sunscreen and "sun-smart" clothing). His wake-up time was set by the sleep restriction routine at 6:30 am. The purpose of these three behavioral strategies was to reinforce and maintain a constant circadian phase position. The literature on the benefits of exercise for sleep in older adults with insomnia is currently weak but positive (Montgomery & Dennis, 2002). Increased daily activity may be a protective factor against insomnia in older adults (Morgan, 2003). Most older adults attending our clinic do not engage in much formal exercise, and many have limited incidental exercise (Smith et al., 2008). Mr. Albert had no physical impediments to exercise, but he didn't engage in any exercise apart from ordinary daily activities. He did owned a stationary bicycle, consistent with some contemplation or willingness to engage in exercise. His preference though was to go for a walk around his neighborhood in the morning, or to walk around his local shopping center on very hot or rainy days. Both Mr. Albert and his wife were overweight by current NHMRC guidelines, and they agreed that walking would be of benefit to both of them. There is some evidence that exercise, with or without any change to body fat, can improve clinical indices of OSA. If this is the case, exercise could be of particular benefit to Mr. Albert and his wife.

This exercise prescription also provides a natural mechanism for increased light exposure in the morning. The use of light as a time setter (or zeitgeber) for the human circadian clock is now well understood. In short, timed exposure to bright light in the late evening acts to phase delay the circadian rhythm (driving a later sleep onset and later wake time), while light exposure first thing in the morning acts to phase advance the circadian rhythm (driving an earlier sleep-onset time and earlier wake time). There is evidence that some patients with sleep-onset insomnia have a relative phase delay in their circadian rhythm (Morris, Lack, & Dawson, 1990), and evidence for the benefit of morning bright light to advance this rhythm (Lack, Wright, & Paynter, 2007). Remarkably, bright light treatment alone has been found to reduce pre-sleep anxiety and improve daytime functioning in patients with sleep-onset insomnia (Lack et al., 2007). There is further evidence that circadian function may be disrupted in older adults (Gibson, Williams, & Kriegsfeld, 2009), and a relative advance of the rhythm (with early bedtimes and early wake times) is also a common pattern (Monk, 2005). Despite this rationale, the current evidence for the efficacy of bright light to improve insomnia in older adults is currently mixed at best (Gammack, 2008; Friedman et al., 2009), but has better support for use in older adults with a diagnosis of dementia (Sloane et al., 2007). A wide variety of artificial light sources are now available for use in circadian re-setting and as a treatment for seasonal affective disorders, but we have demonstrated that natural sunlight in the morning can phase advance the circadian rhythm (Smith & Trinder, 2005). In Queensland, Australia, where our clinic is located, morning sunlight is almost always available. Because the state hasn't embraced daylight saving, the sun rises as early as 5:00 am in midsummer. This raises a potential problem of inadvertent light exposure before the circadian nadir causing a paradoxical circadian phase delay. Because of this possibility, Mr. Albert was instructed to ensure minimal light intrusion into his bedroom before 6:30 am.

The relationship between insomnia and depression was also discussed with Mr. Albert in light of his ongoing pharmacological treatment for depression. There is a growing consensus that treatment of insomnia has specific benefits for depression. Morawetz (2003) reported that level of mood improved substantially in depressed patients whose sleep was improved by a self-help program. Other studies have found augmenting antidepressant medication with CBTi promising for individuals with MDD and co-morbid insomnia, alleviating both depression and insomnia (Manber et al., 2008). Further, greater levels of sleep disturbance and depression may predict better outcomes from CBTi (Espie et al., 2001).

Follow-up

Mr. Albert was seen for follow-up 3 months after his initial sessions. He was sent a questionnaire pack to complete prior to the follow-up session, again containing the ISI, DBAS, and DASS measures. The intent of the follow-up session was to review symptom levels, progress, and adherence to the behavioral strategies, and also to provide reinforcement of these strategies to minimize the impact of future lapses in adherence. Mr. Albert reported an overall reduction in insomnia severity. He had found the stimulus control requirements difficult, preferring instead to "try harder" to fall asleep. Although this maladaptive strategy had been addressed in the patient manual, it was addressed more specifically during this session. In any case, he had stuck closely to the sleep restriction protocol, and had not made any changes to the original schedule. He reported a significant reduction in sleep-onset latency, from up to 2 hours, down to 30 minutes on average.

A reduction in sleep-onset latency of this magnitude is very large. Most reports suggest small to medium effect sizes for changes in sleep quantity in response to either CBTi or pharmacological treatments. Self-report of improvement in sleep quality and daytime functioning, on the other hand, is typically greater. This has led to recent interest in directly addressing daytime functioning as a focus of treatment, including the use of mindfulness meditation and third wave therapies (Ong, Shapiro, & Manber, 2008). Mr. Albert felt that his sleep had become a lot more "predictable," and that he now had much less concern regarding his ability to achieve sleep. This report was reflected in his DBAS scores, which had reduced for most of the items (Carney & Edinger, 2006). Changes in level of mood on the DASS were not significant (still in the moderate range), although Mr. Albert felt that his concerns about "loss of control" and anticipation or poor sleep had reduced.

Mr. Albert had managed to exercise as prescribed on most days. This behavior was less consistent on the weekends, despite the fact that he no longer worked during the weekdays. Mr. Albert had apprehensions about continuing his morning exercise in the cold of winter. This was addressed through a discussion, together with his wife, of the costs and benefits of exercise for him, and he agreed to adopt some simple strategies and continue with the exercise. Mrs. Albert had found daily exercise difficult in terms of the exertion required, but was otherwise quite enthusiastic about its benefits. Mr. Albert found the sleep diary a very useful way to track patterns in his sleep. We had discussed the need to focus on changes in sleep over a period of weeks, rather than reacting to night-to-night changes, and this strategy had provided him with a sense of progress. He was able to articulate a strategy to use in the event of acute sleeplessness; essentially based on sticking to his regular sleep-wake routine as much as possible. The evidence for the durability of CBTi over at least 12 months is now strong (Harvey et al., 2002; Sivertsen et al., 2006; Morin et al., 2009). Mr. Albert was returned to the care of his GP for follow-up.

Conclusions

Changes in sleep quality with age are often seen as natural and unremarkable, but all evidence suggests strong benefits from improved sleep quality. There appear to be no physical or psychological impediments to older adults engaging fully in CBTi, and the intervention has demonstrated effectiveness in that cohort. The rationale for treatment is stronger, rather than less strong, where insomnia is co-morbid with other medical or psychiatric disorders. The mainstream interventions exploit natural biological processes, and these are in turn directly reinforced by behavioral change. This reinforcing cycle means that it gets easier to sleep better. A pragmatic approach to most presentations is to stabilize and reinforce the circadian rhythm by encouraging regular sleep-wake habits, to ensure that the homeostatic drive for sleep is focused onto consolidated nighttime sleep, and to remove obvious barriers to sleep onset. The emphasis on exploiting the biological drive for sleep, the routine use of standardized CBTi in therapy, and the view that sleep is a positive health behavior, is emerging as a consensus approach. This approach fits well with other contemporary positive health promotion perspectives. The nature of these interventions is such that patients are armed against future relapse, and know how to self-manage in the inevitable event of an acute interruption to sleep.

Post-case conclusions and reflections

There is a community belief that poor sleep is an inevitable consequence of aging. Although it may be the case that aspects of sleep duration and sleep architecture change with increasing age, satisfaction with sleep quality is still an important aspect of general health and well-being. How might the therapist go about challenging these stereotypical age-related beliefs in patients? In other health professionals?

Medical intervention with sedative-hypnotic medication is by far the most common treatment modality offered to older adults presenting in primary care environments with a sleep complaint. The potential for increased risk for falls, and for driving crashes, that may be associated with sedative-hypnotic use by older adults should always be considered. The potential risks or benefits of adding a sedative-hypnotic drug to an existing medication regime in the case of co-morbid medical conditions should be taken into account. What then are the implications of this for practitioners across a range of settings?

1. It is often important to recruit spouses or partners to assist (or at least not hamper) sleep hygiene and insomnia treatments. In the case presented the wife was a willing partner; what steps might need to be taken if the cooperation of the spouse or partner was not assured? What about the situation of well-meaning friends and family providing advice in contrast to the treatment regime?

References

Åkerstedt, T., Hume, K., Minors, D., & Waterhouse, J. (1994). The subjective meaning of good sleep, an intraindividual approach using the Karolinska Sleep Diary. *Perceptual and Motor Skills, 79*(1 Pt 1), 287–296.

American Academy of Sleep Medicine (2005). *The International Classification of Sleep Disorders: Diagnostic and coding manual*. Westchester, IL: American Academy of Sleep Medicine.

American Psychiatric Association (2000). *Diagnostic and Statistical Manual of Mental Disorders, Fourth Edition, Text Revision (DSM-IV-TR)*. Washington, DC: American Psychiatric Association.

Bastien, C.H., Vallieres, A., & Morin, C.M. (2001). Validation of the Insomnia Severity Index as an outcome measure for insomnia research. *Sleep Medicine, 2*(4), 297–307.

Berdot, S., Bertrand, M., Jean-François, D., Annie, F., Béatrice, T., Karen, R., et al. (2009). Inappropriate medication use and risk of falls—A prospective study in a large community-dwelling elderly cohort. *BMC Geriatrics, 9*(1), 30.

Bixler, E.O., Kales, A., Soldatos, C.R., Kales, J.D., & Healey, S. (1979). Prevalence of sleep disorders in the Los Angeles metropolitan area. *American Journal of Psychiatry, 136*(10), 1257–1262.

Bootzin, R.R., Epstein, D., & Wood, J.M. (1991). Stimulus control instructions. In P.J. Hauri (Ed.), *Case studies in insomnia* (pp. 19–28). New York, NY: Plenum Medical Book Company.

Broman, J.E., Lundh, L.G., & Hetta, J. (1996). Insufficient sleep in the general population. *Clinical Neurophysiology, 26*(1), 30–39.

Cacioppo, J.T., & Hawkley, L.C. (2003). Social isolation and health, with an emphasis on underlying mechanisms. *Perspectives in Biology and Medicine, 46*(3 Suppl), S39–S52.

Cajochen, C., Münch, M., Knoblauch, V., Blatter, K., & Wirz-Justice, A. (2006). Age related changes in the circadian and homeostatic regulation of human sleep. *Chronobiology International, 23*(1–2), 461–474.

Carney, C.E. & Edinger, J.D. (2006). Identifying critical beliefs about sleep in primary insomnia. *Sleep, 29*(4), 444–453.

Chung, K.-F., Krakow, B., Melendrez, D., Warner, T.D., & Sisley, B.N. (2003). Relationships between insomnia and sleep-disordered breathing. *Chest, 123*(1), 310–313.

Dijk, D.-J., Duffy, J.F., Riel, E., Shanahan, T.L., & Czeisler, C.A. (1999). Ageing and the circadian and homeostatic regulation of human sleep during forced desynchrony of rest, melatonin and temperature rhythms. *The Journal of Physiology, 516*(2), 611–627.

Edinger, J.D., Fins, A.I., Goeke, J.M., McMillan, D.K., Gersh, T.L., Krystal, A.D., et al. (1996). The empirical identification of insomnia subtypes: A cluster analytic approach. *Sleep, 19*(5), 398–411.

Edinger, J.D., Wohlgemuth, W.K., Radtke, R.A., Marsh, G.R., & Quillian, R.E. (2001a). Cognitive behavioral therapy for treatment of chronic primary insomnia: A randomized controlled trial. *JAMA, 285*(14), 1856–1864.

Edinger, J.D., Wohlgemuth, W.K., Radtke, R.A., Marsh, G.R., & Quillian, R.E. (2001b). Does cognitive-behavioral insomnia therapy alter dysfunctional beliefs about sleep? *Sleep*, *24*(5), 591–602.

Edinger, J.D., Bonnet, M.H., Bootzin, R.R., et al. (2004). Derivation of research diagnostic criteria for insomnia: Report of an American Academy of Sleep Medicine Work Group. *Sleep*, *27*(8), 1567–1596.

Edinger, J.D., Wohlgemuth, W.K., Radtke, R.A., Coffman, C.J., & Carney, C.E. (2007). Dose-response effects of cognitive-behavioral insomnia therapy: A randomized clinical trial. *Sleep*, *30*(2), 203–212.

Espie, C.A., Inglis, S.J., Tessier, S., & Harvey, L. (2001). The clinical effectiveness of cognitive behaviour therapy for chronic insomnia: Implementation and evaluation of a sleep clinic in general medical practice. *Behaviour Research and Therapy*, *39*(1), 45–60.

Foley, D.J., Monjan, A., Simonsick, E.M., Wallace, R.B., & Blazer, D.G. (1999). Incidence and remission of insomnia among elderly adults: An epidemiologic study of 6,800 persons over three years. *Sleep*, *22*(Suppl 2), S366–S372.

Foley, D., Ancoli-Israel, S., Britz, P., & Walsh, J. (2004). Sleep disturbances and chronic disease in older adults: Results of the 2003 National Sleep Foundation Sleep in America Survey. *Journal of Psychosomatic Research*, *56*(5), 497–502.

Friedman, L., Zeitzer, J.M., Kushida, C., Zhdanova, I., Noda, A., Lee, T., et al. (2009). Scheduled bright light for treatment of insomnia in older adults. *Journal of the American Geriatrics Society*, *57*(3), 441–452.

Gammack, J.K. (2008). Light therapy for insomnia in older adults. *Clinics in Geriatric Medicine*, *24*(1), 139–149.

Gibson, E.M., Williams, W.P., & Kriegsfeld, L.J. (2009). Aging in the circadian system: Considerations for health, disease prevention and longevity. *Experimental Gerontology*, *44*(1–2), 51–56.

Harvey, A.G. (2001). Insomnia: Symptom or diagnosis? *Clinical Psychology Reviews*, *21*(7), 1037–1059.

Harvey, A.G. (2002). A cognitive model of insomnia. *Behaviour Research and Therapy*, *40*(8), 869–893.

Harvey, A.G., & Tang, N.K.Y. (2003). Cognitive behaviour therapy for primary insomnia: Can we rest yet? *Sleep Medicine Reviews*, *7*(3), 237–262.

Harvey, L., Inglis, S.J., & Espie, C.A. (2002). Insomniacs' reported use of CBT components and relationship to long-term clinical outcome. *Behaviour Research and Therapy*, *40*(1), 75–83.

Katz, D.A., & McHorney, C.A. (1998). Clinical correlates of insomnia in patients with chronic illness. *Archives of Internal Medicine*, *158*(10), 1099–1107.

Krakow, B., Melendrez, D., Ferreira, E., Clark, J., Warner, T.D., Sisley, B., et al. (2001). Prevalence of insomnia symptoms in patients with sleep-disordered breathing. *Chest*, *120*, 1923–1929.

Lack, L., Wright, H., et al. (2003). *Insomnia: How to sleep easy*. Double Bay, NSW: ACP and Media 21.

Lack, L.C., Wright, H., & Paynter, D. (2007). The treatment of sleep onset insomnia with bright morning light. *Sleep and Biological Rhythms*, *5*(3), 173–179.

Lavie, P. (2007). Insomnia and sleep-disordered breathing. *Sleep Medicine*, *8*, 21–25.

Lichstein, K.L., Riedel, B.W., Lester, K.W., & Aguillard, R.N. (1999). Occult sleep apnea in a recruited sample of older adults with insomnia. *Journal of Consulting and Clinical Psychology*, *67*, 405–410.

Lichstein, K.L., Durrence, H.H., Bayen, U.J., & Riedel, B.W. (2001). Primary versus secondary insomnia in older adults: Subjective sleep and daytime functioning. *Psychology and Aging*, *16*(2), 264–271.

Lichstein, K.L., Durrence, H.H., Taylor, D.J., Bush, A.J., & Riedel, B.W. (2003). Quantitative criteria for insomnia. *Behaviour Research and Therapy*, *41*(4), 427–445.

Lovibond, S.H., & Lovibond, P.F. (1995). *Manual for the depression anxiety stress scales*. Sydney: Psychology Foundation.

Manber, R., Edinger, J.D., Gress, J.L., San Pedro-Salcedo, M.G., Kuo, T.F., & Kalista, T. (2008). Cognitive behavioral therapy for insomnia enhances depression outcome in patients with comorbid major depressive disorder and insomnia. *Sleep*, *31*(4), 489–495.

Martin, S.K., & Eastman, C.I. (2002). Sleep logs of young adults with self-selected sleep times predict the dim light melatonin onset. *Chronobiology International*, *19*(4), 695–707.

Means, M.K., Lichstein, K.L., Epperson, M.T., & Johnson, C.T. (2000). Relaxation therapy for insomnia: Nighttime and day time effects. *Behaviour Research and Therapy*, *38*(7), 665–678.

Monk, T.H. (2005). Aging human circadian rhythms: Conventional wisdom may not always be right. *Journal of Biological Rhythms*, *20*(4), 366–374.

Monk, T.H., Reynolds, C.F., 3rd, Kupfer, D.J., Buysse, D.J., Coble, P.A., & Hayes, A.J. (1994). The Pittsburgh Sleep Diary. *Journal of Sleep Research*, *3*, 111–120.

Monk, T.H., Buysse, D.J., Rose, L.R., Hall, J.A., & Kupfer, D.J. (2000). The sleep of healthy people—a diary study. *Chronobiology International*, *17*(1), 49–60.

Montgomery, P., & Dennis, J. (2002). Physical exercise for sleep problems in adults aged 60+. *Cochrane Database of Systematic Reviews*, (4), CD003404.

Morawetz, D. (2003). Insomnia and depression: Which comes first. *Sleep Research Online*, *5*(2), 77–81.

Morgan, K. (2003). Daytime activity and risk factors for late-life insomnia. *Journal of Sleep Research*, *12*(3), 231–238.

Morgan, K., Dixon, S., Mathers, N., Thompson, J., & Tomeny, M. (2003). Psychological treatment for insomnia in the management of long-term hypnotic drug use: A pragmatic randomised controlled trial. *British Journal of General Practice*, *53*(497), 923–928.

Morgenthaler, T., Kramer, M., Alessi, C., Friedman, L., Boehlecke, B., Brown, T., et al. (2006). Practice parameters for the psychological and behavioral treatment of insomnia: An update. An American academy of sleep medicine report. *Sleep*, *29*(11), 1415–1419.

Morin, C.M. (1993). *Insomnia: Psychological assessment and management*. New York, NY: Guilford Press.

Morin, C.M., & Espie, C.A. (2003). *Insomnia: A clinical guide to assessment and treatment*. New York, NY: Kluwer Academic Publishers.

Morin, C.M., Kowatch, R.A., Barry, T., & Walton, E. (1993). Cognitive-behavior therapy for late-life insomnia. *Journal of Consulting and Clinical Psychology*, *61*, 137–147.

Morin, C.M., Blais, F., & Savard, J. (2002). Are changes in beliefs and attitudes about sleep related to sleep improvements in the treatment of insomnia? *Behaviour Research and Therapy*, *40*(7), 741–752.

Morin, C.M., Bootzin, R.R., Buysse, D.J., Edinger, J.D., Espie, C.A., & Lichstein, K.L. (2006). Psychological and behavioral treatment of insomnia: Update of the recent evidence (1998–2004). *Sleep*, *29*(11), 1398–1414.

Morin, C.M., Vallières, A., & Ivers, H. (2007). Dysfunctional beliefs and attitudes about sleep (DBAS): Validation of a brief version (DBAS-16). *Sleep*, *30*(11), 1547–1554.

Morin, C.M., Vallieres, A., Guay, B., Ivers, H., Savard, J., Merette, C., et al. (2009). Cognitive behavioral therapy, singly and combined with medication, for persistent insomnia: A randomized controlled trial. *JAMA*, *301*(19), 2005–2015.

Morris, M., Lack, L., & Dawson, D. (1990). Sleep-onset insomniacs have delayed temperature rhythms. *Sleep*, *13*(1), 1–14.

National Institutes of Health (2005). State of the Science Conference Statement on Manifestations and Management of Chronic Insomnia in Adults, June 13–15, 2005. *Sleep*, *28*, 1049–1057.

Nau, S.D., McCrae, C.S., Cook, K.G., & Lichstein, K.L. (2005). Treatment of insomnia in older adults. *Clinical Psychology Reviews*, *25*(5), 645–672.

Ohayon, M.M. (2002). Epidemiology of insomnia: What we know and what we still need to learn. *Sleep Medicine Reviews*, *6*(2), 97–111.

Ohayon, M.M., Zulley, J., Guilleminault, C., Smirne, S., & Priest, R.G. (2001). How age and daytime activities are related to insomnia in the general population: Consequences for older people. *Journal of the American Geriatrics Society*, *49*(4), 360–366.

Olsen, S., Smith, S., & Oei, T.P. (2008). Adherence to continuous positive airway pressure therapy in obstructive sleep apnoea sufferers: A theoretical approach to treatment adherence and intervention. *Clinical Psychology Review*, *28*(8), 1355–1371.

Ong, J.C., Shapiro, S.L., & Manber, R. (2008). Combining mindfulness meditation with cognitive-behavior therapy for insomnia: A treatment-development study. *Behavior Therapy*, *39*, 171–182.

Ozminkowski, R.J., Wang, S., & Walsh, J.K. (2007). The direct and indirect costs of untreated insomnia in adults in the United States. *Sleep, 30*(3), 263–273.

Pace-Schott, E.F., & Hobson, J.A. (2002). The neurobiology of sleep: Genetics, cellular physiology and subcortical networks. *Nature Reviews Neuroscience, 3*(8), 591–605.

Pincus, H.A., Vettorello, N.E., McQueen, L.E., First, M., Wise, T.N., Zarin, D., et al. (1995). Bridging the gap between psychiatry and primary care. The DSM-IV-PC. *Psychosomatics, 36*(4), 328–335.

Prakash, K., Nissen, L., et al. (2007). Efficacy of Medication Histories for the diagnosis of Sleep Disorders in Hospital and Community Settings. *Australasian Pharmaceutical Science Association (APSA)—Annual Conference. Medicines Design to Delivery*. Sydney, NSW: APSA.

Rebbapragada, V., Subramanian, S., Chanamolu, S., Guntupalli, K., Patel, B., Casturi, L., et al. (2006). Insomnia in obstructive sleep apnea: Prevalence and gender and ethnic variance. *Sleep Medicine, 7*, S118–S119.

Riemann, D., & Voderholzer, U. (2003). Primary insomnia: A risk factor to develop depression? *Journal of Affective Disorders, 76*(1–3), 255–259.

Roehrs, T., & Roth, T. (2001). Sleep, sleepiness, and alcohol use. *Alcohol Research & Health, 25*(2), 101–109.

Scharf, S.M., Tubman, A., & Smale, P. (2005). Prevalence of concomitant sleep disorders in patients with obstructive sleep apnea. *Sleep and Breathing, 9*(2), 50–56.

Schramm, E., Hohagen, F., Grasshoff, U., Riemann, D., Hajak, G., Weess, H.G., et al. (1993). Test-retest reliability and validity of the structured interview for sleep disorders according to DSM-III-R. *American Journal of Psychiatry, 150*(6), 867.

Schutte-Rodin, S., Broch, L., Buysse, D., Dorsey, C., & Sateia, M. (2008). Clinical guideline for the evaluation and management of chronic insomnia in adults. *Journal of Clinical Sleep Medicine, 4*(5), 487–504.

Scrima, L., Broudy, M., Nay, K.N., & Cohn, M.A. (1982). Increased severity of obstructive sleep apnea after bedtime alcohol ingestion: Diagnostic potential and proposed mechanism of action. *Sleep, 5*(4), 318–328.

Shochat, T., Umphress, J., Israel, A.G., & Ancoli-Israel, S. (1999). Insomnia in primary care patients. *Journal of Sleep Research & Sleep Medicine, 22*, S359–S365.

Sivertsen, B., Omvik, S., Pallesen, S., Bjorvatn, B., Havik, O.E., Kvale, G., et al. (2006). Cognitive behavioral therapy vs zopiclone for treatment of chronic primary insomnia in older adults: A randomized controlled trial. *JAMA, 295*(24), 2851–2858.

Sloane, P.D., Williams, C.S., Mitchell, C.M., Preisser, J.S., Wood, W., Barrick, A.L., et al. (2007). High-intensity environmental light in dementia: Effect on sleep and activity. *Journal of the American Geriatrics Society, 55*(10), 1524–1533.

Smith, M.T., Perlis, M.L., Smith, M.S., Giles, D.E., & Carmody, T.P. (2000). Sleep quality and presleep arousal in chronic pain. *Journal of Behavioral Medicine, 23*(1), 1–13.

Smith, M.T., Perlis, M.L., Park, A., Smith, M.S., Pennington, J., Giles, D.E., et al. (2002). Comparative meta-analysis of pharmacotherapy and behavior therapy for persistent insomnia. *American Journal of Psychiatry, 159*(1), 5–11.

Smith, M.T., Huang, M.I., & Manber, R. (2005). Cognitive behavior therapy for chronic insomnia occurring within the context of medical and psychiatric disorders. *Clinical Psychology Reviews, 25*(5), 559–592.

Smith, S., & Trinder, J. (2001). Detecting insomnia: Comparison of four self-report measures of sleep in a young adult population. *Journal of Sleep Research, 10*(3), 229–235.

Smith, S., & Trinder, J. (2005). Morning sunlight can phase advance the circadian rhythm of young adults. *Sleep and Biological Rhythms, 3*, 39–41.

Smith, S., Sullivan, K., Hopkins, W., & Douglas, J. (2004). Frequency of insomnia report in patients with obstructive sleep apnoea hypopnea syndrome (OSAHS). *Sleep Medicine, 5*(5), 449–456.

Smith, S., Dingwall, K., Jorgenson, G., & Douglas, J. (2006). Associations between the use of common medications and sleep architecture in patients with untreated obstructive sleep apnea. *Journal of Clinical Sleep Medicine, 2*, 156–162.

Smith, S.S., Doyle, G., et al. (2008). Intention to exercise in patients with obstructive sleep apnoea. *Journal of Clinical Sleep Medicine*, *328*(17), 1230–1235.

Spiegel, K., Leproult, R., & Van Cauter, E. (1999). Impact of sleep debt on metabolic and endocrine function. *Lancet*, *354*(9188), 1435–1439.

Spielman, A.J. (1986). Assessment of insomnia. *Clinical Psychology Review*, *6*(1), 11–25.

Spielman, A.J., Caruso, L.S., & Glovinsky, P.B. (1987). A behavioral perspective on insomnia treatment. *Psychiatric Clinics of North America*, *10*(4), 541–553.

Spielman, A.J., Saskin, P., & Thorpy, M.J. (1987). Treatment of chronic insomnia by restriction of time in bed. *Sleep*, *10*(1), 45–56.

Strogatz, S.H., Kronauer, R.E., & Czeisler, C.A. (1987). Circadian pacemaker interferes with sleep onset at specific times each day: Role in insomnia. *American Journal of Physiology. Regulatory, Integrative and Comparative Physiology*, *253*(1), R172–R178.

Van Cauter, E., Leproult, R., & Plat, L. (2000). Age-related changes in slow wave sleep and REM sleep and relationship with growth hormone and cortisol levels in healthy men. *JAMA*, *284*(7), 861–868.

Verster, J.C., Mets, M.A.J., Leufkens, T.R.M., & Vermeeren, A. (2008). Insomnia, hypnotic drugs and traffic safety. In J.C. Verster, S.R. Pandi-Perumal, J.G. Ramaekers & J.J. de Gier (Eds.), *Drugs, Driving and Traffic Safety* (pp. 233). Basel: Springer.

Vincent, N., & Lionberg, C. (2001). Treatment preference and patient satisfaction in chronic insomnia. *Sleep*, *24*(4), 411–417.

Walker, M.P., & Stickgold, R. (2004). Sleep-dependent learning and memory consolidation. *Neuron*, *44*(1), 121–133.

Walsh, J.K. (2004). Clinical and socioeconomic correlates of insomnia. *Journal of Clinical Psychiatry*, *65*(8), 13–19.

Wang, M.Y., Wang, S.Y., & Tsai, P.S. (2005). Cognitive behavioural therapy for primary insomnia: A systematic review. *Journal of Advanced Nursing*, *50*(5), 553–564.

Wittchen, H.U., Krause, P., Hofler, M., Pittrow, D., Winter, S., Spiegel, B., et al. (2001). NISAS-2000: Die Nationwide Insomnia Screening and Awareness Study. Pravalenz und Verschreibungsverhalten in der allgemeinarztlichen Versorgung.[NISAS-2000: The Nationwide Insomnia Screening and Awareness Study. Prevalence and interventions in primary care]. *Fortschritte der Medizin. Originalien*, *119*(1), 9–19.

Zhou, J.N., Liu, R.Y., van Heerikhuize, J., Hofman, M.A., & Swaab, D.F. (2003). Alterations in the circadian rhythm of salivary melatonin begin during middle-age. *Journal of Pineal Research*, *34*(1), 11–16.

Chapter 12

Personality disorders in later life

Erlene Rosowsky and Daniel L. Segal

Introduction

Personality disorders (PDs) are among the most misunderstood and poorly researched forms of mental illness, especially as the PDs present in later life (Abrams & Bromberg, 2006; Agronin & Maletta, 2000; Molinari & Segal, in press; Segal, Coolidge, & Rosowsky, 2006; Zweig, 2008; Zweig & Agronin, 2006). In contrast to the meager knowledge base, the deleterious impact of the PDs in later life is substantial, as PDs are known to complicate case formulation, create barriers to the formation of a therapeutic alliance, and generally make all types of treatments more arduous and less effective (Segal et al., 2006). Indeed, those with PDs are highly troubled people, frequently characterized by a host of pejorative terms, such as *difficult, hateful, toxic, aggravating, intolerable*, and *insufferable*. But what exactly is a Personality Disorder?

In essence, a PD is diagnosed clinically when a person's personality traits (defined as one's characteristic pattern of thinking, feeling, behaving, and relating to others) become inflexible and maladaptive. More formally, according to the *DSM-IV-TR* (Diagnostic and Statistical Manual of Mental Disorders, fourth edition, text revision), a PD is defined as "an enduring pattern of inner experience and behavior that deviates markedly from the expectations of the individual's culture, is pervasive and inflexible, has an onset in adolescence or early adulthood, is stable over time, and leads to distress or impairment" (American Psychiatric Association, 2000, p. 685). Although this definition of PD requires an onset no later than early adulthood, it commonly occurs that some people with a PD are not diagnosed or treated until later life, reflecting the general difficulty in diagnosing this class of mental illness (Balsis, Segal, & Donahue, 2009; Segal et al., 2006).

The 10 heterogeneous PDs in the *DSM-IV-TR* are organized into three superordinate clusters based on presumed common underlying themes. Cluster A includes three disorders in which individuals often appear odd, eccentric, suspicious, or withdrawn: paranoid, schizoid, and schizo-typal PDs. Cluster B includes four disorders in which individuals appear to be dramatic, emotional, or erratic, often with intense interpersonal conflicts: antisocial, borderline, histrionic, and narcissistic PDs. Cluster C contains three disorders in which individuals often appear fearful or anxious: avoidant, dependent, and obsessive-compulsive PDs.

Several prominent research and conceptual issues regarding PDs and later life exist and are discussed here as a backdrop to the presentation of cases. First, many researchers (Agronin, 2007; Agronin & Maletta, 2000; Balsis et al., 2009; Segal et al., 2006) have raised serious concerns about the adequacy of the current diagnostic criteria to accurately capture the expression of PD pathology in the context of later life. Indeed, many of the PD diagnostic criteria have poor face validity for older adults, often measuring some aspect of aging rather than PD pathology. This problem with face validity has cascading detrimental effects for all other aspects of validity of the PD criteria (Tackett, Balsis, Oltmanns, & Krueger, 2009). A serious implication of poor face validity is that studies measuring the prevalence of PDs across the lifespan may suffer from *measurement bias*. A second and especially important conceptual issue is whether the field will move toward an age-specific measurement system for PDs (e.g. a new geriatric subclassification of PDs) or develop an age neutral system (in which specific criteria would work equivalently well across all age groups). Both approaches have their advantages and disadvantages and in fact are exceptionally difficult to achieve. For a full discussion of these issues, the interested reader is referred to Tackett et al. (2009), Balsis et al. (2009), and Balsis, Gleason, Woods, and Oltmanns (2007).

In this chapter, as an organizational expedient, we present three cases of older adults with a personality disorder (one case from each PD cluster). After each case, we provide some key points about this important type of psychopathology in later life and offer some questions and reflections for further discussion. We conclude this chapter with some general discussion points to further assist the reader in understanding PDs in older adults.

Cluster A: schizoid personality disorder

Case example: Mr. Everett P

History

Mr. Everett P came from a small New England town, the third child and second son born into a middle class family. His father was a civil servant who worked for the Postal Service, and was also active in town politics. Everett's mother was a housewife and attentive mother. Although her husband was outgoing and a popular local citizen, she herself was reserved, clearly preferring to be in her own home rather than out and about. She came from a farm family and was one of six children. Two of her brothers were considered "a bit strange." They were extremely remote, taciturn, and did not go past grammar school, but were able to help on the farm and were accepted as "that's just the way they are" by their family and rural community. Everett's mother completed a secretarial course in high school and soon after graduation she left the farm and moved to an office job in the city where she met Everett's father who was just beginning his career as a young clerk with the Postal Service.

Everett himself had always been thought of as "odd," and as taking after his uncles. He made no friends at school, preferring to spend time at his hobbies, which reflected a mechanical interest or a collection of one sort or another. He did not seek, nor especially respond to, feedback from others. His relationships with others were limited to his parents and siblings and marginally extended to his nieces and nephews. Although a poor student, he was quiet and "not a problem" in the classroom and so was passed along, one grade to the other, through grammar school, after which he was placed in a trade curriculum, ultimately earning a high school diploma. Through his father's local connections, Everett was able to land a job as a night watchman for a nearby factory. He continued to live at home with his parents while his siblings went on with their educations and careers, married, and began to raise their own families. Working at night, and sleeping during the day, suited Everett very well. The world was quieter at night and being alone in the factory felt right to him. He was a true loner and the minimal time he needed to "socialize" with his parents, his siblings, and their families was usually about what he could tolerate. On a few occasions, when too many demands were placed upon him to "mix more," "talk more," or "be more friendly," he would disappear for a day or two. When asked where he was he would answer that he went to the woods.

Over the years, Everett was able to buy a small cabin in about 2 hours drive from his parents' home, in a very remote area. During this time he also developed a drinking habit. He became known to the proprietors of a general goods store close by his cabin as the nearly silent "odd duck" who stopped by regularly to purchase beer and vodka. He left his job, retiring himself in his 50s, and moved to his cabin full time. His family continued to send him money to "get by on" and always knew of his whereabouts. Everett was notified when first one, and then the other, of his parents died, and that they had bequeathed him the house. Everett soon after walked away from his small cabin in the woods, and took up residence in the family home, attempting there to replicate his reclusive existence, which he was able to do for a number of years. During this time, his nephew maintained some oversight, attending to home maintenance and checking in on his uncle from time to time.

When Everett was in his early 70s, he had a serious fall after a bout of drinking, and he fractured his leg. He was admitted as a patient to a skilled nursing facility for rehabilitation. There he was found to be grossly malnourished and in need of alcohol detoxification. His sister and her son, Everett's nephew, facilitated his admission into the facility as a permanent resident. Learning of this, Everett bolted and found his way back to his cabin in the woods. Intermittently, he would return for a brief time to the family house to access what supplies and money he needed. Neighbors and the postal worker recognized these returns by the lights having been turned on inside the house. During the periods when Everett was living in his cabin, his nephew would see to it that the exterior of the family house was kept up and that mail was collected so the house did not appear abandoned or neglected. Everett gradually moved back into the family residence full time.

Index event

One day the postman noticed that the mail had not been retrieved from the mailbox as usual. When he peeked through a front window, he observed someone lying on the floor and called the police. When the police entered the house, they found Everett (now 81 years old) lying unconscious in vomit and blood, and transferred him to the community hospital where he was directly admitted to the ICU. After a few days, when he was cleaned, hydrated, and stabilized, Everett was transferred to the general medical unit. There upon admission he would not interact with the staff or cooperate in his care. He refused to eat and refused physical therapy.

The culture of the hospital is of relevance here. This community hospital is small and most of its patients are older adults. The staffs of all departments, from administration through direct clinical care, take enormous pride in being kind, patient, and respectful, providing whatever services are needed to help their patients get better. When, despite their best efforts, Everett would not respond, they became concerned. Recognizing that he had no visitors, they felt badly for him and assumed that his sadness and loneliness were contributing to his lack of appetite and responsiveness. Acting on this assumption, they enlisted the help of a kindly woman volunteer to sit with him at mealtime. Everett was assigned to a triple room, but as there was only one other man in the room, his bed and Everett's bed were set at opposite ends of the room. Thinking that Everett would also benefit from closer proximity to a roommate with a healthy appetite, watching him enjoying his food, staff moved the other gentleman's bed closer to Everett's bed. Although Everett would drink some of the fluids on his tray, he continued to refuse to eat his meals or even to indicate which foods from the menu he would prefer.

Another aspect of his treatment plan was physical therapy for ambulation and general strength conditioning. Everett was transported by wheelchair to the physical therapy suite where several therapists and patients worked in pairs but often interacting as a group to offer encouragement and appreciation of hard-won gains. Everett refused to get out of the wheelchair. The staff would keep him in the suite until the session was over and then return him to his room. They were hopeful that by observing the efforts and progress of others, most of whom were significantly more physically impaired than Everett, he would ultimately come around and be willing to participate.

The aides assigned to assist Everett with his showering and hygiene chores soon understood that this would be a regular battle. He didn't want them near him and became agitated when they tried to help. He struck out at one aide assigned to help him soap up in the shower. When a second aide reported that he tried to push her away when she attempted to towel dry his back, the nurse in charge had to acknowledge that kindness, patience, and respect were clearly not enough, or not right, for this patient in their care. She had on her hands a defiant, treatment-resistant patient and a frustrated staff. Everett's primary care doctor, the admitting physician, was annoyed with all the complaints from the hospital about Everett and was himself becoming agitated. In desperation, he called for a mental health consult concluding the request with "I don't know what you can do but you better be able to do something before this guy dies, escapes, or is thrown out of the window by the staff."

Consultation process

The consulting mental health clinician began the process by reviewing the notes from the current hospitalization as well as the discharge summary from Everett's previous, aborted stay in the rehabilitation facility. She met with Everett (a brief and focused meeting) for the purpose of explaining to him that she appreciated how difficult it was for him to be in the hospital and that she would work with the staff to arrange for his discharge as soon as possible. She would report back to him as soon as she learned what steps he had to take to allow them to discharge him. She then met three times with each of the staff identified in the patient's chart as having had difficulties with him (nurses, physical therapist [PT], nursing aides, volunteer, dietary aides, social worker, and physician). The initial meeting was intended to gather information, to hear first hand their experiences with Everett and, in the case of the physician, his history with him. The consultant then wrote the "story of Everett" incorporating his pertinent history and detailing how he thinks, feels, and behaves.

The second meeting involved sharing the "story" and clarifying what, from their perspective, the patient would need to do (in terms of observable, measurable behaviors) for him to be discharged to home (the goal) as well as what they believed would need to be put in place for his post-discharge care. The third and last meeting was a group meeting during which a "final report" was presented including what would need to be done to enable the discharge and what would need to be put in place for post-discharge. The consultation with the staff concluded with praise for their flexibility. It was explained that when the patient's "way of being" does not fit with the culture of the system of care, no matter how benevolent the system, and when the patient is unable to be flexible, the burden of flexibility falls more upon the system. This final plan was then presented to Everett and his agreement was secured. A copy of the plan was given to him and a copy was placed in the hospital chart.

Treatment plan

In-patient: Everett would need to show that he would eat the meals provided. The volunteer who was assigned to sit with him during meals was removed. The dietary menu was left on his breakfast tray, with no discussion. His roommate was returned to the opposite side of the room and the privacy curtain was left closed at Everett's bedside.

Everett would need to show that he could safely climb up and down stairs (there were four leading into his house and his house was a two-story house). He would work with the PT on this at a time when they were the only ones in the PT suite. Everett would be taken to the shower room in the evening, after visitors to the hospital had left and the corridor was quiet. The aide would stand outside the shower, only to oversee his safety, and would not engage in unnecessary conversation.

Post-discharge: Meals-On Wheels would deliver a main meal daily. The Visiting Nurse Association (VNA) would visit three times per week, to be reduced to two times per week, and then to one time per week. This decline in services and contact would be contingent upon Everett appearing clean, sober, and well nourished during visits. Everett agreed that he would not purchase alcohol.

His nephew would bring him a limited amount each week. (Everett refused to connect with Alcoholics Anonymous.)

Social Service (Hospital aftercare) would check in after a month to see how the patient was faring with this program. Elder Protective Services was assigned his case to monitor him as an elder living alone in the community who was potentially at risk. It was decided that Everett would see his primary care physician every 3 months or as needed. Beyond these contracted points, Everett would be left alone.

Questions for reflection and discussion

Cluster A includes paranoid PD, schizotypal PD, and schizoid PD. The core organizing feature for paranoid PD is a pervasive pattern of suspiciousness and distrust of the motives of others. The core features of schizotypal PD and schizoid PD are a pattern of detachment from relationships with others and a restricted range of expression. The schizotypal PD in addition evidences eccentric behaviors and perceptual distortions. Mr. Everett showed evidence of all of the dominant features of schizoid PD.

Some questions generated by this case include the following:

◆ What are this person's privacy needs? How might they be met in a hospital setting?

◆ How can he be encouraged to accept help for his medical management and for his instrumental activities of daily living (IADLs)?

◆ How can the staff get close enough to help?

◆ How is this very private person likely to experience the need for mutual interdependence?

◆ What feelings do people with this PD tend to engender in care providers? How might care providers be expected to respond to these feelings?

It is relevant for this type of case to appreciate that people with schizoid PD have a low need for emotional support and connections to other people, nor do they need or desire much feedback from others no matter how concerned or benevolent they may be. As such, the therapeutic relationship with this type of patient is not expected to be intense or emotional. Rather, a focus on pragmatics and helping the patient achieve his goals of maintaining or maximizing independence and privacy is advised. Pushing for an emotional closeness may in fact push the client away as closeness is not what the patient is needing from the clinician. This point was illustrated in the case as the clinician helped the medical staff appreciate the patient's important need for privacy and his distinct aversion to emotional interactions.

Cluster B: narcissistic personality disorder

Case example: Mr. Karl R

History

Mr. Karl R, age 84, entered the skilled nursing facility a year ago. For the first few months he was an agreeable resident, highly socially skilled, undemanding, and always behaving like a gentleman. However, he gradually became irritable and ultimately aggressive. The staff mirrored this progression by, at first, being charmed by Karl, then feeling irritated by his behavior, and finally becoming angry and verbally lashing out at him. More than anything they were baffled by this apparent change in Karl's personality. They felt they did not know how to care for him and requested a consultation.

Karl was the only child of Rita and Karl Sr. His father was a physician, raised in a prestigious suburban community, receiving an elite, private education. After university, before medical school, Karl Sr. proposed to Rita and soon after left for military service. When he returned to civilian life, the couple married and Karl Sr. attended medical school. Following graduation, he accepted a post-degree training assignment in a semi-rural area far away from their families and cosmopolitan roots. It was here where Karl was born and lived until age 12.

Rita did not transplant well in the move from the city to the country. She missed her family and she, unlike her husband, did not have a work life to distract her from her loneliness and boredom. Also, unlike her husband, she was by nature shy and reserved, and did not make friends easily. A large family might possibly have helped, but this was not to be. Rita had experienced a difficult pregnancy, a protracted labor, and complicated delivery with Karl. She was told not to have more children.

As was customary in both their families of origin, Rita and Karl engaged a nursery nurse to care for little Karl directly after his birth. Karl was a gentle, contented baby who grew into an intelligent young child. He was reading at age 3, much to the delight of his "audience." His curiosity was unbounded and the dinner table became a stage for his endless questions. His father encouraged his precocious son especially in the domains of science. He anticipated having another physician in the family. His mother saw in him a handsome lad who learned quickly how to charm and woo her. "Mama, you are so pretty." "Mama, your hands are so soft." "Mama, I love you with all my heart." His nurse, in time, was able to see another side developing in the child. With her Karl was often rude and hurtful. If she dared to confront him or to challenge him too harshly, Karl would run to his mother bearing exaggerated tales of mistreatment, and the nurse would be reprimanded.

Karl was educated at home. There was no private academy near to where they lived, and the local public schools were not acceptable to his parents, thus tutors were engaged. Karl was an apt student and used to being the singular focus of attention, so this arrangement suited him well. His exposure to and experience with other children continued to be limited to social visits between families and summer holidays with the extended families. He found children of his own age to be intellectually inferior and culturally deprived. He clearly preferred the company of adults who found him to be generally charming, referring to him as "the little man."

Progressively, during Karl's early childhood, Rita became depressed and increasingly withdrawn. She would spend most of her days in her room, resting with her eyes closed or reading on a chaise. She came to avoid the dinner table, preferring instead to take her meals in her room. Karl, for his part, continued to seek her attention, but needed to work harder for it. He increased his display of charm and was the only one who could make his mother smile. He entertained her with stories of life outside the bedroom, with anecdotes about the nurse, his father, others in their employ, and visitors to the household. Karl would embellish and fabricate what had occurred, bending and shaping the facts, or creating them. It didn't matter to him. What did matter was to be able to see him reflected in his mother's eyes as a grand and wonderful human being.

Karl Sr., hoping to help his wife recover from her malaise, decided to move the family near to their extended families. He never practiced as a physician again. Financially secure through inheritance, he chose to make changes in his own life. He bought a gentleman's farm and took a post as a biology teacher at a private boys' school. Karl Jr. entered that same school, marking the first time, at nearly 13, that he had ever been in a classroom. He suffered terribly that first year. He was small for his age, not especially athletic, presented as haughty and standoffish, and was the son of a teacher there. The school was situated on the water and sailing was a highly esteemed activity and sport at the school. Karl took to this quickly and, through the sailing club and ultimately the sailing team, he earned an acceptable position at the school. He made no close friends, but between sailing and excelling in his classes, he was tolerated by his classmates, albeit known to them as a braggart, prone to inflate his accomplishments and abilities. Although this behavior interfered with the development of intimate relationships, it made him a somewhat colorful fellow on the campus.

When Karl went on to attend a prestigious university, he developed and refined his persona. His years there allowed him to become an elite gentleman on campus; a bon vivant often at the expense of others. Wealthy, well dressed, charming, with a reputation of being "hard to catch," Karl became a sought after escort for the co-eds. His relationship with his mother had trained him well in how to please, charm, and make a girl feel special. His sailing also earned him recognition, and he continued to excel at his studies. Indifferent to planning his future, which he knew was financially secure no matter what he chose to do, he decided to take the path of going to medical school, thereby continuing a three generation tradition among the men in his family.

At this time, war had broken out and Karl joined his peers presenting himself to enlist, but was rejected. The mandatory physical examination revealed a heart murmur that had not previously been detected. A relatively benign condition (indeed it had never interfered with his sailing or other activities), it was nonetheless cause for rejection by the military. Karl presented himself three times requesting to enlist, even asking to be assigned to desk duty, but was unsuccessful in these efforts. Karl, deeply wounded, demoralized, and ashamed, entered into a serious depression. He spent the next 2 years at home, repeating his mother's behavior a decade earlier. He stayed to himself, mostly in his bedroom where he read and re-read literary classics. He walked the family dog, but kept a low profile in the community, lest he be recognized and identified as an inferior specimen of manhood. After the war, he emerged from his despair and self-imposed exile and began medical school. His old presentation quickly returned, but now a fault line of shame and hostility came to underlie a patina of ease and charm.

Karl did moderately well in his coursework, but was a clinical star as his bedside manner was exemplary. He married the daughter of a family friend, as had his father. His wife was less interested in Karl—his career and love of sailing—than in her horses. The marriage produced no children and ended in divorce after 6 years. Karl went on to have a series of relationships with women, some brief, others lasting years, but never married again. He considered himself a lover of women, but never really loved a woman. He would pursue the most idealized image of a woman, would woo her, win her heart, and thrive on her adulation. When this would wane, as it inevitably did, Karl would become hostile, demeaning, even cruel, and ultimately provoke the end of the relationship. If the woman's feelings were hurt, it did not matter to him. What did matter was that he was recognized as a superior individual and of central importance in her life. This feedback was more easily achieved in his medical practice where his patients did indeed idolize him, perhaps especially the women who sought his attentions and ministrations, contributing both to the robustness of his practice and his sense of self-worth.

As he became older, Karl was looked upon as a nice looking, nattily dressed, and well-to-do sportsman-physician, a prominent figure in the community. Karl's major passion remained his love of sailing, and the friends he claimed were also those involved in the sport. He was a fierce racing competitor and he relished the admiration this brought. When he failed and placed poorly in a race, he would blame the failure on others. He believed that anyone who criticized him was jealous of his accomplishments and superior talents. Clearly not a team player, most of his races were in the solo class.

Karl closed his medical practice when he was in his 70s, selling it to a younger doctor. He was privately pleased to learn that the "new doc" was not able to replace him in the hearts of his former patients. Soon after retiring he developed some worrisome physical signs and symptoms including hand tremors and a significant gait disturbance. His fine motor coordination and especially his mobility became curtailed and he required increasing assistance with activities of daily living. He managed, marginally, with day help until he was 82 when he was hospitalized with a life-threatening pneumonia. He recovered but was left in a very weakened state. At Karl's insistence, upon discharge he was transferred to the finest skilled nursing facility in the region.

Although ostensibly this was for a short recuperative stay, Karl knew that this would become his "final home" and wanted to make certain that it was fitting to his station and style.

Index event

Karl was a delightful resident early on. He occupied a large, private room and would use it much as a salon, engaging the mostly female staff with his stories, displaying what appeared to be genuine interest in their lives. Ever the gentleman, he would always say "please," and "thank you," and smile endearingly when well served, and he expected to be well served. He insisted upon being addressed as Dr. R, politely but firmly correcting anyone who made the mistake of addressing him as Karl. He felt that the other residents were not up to his standards. Many appeared comparatively disheveled. Others talked too softly for him to hear. He dismissed the suggestion that he be fitted for hearing aid, convinced that if others would speak up he would be able to hear perfectly well. He also had problems remembering the names of those to whom he was introduced, or what information they shared about themselves in an effort to strike up a friendship. In reaction to this, he became more isolated in his room, more likely to refuse participation in activities, and more dependent on the sociability and reflected glory of the staff. They could not always give Karl the attention he felt he deserved, and so, over time, he became irritated and then angry. He resorted to the pattern of behaviors he had used all his life, especially with women: at first to engage, charm and win their adulation; when that was waning, to demean them, in order to restore his more powerful position relative to them; express an entitled demanding attitude; and ultimately to behave cruelly and abusively toward them.

Consultation process

Staff: The consultant met with staff before beginning with the patient. At the first meeting, they were asked about how they see him and to identify what they considered the major problems. They were then asked to rank these problems according to their relative salience, and to identify which issues they felt might be the easiest ("least difficult") to address. Discussion ensued about their role in the treatment plan and the critical element of consistency. Their willingness to participate was requested and secured. They all had to be on-board for the care plan to succeed.

The next step was to identify who else might need to be included in the plan. For Karl, this included:

- A psychopharmacologist to assess the role of medication to treat his agitation, anxiety, and probable depression.
- A neuropsychologist to administer testing to assess the degree and type of his probable dementia.
- A neurologist to order and interpret neuroradiologic studies (e.g. magnetic resonance imaging [MRI]).

Treatment plan

Two conceptual models were used to inform the treatment/intervention plan: the goodness of fit (GOF) model and the ABC model. The core premises of the GOF model (Segal et al., 2006) are: (1) personality traits, and their expressions, lie along continua where they can be identified as a style or as a disorder and (2) the identification depends on facets outside of the individual. The dominant factors are: what is being asked of the personality (task), and where is this being asked (context). Each context (actual or the culture of a system) values and devalues specific (manifestations of) personality traits. How well the individual's dominant traits correspond to the traits valued or devalued by the system informs the movement along the style/disorder continuum and defines the GOF with that system. The GOF between the individual and the system affects adaptation to the system, how the individual is experienced and labeled by the system, and the actual care received. The system is in position to shape the expressions of the personality so that it appears less like a disorder and more like a personality style, reflecting a more positive adaptation to the system.

The ABC model, from the behavioral paradigm, includes the identification of **A**ntecedents, **B**ehaviors, and **C**onsequences of the target problem(s).

Patient: The initial meeting with the resident was to establish a relationship and to understand his perceptions of what is working and not working for him in the facility. An additional purpose was to identify if there were any staff members with whom he had an especially positive connection as well as any with whom he felt in conflict. The next step was the identification of goals ("changes") that would help him, what his role as an agent of the change could be, and to get his commitment to the process. He would be asked what pleases him? What does he need that he is not getting or not getting enough of? What disturbs him? The goal was to identify reinforcers that could be used to motivate and reward the efforts he makes to change.

Using both patient and staff reports, the behavior change plan was designed and then presented to the patient and the staff liaison for fine-tuning and contractual agreements. Karl and the staff agreed on two goals: (1) he would participate in one group activity daily (of his choosing) and (2) he would refrain from scolding and cursing the staff. At the end of each "successful" day, he would meet with a staff person (one of his identified "favorites," for a private conversation for about 15 minutes). An activities aide would be assigned to work with him on a special project, designing a guided autobiography ("history of remembrances") of his life.

At the end of a month, the consultant would meet with Karl and with the staff liaison to assess the how well the plan met the intervention goals, where resistance (patient or staff) was encountered, and which reinforcers appeared to be most effective. The consultant would meet with the staff to review whether these changes in the patient's behavior relieved the system adequately or whether additional goals needed to be identified and addressed. Karl would be asked about this as well. This might in time lead to the identification of specific staff in-service trainings that needed to be offered.

Questions for reflection and discussion

Cluster B includes antisocial PD, borderline PD, histrionic PD, and narcissistic PD. The core organizing feature of antisocial PD is a pervasive pattern of disregard for social norms and the absence of empathy and guilt. The core feature of borderline PD is a constellation of extreme instability of relationships, self-image, and affective dyscontrol. The core feature of histrionic PD is a combination of high emotionality and attention-seeking behaviors. The core feature of narcissistic PD is a grandiose sense of self-importance and an illusion of specialness. Karl evidenced all of the dominant features of narcissistic PD.

Some questions produced by this case include the following:

- How might age-related changes affect the presentation?
- What feelings do people with this PD tend to engender in care providers? How might they be expected to respond to those feelings?
- What is a narcissistic injury? Where is this patient's vulnerability?
- What can be done to minimize such injury to people presenting with this type of vulnerability?

Despite the fact that his sense of entitlement came to exasperate the staff, there was also his ability to be charming and engage others on his behalf to be considered. The ultimate goal of the plan, beyond reducing stress in the system and reversing the direction of the patient-staff interactions, was to put his adaptive skills to good use, while diminishing the maladaptive ones.

When he is engaging and endearing, using his considerable wit and a wealth of stories, he is able to get what he needs from those who care for him—namely attention, time, and admiration—and to avoid what is toxic, especially to the narcissistic character, namely shame and indifference.

It is particularly important for clinicians to understand and manage their emotional reactions to patients with this type of pathology. Because of the patient's angry, blaming, dismissive, and interpersonally manipulative and exploitative behaviors, it is likely that patients with narcissistic PD engender in the clinician some degree of frustration, anger, and often frank dislike. Although it may be tempting to supportively challenge the patient and offer corrective feedback, one must first develop an alliance with the patient by aligning with his strengths and acknowledging his accomplishments before he is likely to be able to correct his behavior without perceiving change to be in response to intolerable, shaming criticism. This point was illustrated in the case as the clinician helped the patient to use his adaptive skills to get *what he wants*, without responding angrily to the patient or challenging him too early in the process.

Cluster C: avoidant personality disorder

Case example: Ms. Emma T

History

Ms. Emma T, age 73, was referred by her primary care physician for outpatient psychotherapy. Born and raised in the United Kingdom, Emma was inclined to believe that any trouble with feelings, problems rising from emotions, were to be summarily checked and held close to the vest. Such troubles and problems were shameful. People who suffered these were weak and flawed and were best off to hide this sad fact. The hardest part was that Emma knew at her deepest core that people could tell how very inadequate she was.

Emma had been born in England to older parents. Her mother, Megan, was from Ireland but moved to England to take advantage of a job opportunity. Moving to another country had been especially challenging for her, but she was motivated by the prospect of the increase in wages, as she was the sole support of her mother who experienced poor health and was becoming frail. A quiet and painfully shy soul, Megan's entire life revolved around work, the Church, and her mother. She worked hard at her office job and lived frugally, sending money home regularly to her mother. She did not have the courage to pursue a social life, and thus spent most of her non-work hours alone in her flat. One time a co-worker, a lively young woman, was successful in insisting that Megan go with her to a church social. It was there that Megan met Emma's father, Michael.

Michael came from a hard working family in a city in the north. He, too, came to the London area for work opportunities. His father and uncles owned and ran a small market, and Michael had grown up working at the store, learning all aspects of the business. He was not an apt student, leaving school before entering high school to work with his family at the store. As he came of age to find a wife and "settle down," it was apparent that the store could not support another family. Nearing 30, Michael learned of an opportunity to buy a small store in the East End. Having been a good saver, Michael was able to buy the store outright. It was in dreadful shape and Michael worked endless hours to clean it up, restock the shelves, aiming to reopen it and achieve the attention and ultimately the loyalty of neighborhood customers. It was at this point—relieved, excited, optimistic, and scared—that Michael allowed himself a carefree evening at the church social. Being naturally reserved and cautious, he was able to recognize these same traits in a petite redhead he saw standing at the edge, nearly behind, the refreshments table. He asked her to dance, and over the course of the evening he told her all about his new store which was just at the brink of becoming a reality. Megan listened, so appreciative that she did not need to talk very much. Over the next few months they met after church on Sunday, and walked and talked. Megan felt safe with Michael and told him her story. Through his eyes she felt interesting, appealing, and not at all ashamed.

When they married, Megan left her job and worked keeping books and inventories at the store "just until" the babies started to arrive. They did not for many years when at last, both now nearly 40, Megan and Michael found themselves new parents when first Emma was born and 1 year later her sister, Kate.

Megan stayed at home with the girls and tried to protect these precious beings, so long awaited, from anything that could harm them. They were rarely allowed to play with other children for fear of germs. They were only allowed outdoors to play at a nearby park if the weather was ideal for fear of catching a cold, if it was too cold, or becoming overheated, if it was too warm. They were always well dressed and trained to be quiet and polite at church where they would go as a family every week. The messages were "People are watching and judging," and "The world is an unsafe place so be careful." This very restricted lifestyle suited little Emma's temperament well. She was painfully shy, and would hide behind her mother or father whenever someone would approach her. She would not meet their eyes and became even shyer knowing that others could see her faults and weaknesses. Kate was quite the opposite. A bit of a "handful" and physically larger than Emma, she was usually taken as the older of the two sisters. Emma came to depend on Kate for protection from the outside world. Kate always had many friends, even boyfriends when the she became older, but Emma did not. Emma envied Kate, and longed for the friends and the fun times her sister had, wishing fervently that she were different and that these relationships and experiences could be hers too.

Life progressed unremarkably for both girls until the war years. Everyone during that time was deeply anxious especially during the attacks on the city. Emma, inherently timid and fearful, suffered perhaps even more than those who were hardier. The family lived almost directly across the street from the church and would take cover there during the air raids. Tragedy struck during one such raid, an event which marked Emma's life. She was in the house with her father when the sirens began to wail. Her father wanted to finish something he was doing, so they didn't leave right away, instead waiting until the sirens announced an imminent alert. At that point her father ran from the house, dashing across the street and was struck down by a car, killed on the spot. Emma, following behind, witnessed the horror of this tragedy, and became immobilized at the scene, torn between attending to her father and taking cover in the church.

At the end of the war, Emma's mother sold the store and returned to Ireland where she lived for the remainder of her life. Kate, seeking adventure and to break away from the sadness and trauma of the war years, encouraged Emma to join her moving to the United States. They were able to get good jobs and lived together until Kate became married. Emma then took up living alone, but nearby, and added a cat into her life. She visited Kate often and came to accept Kate's husband as a trusted other with whom she could be at ease. Emma married late in life to an older man she had known for many years through work. When he retired, she retired along with him. Her husband was more socially confident than Emma and would protect her as much as possible from the outside world, as her sister had done.

Index event

Just before her 70th birthday, Emma's husband suffered a sudden, fatal heart attack. Now all the "errands of life" they had previously done together fell to Emma alone. Emma had never learned to drive, but was a sturdy walker and was able to walk to shops or whatever errands she needed to do or to use public transportation if her destination was beyond walking distance. Feelings of panic however began one time when she was crossing a main street. In response, she began to avoid the larger streets in favor of smaller ones, even if this meant extending the route. In time, she felt panic rising while crossing the smaller streets, and so limited herself to the back roads. Arriving at a market after one such journey, Emma hyperventilated and passed out. This led to her being transported to the emergency room of the community hospital where, still anxious and tremulous, she was mortified at being seen in this condition. Emma was no longer able to use the bus because the bus stop was on a main road, which she would of necessity have to cross. She was hemmed in by her fears. Her anxiety escalated to the point where it interfered with her sleep, and she developed an anxiety-related cough, which lead to urinary leakage. Because of this she gave up going to weekly mass at church, to which she could "safely" walk, out of concern that she would smell bad and that she would be shamed. Her sister, alarmed at the changes in Emma's behaviors since becoming widowed, insisted on Emma making an appointment with her primary care physician and accompanied her there, to make certain that what was going on was conveyed accurately to the doctor.

Treatment plan

Establishing a therapeutic alliance with an individual with avoidant PD poses unique challenges. Although nearly desperate for help with her anxiety and fears, Emma would also be exquisitely sensitive to any perceived judgment, feeling exposed and vulnerable and found wanting. Patience and pacing are keys to the establishment of the alliance.

Pharmacology: Emma was referred to a psychopharmacologist who met with her and consulted with her primary care physician. An anxiolytic was prescribed to offer some early symptomatic relief, with the understanding that the psychotherapy benefits would take time. An antihistamine was prescribed to help with a post-nasal drip that was possibly contributing to the "nervous cough." This was taken at night so had the useful side effect of promoting sleep.

Psychotherapy: The sessions were mostly focused on leisurely encouraging and hearing the patient's story deriving her history, symptoms, and the effect these had on her life. The sessions also incorporated simple stress reduction techniques, offered at the beginning and end of the sessions, including for example, breathing techniques, guided imagery, and progressive muscle relaxation. A subjective unit of distress (SUDS) 1–10 scale was introduced to Emma and used in the sessions. The patient was encouraged to practice stress reduction as homework between sessions and to record the impact these had on her perceived distress.

Psychoeducational components included:

1. Construction of a genogram that clearly revealed the hereditable contribution of the constellation of traits and features describing the avoidant personality.

2. Identification of social learning contributions and the contributions of her protective upbringing. Specifically, Emma was able to recognize how the messages from her mother were "absorbed" and how they led to apprehension (before the fact) and self-statements supporting these presumed "facts."

3. Education about the cognitive model, specifically how one's thoughts affect feelings, how feelings affect behaviors, and how behaviors affect our thoughts.

A psychodynamic component was also included in the treatment. When the alliance felt secure and the level of her distress had lessened, Emma was able to explore the core fear of "the road" and how that related to her original traumatic experience of witnessing her father's death. Its meaning of the loss of protection (necessary because she would be recognized as being inadequate), and the validation that the world was indeed an unsafe place were identified as the core message she internalized as a child.

To address the patient's complaints of feeling terribly hemmed in and lonely, a cognitive behavioral plan was proposed and accepted by her incorporating two hierarchies. The first was a hierarchy of the road, progressing from small lanes and roads to main roads, using stress reduction techniques and monitored by SUDS. The patient was in control of the movement from one step to the next along the hierarchy. The second was a hierarchy of the social encounter. This hierarchy was established by the patient, beginning with what she found the easiest (i.e. least anxiety provoking) and progressing to the most challenging social encounter. Her self-statements contributing to her distress, and "disabling" versus "enabling" thought patterns were identified. She was trained to challenge each of these and counter them with new, more adaptive beliefs.

At each session the efficacy of the plan was appraised. There was also a regular check-in time focusing on what was currently going on in Emma's life. Where relevant, these experiences were linked to the hierarchies and to Emma's evolving (changing) image of herself, creating new, positive cognitions. Where progress along the steps of a hierarchy was problematic, either substeps were designed and introduced or repetitions of the last successfully negotiated task were increased.

Questions for reflection and discussion

Cluster C PDs includes dependent PD, obsessive-compulsive PD, and avoidant PD. The core organizing feature of dependent PD is an excessive need to be directed by and taken care of by others. The core feature of obsessive-compulsive PD is an extreme preoccupation with details, for example regarding organization, rules, routine, orderliness, or cleanliness. The core feature of avoidant PD is a pervasive pattern of feelings of inadequacy and hypersensitivity to the judgments and negative evaluations of others, leading to extreme social inhibition. Emma evidenced the features of Cluster C PDs in general (underlying anxiety, fearfulness, and need for control), as well as those specific to avoidant PD: fear of being shamed or attracting the criticism of others, and deep feelings of inadequacy and social ineptness resulting in *avoidance* of relationships or participation in social activities where they might be judged. Emma functioned quite well for most of her life, albeit objectively limited, including coping with war-related hardships and tragedy. However, later in life, with the loss of her protectors, and faced with the necessity of having to alone negotiate "the road," both metaphorically and physically, she became significantly distressed, symptomatic, and came to clinical attention. Her diagnosis of avoidant PD shared features with another Cluster C PD, namely dependent PD, and this is not unusual. However, the core distinguishing feature for Emma was her longing for intimate relationships even as she avoided opportunities to establish these, so great was her fear of being scrutinized, found wanting, and shamed.

Questions for further reflection generated by this case include the following:

◆ What dominant personality traits would you want to recruit/align within the treatment plan?

◆ With this kind of patient, what might be some of the emotional responses of the patient to the therapist reflecting, early important relationships?

◆ With this kind of patient, what might be some of the emotional responses of the therapist to the patient reflecting early, important relationships?

◆ Which evidenced-based treatments should be included in the treatment plan?

As noted earlier, development of the therapeutic alliance with this type of patient presents significant challenges, perhaps most importantly the patient's exquisite sensitivity to any signs of rejection or criticism. Unlike the previous case with the narcissistic patient, the patient with avoidant PD will likely not respond angrily or aggressively to such perceived criticisms but will rather likely withdraw (perhaps flee treatment). This point was illustrated in the case as the clinician did not push hard for change, but rather allowed the patient to set the pace of her changes. In contrast, some clinicians may also respond to this type of patient with feelings of needing to protect the patient and to take care of her. This pull toward nurturance of the patient should be balanced by encouragement of the patient's ability to take care of herself, with a goal of tolerating appropriate independence.

General discussion points

1. Personality disorder symptoms are often ego-syntonic meaning that people with a PD typically do not recognize that their maladaptive traits are part of a disorder. According to O'Connor and St. Pierre (2010), "people with PDs feel normal and at home with their conditions. Their disordered personalities and self-concepts are all they know and remember, and they may value the traits in themselves that are problematic for those around them" (p. 201). The ego-syntonic nature of PDs may be further exacerbated in later life, because the older person has had a much longer history of acting in the dysfunctional way, with the perception that "this is who I am and who I have always been." There is a lifelong press for each individual to "feel like me" even if the supporting thoughts, feelings, and behaviors are maladaptive.

2. People with PDs are not like robots, emitting the same dysfunctional behavioral response over and over again without variation. Although not automatons, older adults with a PD do present with an innate and practiced rigidity, with a narrow repertoire of responses to situations and feelings on which to call. Despite this limited range of responses, the behavioral expressions of PDs are influenced by the context in which the person finds himself or herself. In later life, the challenges and environmental changes may be highly significant (e.g. loss of independence, ill-health, death of a spouse) thereby engendering an emergence of PD symptoms that previously were not present or exacerbating existing PD features.

3. People with PDs are notable for their impairment in the social domain, especially in regard to intimate relationships. In later life, many people with PDs have "worn-out" family and friends and find themselves particularly vulnerable to the challenges of later life, lacking the buffering effects of social support from intimate others.

4. People with PDs usually suffer from co-morbid Axis I clinical disorders, most notably depression and anxiety. The symptoms of the clinical disorders typically precipitate entry into mental health treatment and must be addressed in the treatment plan. Successful interventions directed at clinical symptoms may instil some hope and confidence in the client so that later, more deep, therapeutic work can begin to focus on the underlying PD symptoms. One should also expect some co-morbidity among the PDs, as individuals rarely present with the prototypical signs and symptoms of one PD without having features of other PDs. Co-morbidity is the rule and not the exception.

5. Goals for treatment of the older adult with a PD should be modest and directed more toward helping the person move "from personality disorder to personality style" rather than complete remission of the PD. This implies that in some cases, changes in the environment may be what are indicated rather than directing treatment toward changes in the behavior of the older person with PD. Although the individual's dominant personality traits remain generally constant, how these mesh with the later life context or with what is being asked of them can make these traits either be identified as pathological (as a PD) or as idiosyncratic (as a personality style). The environment has the increased obligation of flexibility as it functions synergistically with the patient/resident who is pathologically inflexible (e.g. with a lifelong PD).

6. Development of the therapeutic alliance between the older adult with PD and the mental health professional is a priority. The wise clinician should expect challenges to the development of rapport and threatened ruptures to the alliance over the course of treatment. The clinician should expect that the client will relate to her in a similarly dysfunctional manner that the client relates to other people in the client's life.

7. Clinicians should pay close attention to the emotional reactions engendered in them by the older client with PD. To do so often provides valuable insights into the types of reactions that other people are likely to have in response to the client and can inform diagnostic hypotheses and therapeutic interventions.

8. The diagnosis of individuals with PDs is more closely tied to cultural expectations than most other types of mental disorders (O'Connor & St. Pierre, 2010). Diagnosing PDs requires that judgments of personality deviance be made with a full understanding of the person's social and cultural context. As such, sensitivity to different cultures is imperative when diagnosing PDs to avoid either overpathologizing normal behaviors or underpathologizing maladaptive behaviors. The understanding of stage of life and cohort effects is also imperative to understand PDs as they present in later life.

References

Abrams, R.C., & Bromberg, C.E. (2006). Personality disorders in the elderly: A flagging field of inquiry. *International Journal of Geriatric Psychiatry, 21,* 1013–1017.

Agronin, M.E. (2007). Personality is as personality does. *American Journal of Geriatric Psychiatry, 15,* 729–733.

Agronin, M.E., & Maletta, G. (2000). Personality disorders and later life: Understanding the gap in research. *American Journal of Geriatric Psychiatry, 8,* 4–18.

American Psychiatric Association (2000). *Diagnostic and statistical manual of mental disorders* (4th edition, text revision). Washington, DC: American Psychiatric Association.

Balsis, S., Gleason, M.E.J., Woods, C.M., & Oltmanns, T.F. (2007). An item response theory analysis of DSM-IV personality disorder criteria across younger and older age groups. *Psychology and Aging, 22,* 171–185.

Balsis, S., Segal, D.L., & Donahue, C. (2009). Revising the personality disorder diagnostic criteria for *Diagnostic and Statistical Manual of Mental Disorders – Fifth edition (DSM-V)*: Consider the later life context. *American Journal of Orthopsychiatry, 79,* 452–460.

Molinari, V., & Segal, D.L. (in press). Personality disorders: Description, etiology, and epidemiology. In M. Abou-Saleh, C. Katona, & A. Kumar (Eds.), *Principles and practice of geriatric psychiatry*. Third edition. New York, NY: John Wiley & Sons.

O'Connor, B.P., & St. Pierre, E.S. (2010). Personality disorders. In D.L. Segal, & M. Hersen (Eds.), *Diagnostic interviewing*. Fourth edition (pp. 201–226). New York, NY: Springer.

Segal, D.L., Coolidge, F.L., & Rosowsky, E. (2006). *Personality disorders and older adults: Diagnosis, assessment, and treatment*. Hoboken, NJ: John Wiley & Sons.

Tackett, J.L., Balsis, S., Oltmanns, T.F., & Krueger, R.F. (2009). A unifying perspective on personality pathology across the lifespan: Developmental considerations for the fifth edition of the *Diagnostic and Statistical Manual of Mental Disorders. Development and Psychopathology, 21,* 687–713.

Zweig, R.A. (2008). Personality disorder in older adults: Assessment challenges and strategies. *Professional Psychology: Research and Practice, 3,* 298–305.

Zweig, R.A., & Agronin, M.E. (2006). Personality disorders in late life. In M.E. Agronin & G.J. Maletta (Eds.), *Principles and practice of geriatric psychiatry* (pp. 449–469). Philadelphia, PA: Lippincott, Williams, & Wilkins.

Chapter 13

Bereavement issues in later life

Gerard J. Byrne

Introduction

Although bereavement and grief are normal accompaniments to later life, they can nevertheless lead to considerable distress for many older people and are sometimes complicated by mental disorder. This chapter deals with the psychological aspects of bereavement in later life and describes assessment and management options. Two illustrative case studies will highlight common presentations.

At the outset, it is worth considering some definitions. *Bereavement* can be defined as the objective state of having lost someone significant as a result of their death. Thus, death of spouse leads to conjugal or spousal bereavement. By contrast, *grief* is defined as the emotional reaction to loss. Grief is a common, although not universal, accompaniment to bereavement. However, grief may occur in many situations involving loss, not just bereavement. *Mourning* is the public expression of grief. Spousal bereavement is a common phenomenon in older people. For example, in the United States, the Census Bureau reported that among persons aged 65 years and over in 2008 there were 2.2 million males (13.8%) and 8.8 million females (41.8%) who were widowed (U.S. Census Bureau, 2008). Thus, there were more than 11 million older U.S. residents who had experienced spousal bereavement at least once. Bereavement is associated with excess *all causes* mortality in both men and women (Schaefer, Quesenberry, & Wi, 1995) and suicide rates are significantly increased in widowed males but not females (Li, 1995).

Attachment theory

Attachment theory (Bowlby, 1969, 1973, 1980) posits that affectional bonds develop instinctively between an infant and his or her caregivers in order to ensure that the infant obtains the necessities of life to guarantee their physical survival and emotional security. Over time, a hierarchy of attachments develops and the infant demonstrates a preference for individuals higher up their attachment hierarchy. Loss of an attachment relationship, whether in childhood or in adult life, leads to separation distress and to other symptoms of grief. The nature and severity of the grief reaction relate both to the state of the attachment relationship prior to the loss and the nature of the loss. Bereavement-related losses generate the most severe grief reactions, particularly the death of a spouse or a child.

Bereavement phenomena

The recently bereaved experience a wide variety of symptoms and several inventories have been developed in an attempt to capture the most prevalent of these. Table 13.1 lists the 22 symptoms contained in one such inventory, the Bereavement Phenomenology Questionnaire (Byrne &

Table 13.1 Twenty-two common symptoms of bereavement

1. Intrusive thoughts about the deceased
2. Distressing thoughts about the deceased
3. Preoccupation with images or mental pictures of the deceased
4. Hallucinations of the deceased
5. Sense of presence of the deceased
6. Dreaming of the deceased as though he/she was still alive
7. Yearning or pining for the deceased
8. Looking for the deceased in familiar places
9. Distress when faced with reminders of the deceased
10. Feelings of sadness about the loss
11. Feelings of unreality following the loss
12. Feelings of anger about the loss
13. Feelings of guilt about the loss
14. Feelings of nostalgia when thinking about the deceased
15. Feelings of anxiety following the loss
16. Feelings of depression following the loss
17. Crying about the deceased
18. Acting as though the deceased were still alive
19. Feeling a need to talk about the deceased
20. Searching for the deceased
21. Physical symptoms such as pain or discomfort
22. A reduced ability to organize one's daily life

Source: Adapted from Byrne, G.J., & Raphael, B. (1994). A longitudinal study of bereavement phenomena in recently widowed elderly men. *Psychological Medicine, 24*, 411–421.

Raphael, 1994). Although some of the symptoms listed are similar to those experienced by people with conventional depressive or anxiety disorders, others resonate better with symptoms experienced in post-traumatic stress disorder. Some bereavement phenomena are rather specific to grief and should be directly explored by the therapist. These include the sense of presence of the deceased, hallucinations and dreams of the deceased, pining and yearning for the deceased, and searching for the deceased despite knowing that they are dead. A sense of mental confusion accompanied by executive dysfunction is also often seen in the recently bereaved. Decision-making is often impaired. The recently bereaved of both genders cry frequently, whereas this is much less prevalent in major depressive disorder or generalized anxiety disorder. The recently bereaved sometimes have had no previous experience of strong grief and may not have the benefit of an extended family in which such things are understood. This is particularly likely to be true in individualistic cultures. Some bereaved persons think they are "going crazy" because of the prominence of hallucinations and the sense of presence of the deceased. Many individuals interpret these phenomena as evidence for the supernatural. Thus, in some sociocultural settings the bereaved may benefit from psychoeducation about normal grief symptoms.

Cluster analysis has recently identified three groups of older bereaved spouses based on ratings on the Inventory of Complicated Grief—Revised (Silverman et al., 2000). These have been labeled common (49%), resilient (34%), and chronic (17%) grief (Ott, Lueger, Kelber, & Prigerson, 2007). Using this approach, chronic grief was associated with higher levels of depression and lower overall mental health. Chronic grief more commonly followed sudden spousal deaths and occurred more often when the surviving spouse had scored higher on a measure of spousal dependency. The resilient group did experience grief symptoms but reported being better prepared for the death and having better social support (Ott et al., 2007). Other work has suggested that pre-loss acceptance of the death presages resilience following bereavement (Bonanno et al., 2002).

Although there is substantial individual variation in the time course of bereavement phenomena, there is generally a marked temporal diminution in grief symptoms over time (Byrne & Raphael, 1994). By 6 months after the death of a spouse, most bereaved persons are feeling substantially less distressed than they did shortly after the death. Kübler-Ross (1969) drew attention to the tendency of grief symptoms to evolve over time, often progressing through stages, which she characterized as denial, anger, bargaining, depression, and acceptance. She took care to point out that this sequence was not invariable and that not everyone experienced each of her stages of grief. Despite these qualifications, her work was popular and her five stages of grief became somewhat reified. Some therapists even tried to force the bereaved to move through these stages seriatim.

Certain deaths have been reported to be particularly distressing to the bereaved. These include unexpected deaths, deaths caused by the bereaved, deaths of children, deaths following prolonged illnesses during which the bereaved was a carer for the deceased, deaths by suicide, deaths in which the deceased's body is not recovered (e.g. missing in action, presumed dead), and deaths following an ambivalent or highly dependent relationship. Anticipatory grief is another challenging issue for the mental health worker. Many people grieve in anticipation of a loss.

There are several forms that pathologic grief can take. In some cases, grief may be prolonged or severe. In other cases, grief may be complicated by mental disorder, including depression, anxiety, or post-traumatic stress disorder. The phenomenology and natural history of major depression are quite different from those of normal grief reactions. In particular, the phasic nature of normal grief with so-called "pangs" or waves of grief is quite distinct from the relative constancy of abnormal affect in most cases of major depression. The symptoms of normal grief diminish over time without treatment and within a few months the bereaved are generally starting to feel symptomatically improved.

As already noted, spousal bereavement is commonly associated with hallucinations, which are variably experienced by the bereaved as either distressing or comforting reminders of the deceased. A sense of presence is often experienced. Bereaved spouses often feel the presence of the deceased in the home. They sometimes feel that they are present in the room or in the bed with them. Bereaved adults sometimes experience heightened sexual desire in the absence of their deceased partner. In some instances, this gives rise to feelings of shame or guilt, even though it is a normal phenomenon.

Normal grief

Normal grief is a consequence of normal attachments and resolves spontaneously over time. Customary cultural rituals should be respected and allowed to run their normal course. In some cultures, these will include ritualized wailing or the wearing of black for a prescribed period. Specific funerary practices may also be prescribed. In some cultures, it is expected that the bereaved will view the body of the deceased, whereas in others this is avoided. Normal grief should not be considered a pathological state and diagnostic labels should be eschewed. There is little, if any, place for psychological or medical intervention in normal grief. Grief counseling is not required for normal grief.

People who have been bereaved, or who have suffered grief reactions as a consequence of other losses, generally undertake what has been referred to as "grief work." This consists of "working through" their relationship with the deceased or other lost object. In clinical work with the bereaved it is important to do the usual things well. If there is clearly a depressive or anxiety disorder present it must be treated in the customary way. Medications, exposure therapy, and cognitive work must all be applied. It is inappropriate to neglect the proper treatment of a bereaved individual who is suffering from a mental disorder on the basis that when their grief resolves their mental disorder will too. In fact, grief work may be impossible for them *until* their mental disorder is suitably managed.

Pathologic grief

Several different types of abnormal or pathologic grief are recognized. These include severe or prolonged grief, complicated grief, and absent grief.

Severe grief and prolonged grief are related constructs as most people who experience severe grief also experience prolonged grief. Estimates vary, but between 10% and 20% of the recently bereaved experience severe and prolonged grief reactions. These individuals often report that the frequency and severity of bereavement phenomena 1 year after the death of their loved one are similar to what most people experience 1 month after the loss. Thus, the normal steady diminution of grief symptoms over the first 12 months does not occur or occurs much more slowly than usual. Severe grief reactions may occur when the bereaved had an ambivalent or highly dependent relationship with the deceased, or when the bereaved considered the death to be unexpected. Curiously, deaths can be considered unexpected even when the deceased has died slowly over many months for an inevitably fatal condition. In other words, the degree to which a death is experienced as unexpected is highly subjective.

Complicated grief generally refers to grief reactions complicated by a mental disorder such as a major depressive episode (MDE), generalized anxiety disorder, or a substance use disorder. Spousal bereavement dramatically increases the risk of a mental disorder. In a secondary analysis of the Epidemiologic Catchment Area study, Bruce, Kim, Leaf, and Jacobs (1990) found that major depression was present in 30.8% of widowed persons but in only 3.2% of married persons. Similarly, Zisook, Shuchter, Sledge, and Mulvihill (1993) found that major depression was present in 20% of older widowed persons at 2 months, in 16% at 7 months, and in 10% at 13 months after the death of spouse. In a cohort study restricted to people aged 70 years and over, Turvey, Carney, Arndt, Wallace, and Herzog (1999) found that 15.3% of recently bereaved men and 13.2% of recently bereaved women met diagnostic criteria for major depression.

Thoughts of death and suicide are quite prevalent following spousal bereavement. In a study of older widowers, we found that 12.3% reported wanting to die at 6 weeks after spousal death and 9.6% at 13 months post-loss (Byrne & Raphael, 1999).

Most experienced clinicians who work regularly with the bereaved recognize that a small proportion appears to experience no discernible grief reaction upon loss of a significant other. Sometimes the therapist interprets the absence of an obvious grief reaction as indicative of delayed grief or hidden grief. However, there may be more prosaic explanations. For instance, many bereaved people are observed to be "holding up well" during the first few days of bereavement. This is often when they are busiest dealing with the immediate sequelae of the death—arranging the funeral and greeting well-wishers. Thus, this is merely a culturally sanctioned pause before public mourning and private anguish are allowed to commence. Less commonly, the absence of grief is indicative of a relationship without an affectional bond, perhaps one in which the bereaved had a psychopathic indifference to the deceased.

Exposure to traumatic events is often followed by emotional distress and sometimes by post-traumatic depression or anxiety. Less commonly, such exposure leads to post-traumatic stress disorder. Bereavements that follow traumatic losses are often particularly distressing.

Bereavement in dementia

The bereaved persons who have dementia may pose a particular clinical challenge. The most distressing situation occurs when each day persons with dementia realize, as if for the first time, that their loved one has died. They may wake each morning and look for their deceased spouse. They may disbelieve those who tell them that their spouse died some time ago. They may be reminded of the death of their spouse through letters of condolence or other memorabilia. Occasionally, something similar may occur when older persons with dementia realize that their parents are dead.

The humane handling of such situations requires tact and discretion, together with considerable clinical experience with people with dementia. Interventions should be negotiated with the person's family or substitute decision-makers prior to implementation. A variety of interventions are possible, including distraction techniques, removal of distressing reminders, and even validation of the person's belief that his/her spouse or parent is still alive. Some interventions may appear counterintuitive and may raise ethical questions, and these should be thoroughly discussed with family caregivers prior to implementation.

Institutionalization is another significant issue that arises for some people with dementia upon the death of their spouse. Sometimes this leads to the revelation for the first time of cognitive impairment that had been concealed from the rest of the family by the gradually increasing provision of support by the deceased.

Of course, persons with dementia may also be the deceased and their family caregiver the bereaved. In this circumstance, the bereaved may have to deal with feelings of guilt in the prelude to the death if they find themselves wishing their loved one dead sooner than appears to be happening. Recent work has demonstrated that anticipatory grief adds considerably to caregiver burden in dementia caregivers (Holley & Mast, 2009). A recent 18-month prospective study of the bereaved caregivers of people with dementia (Zhang, Mitchell, Bambauer, Jones, & Prigerson, 2008) described three main depressive symptom trajectories. Syndromal depression was present in 16.5%, subsyndromal depressive symptoms in 34.0%, and no depressive symptoms in 49.5% of the bereaved. Following the death of the person with dementia, the bereaved caregiver may experience high levels of grief (Sanders, Ott, Kelber, & Noonan, 2008). He/she might also experience a sense of relief, which sometimes leads to self-recrimination.

Case study 1

Eleanor was a 67-year-old literary publisher who was referred by her primary care physician (general practitioner) for treatment of persisting depression following the death of her husband, Ted. Shortly after his death, she had abandoned the family home in rural south-east England and fled to Australia to be with her sister, who lived there. For several weeks after her arrival in Australia, Eleanor's sister had been attempting to persuade her to consult a psychiatrist.

Eleanor had married Ted when she was in her late 30s. He had been a little older at 46. It was her first marriage and his second. He had two children from his first marriage, which had ended in divorce. Ted was the general manager of a highly successful orchestra and frequently toured with it. Eleanor had adored Ted and had relied heavily upon him. In their relationship, she saw him as the organized and dependable one, whereas she saw herself as the artistic and "flighty" one.

Eleanor had been brought up in a scholarly family. Her father had been a lecturer at the London School of Economics and her mother a grammar school teacher. Eleanor felt her parents had been mildly eccentric and quite absorbed by their work. As the youngest of five children, Eleanor had been largely left to her own devices.

After completing high school, Eleanor went on to study English and American literature, finishing with a Masters degree. She quickly found employment with a publishing firm and remained in that industry. Eleanor and Ted had no children together, but she reported that they had greatly enjoyed each other's company.

Eleanor reported that Ted had been somewhat of a cycling aficionado and had enjoyed nothing better than spending his Saturday mornings riding with the peloton through the agricultural patchwork of Sussex. Despite the grueling orchestra schedule, he remained physically fit and was free of significant illness through the first three decades of their marriage. It thus came as a complete surprise to Eleanor when Ted developed the first symptoms of the disease that would ultimately kill him.

Eleanor first noticed that Ted seemed uncharacteristically clumsy about 7 years before his death. After a series of mainly negative investigations, he was referred to a neurologist who confirmed that he was suffering from motor neuron disease. His symptoms progressed rapidly and within 18 months he had no option but to retire from his position at the orchestra. Within another 6 months, Ted was dependent upon Eleanor for assistance with dressing and showering. Ted also developed some difficulty with complex decision-making and Eleanor was forced to take over the management of their investments. Fortunately, he remained cheerful and optimistic, despite the progressive deterioration in his physical status and the concomitant increase in his level of dependency.

Eleanor gave up the publishing job; she loved to care for Ted at home. She found the caring role rather difficult, particularly as she had had no prior experience of this. She read all she could find about motor neuron disease and understood the dismal prognosis. Ted's children from his first marriage were generally supportive but lived some distance away and could not provide any practical assistance. Although Eleanor put on a brave front, underneath she felt increasingly distressed and found it impossible to avoid thinking about the inevitability of Ted's further deterioration and death. She slept poorly and lost weight.

Although Ted was wheelchair-bound and unable to swallow safely, he survived longer than Eleanor had expected. Despite this, when Ted finally died Eleanor found herself taken by surprise. She found it hard to comprehend that he was dead, even though she was at his side to the end. She busied herself with the arrangements for his funeral, which was quite an undertaking, given his long connection with the orchestra. There were many visitors to be greeted and an avalanche of letters and cards to be opened.

Once the funeral was over and the detritus from the wake cleared up, Eleanor found herself alone in the house and alone with her thoughts. Over the next few weeks, she tried to deal with the remaining paperwork but found it overwhelming. She was unable to concentrate and still could not sleep properly. She cried frequently and often felt she could hear Ted's footsteps on the stairs. She had guilty thoughts and felt she should have done more to help Ted. She had no appetite and continued to lose weight. She had frequent suicidal thoughts and even made tentative plans to kill herself.

Eleanor saw her U.K. general practitioner who referred her to a grief counselor. She had several sessions with the counselor but continued to find it highly distressing to live in her house alone. She decided to travel to Australia to be with her older sister Charlotte, who had been widowed about 12 years earlier. According to Eleanor, Charlotte had reconstructed her life quite satisfactorily after the death of her own husband and was actively engaged in a variety of cultural and voluntary activities. It seemed that Eleanor was hoping to escape from the memories of Ted and gain support and advice from Charlotte.

When Eleanor arrived in Australia about 6 weeks after Ted's death, Charlotte made her feel welcome and tolerated her distress for several weeks. However, after this initial period Charlotte resumed her usual busy life and was not prepared to tolerate what she felt was Eleanor's self-indulgent immersion in grief. However, Eleanor was still highly symptomatic. She continued to experience strong waves of distressing emotion and was unable to sleep more than 2 or 3 hours at a time. She had little appetite and overwhelming fatigue. She was unable to concentrate sufficiently to read a novel or watch a television program to its conclusion. She felt desperately depressed and intermittently suicidal.

After much badgering by her sister, Eleanor agreed to see a psychiatrist. The psychiatrist noted that, 3 months after the death of her husband, Eleanor was still experiencing a full complement of grief symptoms in the absence of an improving trajectory. She also noted that Eleanor was experiencing the symptoms of a MDE. She thought the MDE was now worthy of treatment in its own right and might actually be making grief resolution difficult. There was no past history of mental illness or substance use disorder.

The psychiatrist negotiated a treatment plan with Eleanor. Although combination treatment with antidepressant medication and psychotherapy was clearly indicated, the psychiatrist recommended starting with medication. This decision was influenced by the severity of the depressive symptoms, including the presence of neurovegetative symptoms and suicidal thoughts. Among the wide range of antidepressants available, the tricyclic nortriptyline was chosen in this instance, on the basis of its known properties and supporting evidence (see Reynolds et al., 1999). In particular, nortriptyline is the tricyclic antidepressant with the best adverse event profile and the one most extensively studied in older people. Although they are generally preferred for the initial treatment of MDEs, selective serotonin reuptake inhibitors (SSRIs) are not ideal for the treatment of depressive episodes associated with marked insomnia, as is usual in depression-complicated bereavement.

After a pre-treatment electrocardiogram (ECG), nortriptyline was commenced at 10 mg taken at night and titrated upward to 60 mg at night over 3 weeks. To minimize the risks associated with overdose, only small quantities of tablets were prescribed initially. Eleanor reported improved sleep once the dose got to 40 mg and she also reported a dry mouth, a common anticholinergic adverse effect. It took approximately 6 weeks for any definite improvement in her symptoms of major depression to occur and during this time the psychiatrist saw Eleanor weekly for supportive work and to monitor her clinical status, particularly her suicidal ideation.

Although the psychiatrist did not think that formal psychotherapy, such as grief-focused interpersonal psychotherapy, was likely to be effective until some symptomatic improvement in Eleanor's depressive symptoms had occurred, she did recommend that she undertake daily light physical exercise as a basic behavioral intervention. After some resistance was overcome, Eleanor commenced walking for 30 minutes daily in the local area. Once some initial improvement in her depressive symptoms was evident, the psychiatrist also recommended that Eleanor schedule regular pleasurable activities as a social reinforcement strategy.

After about 12 weeks of treatment with nortriptyline, Eleanor's MDE had resolved. Her mood was bright, she was sleeping and eating normally, and she was entirely free of suicidal ideation. She had improved concentration and energy. However, she still experienced pangs of grief whenever she encountered reminders of Ted, and cried occasionally. However, the overwhelming sense of presence and the feeling of mental confusion had resolved. She was enjoying social and cultural activities. Interestingly, she was beginning to tire of Australia and felt that she might be ready to return to her home in England.

With Eleanor's approval, the psychiatrist wrote to her general practitioner in Sussex to report on her progress, her current treatment with nortriptyline, and the advisability of some formal psychotherapy upon her return home. About a month after Eleanor's departure for England, the psychiatrist received a letter from her new psychotherapist indicating that Eleanor had commenced a course of grief-focused interpersonal psychotherapy.

Commentary on case study 1

Depressive symptoms and depressive disorders commonly complicate bereavement. For example, Onrust and Cuijpers (2006) undertook a systematic review and found that during the first year of bereavement almost 22% of widowed persons developed a MDE. Recent evidence suggests that MDEs occurring in the context of bereavement are not significantly different to MDEs occurring after non-bereavement adverse life events. The main implication of this is that major depression occurring in the context of bereavement should be treated in the usual way with the same combination of antidepressant medication and psychotherapy that would be applied if the depressive episode were occurring in other circumstances.

The type of antidepressant to be used is likely to vary according to the past treatment history and current medical status of the patient. However, prescribers need to be aware of the high prevalence of insomnia and anxiety symptoms among people with depression in bereavement. Although the best evidence is for the tricyclic antidepressant nortriptyline, there is no reason to think that other sedating antidepressants might not also be suitable. If non-sedating SSRI medications are used, they will often need to be combined with a benzodiazepine to avoid initial worsening of insomnia and anxiety. In the near future, antidepressants with melatonergic effects are likely to be widely available. If early reports are confirmed, depression-related insomnia may respond better to such agents (Kasper et al., 2010).

The choice of psychotherapeutic modality is also likely to vary according to the particular circumstances of the case and as a product of therapist training and patient choice. Although psychodynamic psychotherapy and cognitive behavior therapy are commonly employed, interpersonal psychotherapy is also worth considering as a treatment for older people with depression occurring in the context of bereavement (Reynolds et al., 1999).

Case study 2

Elizabeth was a 73-year-old retired high school teacher who lived with her 79-year-old husband Gerhard in a rural coastal village. Gerhard had had a middle-ranking position in the financial sector. Although they were by no means wealthy, they did have enough savings to get by on, so long as they were prudent with their spending. They had moved to the coastal village 14 years earlier from the large conurbation in which they had spent their working lives. Their three adult children had been educated in the city but were now scattered widely. Their only daughter was a research scientist whose work had taken her abroad and their two sons were living interstate. Elizabeth and Gerhard felt there were few reasons to remain in the city. They generally only saw their grandchildren when they visited with their parents during school vacations, and then generally only in alternate years.

For the first few years of their retirement, Elizabeth and Gerhard enjoyed the relaxing lifestyle of their new coastal setting. They took up some rural pursuits including fishing and bush walking and developed a small circle of new friends. They worked on their own relationship, which at times in the past had been a little strained.

Their lives in retirement were proceeding fairly well until Gerhard started to lose weight for no apparent reason. He also seemed more easily fatigued on their regular walks around the headland. He had no specific concerns about his health and so put these symptoms down to getting older. He told Elizabeth that he did not want to bother their doctor, whose office was situated a 3-hour drive away on a poorly maintained dirt road. Elizabeth had a niggling concern about Gerhard's reluctance to visit the doctor but pushed it out of her mind. She had not wanted to irritate Gerhard by nagging him about seeing the doctor when his symptoms would probably turn out to be nothing to worry about.

About 6 months after the onset of his weight loss, Gerhard discovered a lump in his armpit. He thought he must have been bitten by one of the insects that were prevalent in the village and was not particularly concerned about it. However, a few weeks later the lump seemed a little bigger and Gerhard thought he should see the doctor about it. A biopsy of the lump was taken and a week later Gerhard was contacted by the doctor's receptionist with a request for an urgent appointment. Gerhard and Elizabeth went to see the doctor together. The doctor indicated that the biopsy had been positive for malignancy and that further tests would be required to establish the extent of the disease. Gerhard was mystified because he had no family history of cancer and had never smoked cigarettes.

Gerhard was referred by his doctor to an oncology unit at a major hospital in the city in which they used to live. This hospital was a 5-hour drive away. Imaging studies revealed disseminated cancer and palliative treatment was recommended. Within another 10 weeks Gerhard was dead. He died in a city hospice with Elizabeth at his side and seemed to have had a peaceful, pain-free death. Elizabeth had stayed in temporary accommodation provided by the Red Cross that was adjacent to the hospice.

Elizabeth was highly distressed at Gerhard's death and blamed herself for not insisting that he visit the doctor at the first sign that something was wrong. Her distress was compounded by the fact that her children were not close at hand and that her friends were now a 5-hour drive away. It took several days for her daughter to fly in from her laboratory in France. Meanwhile, her sons had arrived from interstate and had booked rooms in a city hotel when they could all stay while the funeral arrangements were completed.

Elizabeth found the presence of her children very supportive and managed to get through the funeral and a small wake that they held for Gerhard. Within a few days, however, her children had returned to their busy lives elsewhere and she was back in her coastal village by herself. Her children telephoned regularly but Elizabeth found herself feeling anxious and preoccupied. She began obsessing about her own health and despite the long distance to her doctor's office, made the trip at least once a week. Her doctor found Elizabeth to be experiencing a severe grief reaction with marked anxiety and hypochondriacal thoughts.

There was no mental health or counseling service in Elizabeth's village and the only mental health service within hundreds of kilometres was a flying visit from a psychiatrist and a mental health nurse once a month to the small service town in which Elizabeth's doctor worked. These mental health visitors were very busy treating those with chronic psychotic disorders and had a long waiting list for new patients. Elizabeth's doctor felt somewhat out of his depth, and suggested that Elizabeth contact the hospice where her husband had died to see whether they offered a counseling service. Elizabeth conceded that she had already received a card from the hospice offering counseling or referral, but she had felt too embarrassed to contact them. With her doctor's prompting, she agreed to make contact with the hospice counselor.

Elizabeth telephoned the counselor and admitted that she felt awkward calling her. The counselor told Elizabeth that she was pleased she had called and asked her to tell her how she was managing. Elizabeth could not hold back her tears and it was clear to the counselor that she was in the midst of a severe grief reaction. Elizabeth reported that she had marked insomnia and was not able to get to sleep without hypnotic medication or alcohol. She was greatly disturbed by a sense of presence of Gerhard next to her in bed. She was tremulous and cried frequently, particularly when seeing photographs of them together or when trying to sort through his clothes. She wanted to give his clothes to charity but could not bring herself to even sort through them. She needed to answer the letters and cards that had arrived since his death, but these piled up in the spare room. She felt her brain was "damaged" and wondered whether she was becoming demented. She had little appetite and did not want to cook just for herself. She doubted her ability to safely drive the car, because of overwhelming waves of grief. When these occurred, she had to pull over to the side of the road.

The counselor asked Elizabeth to visit her when she next came to the city. She also suggested to Elizabeth that she take the bus rather than drive. In the meantime, she arranged weekly telephone appointments. During the next of these telephone sessions, the counselor purposely reviewed Elizabeth's strengths and current resources. She noted that Elizabeth was a university graduate who had had a satisfying career as a high school geography teacher. She had experienced adversity before, and considered herself to be someone who generally coped well with challenging situations. She had no history of mental illness or substance abuse. She had three supportive, albeit geographically inaccessible, children. She had a small group of friends in the village in which she lived.

For the next session, Elizabeth traveled by bus back to the city and met with the counselor face-to-face. The counselor reviewed the progress of her grief symptoms and noted that these were still very prominent. She gently suggested to Elizabeth that they review the history of her relationship with Gerhard, both the good and the bad aspects of it. She told the counselor that she and Gerhard had married in their early 20s and that she had interrupted her career as a teacher to raise their three children. After the children were all in high school, Elizabeth went back to work as a teacher. Meanwhile, Gerhard had worked long hours in the city and was often home very late. At times, Elizabeth felt quite unsupported in looking after the children and envious of Gerhard's freedom to work without being concerned about when he would get home. On one or two occasions during the time that their children were young, Elizabeth had suspected Gerhard was seeing someone else, although she had never confronted him about her suspicions. However, this was a difficult period in their marriage and she had felt he was becoming emotionally distant. When it became clear that Gerhard would not rise above the middle ranks in his firm, he began spending more time at home and their relationship improved. Despite this, Elizabeth retained her suspicions of Gerhard's previous behavior. She consoled herself with the knowledge that he earned a reliable income and that, in her mother's words, she might have done a lot worse.

The following session was held by telephone and the counselor felt that Elizabeth sounded a little less distressed. They reviewed Elizabeth's early years. She was the only child of immigrants who fled post-war Europe. She had been quite well educated but the war years had been challenging for her parents. Elizabeth had spent several years of middle childhood with her parents in camps for displaced persons while awaiting resettlement. This experience had left her with a tendency toward anxious obsessionality. Although she had no difficulty learning English, she did not have a wide circle of friends in her adopted country. She met Gerhard at University and soon discovered that his family had also been refugees. She found that she did not have to explain her family situation to him. They were attracted to one another and before long were married.

The following week Elizabeth announced that she had managed to sort through Gerhard's clothes and had thrown out those that were not suitable for charity. However, she had not touched the correspondence that was continuing to mount up. The counselor praised Elizabeth's efforts negotiating this difficult task. They next discussed Elizabeth's parents. Elizabeth reported that her relationship with her parents had been rather formal. Their qualifications were not completely accepted in their new country and they had taken jobs of lower skill level and status than they had hoped. On the whole, they put up stoically with this situation, just as they had during the war years in Europe, although it was clear to Elizabeth that the situation in their new country was aggravating for them. They strongly conveyed their stoicism to Elizabeth and made it clear that they expected the same of her. Unfortunately, after smoking heavily for most of their adult lives, both of her parents died in their 60s from cardiovascular disease. Her father died first, followed shortly thereafter by her mother. By this time, Elizabeth was married with three children of her own. She felt a profound sense of loss and emptiness after both of her parents had died, feelings that she felt were strongly recapitulated after Gerhard's death.

After several more weekly telephone sessions, Elizabeth was feeling safe enough to drive herself to the city for another face-to-face session. The counselor noted that Elizabeth was now sleeping better and that the sense of presence of Gerhard was subsiding a little. Elizabeth was still crying frequently and continued to experience waves of emotion that she found hard to handle. However, she was now starting to tackle the correspondence. The counselor asked Elizabeth about whether she was experiencing any feelings of guilt or anger, as these emotions were known to be relatively prevalent among the newly bereaved, particularly those with severe grief. Elizabeth told the counselor about the guilty recriminations that she continued to feel about not having insisted that Gerhard go to the doctor when they had first noticed that he was losing weight. The counselor explored this issue with Elizabeth, and thought to herself that Elizabeth's relationship with Gerhard might have been one in which not too many questions were asked, lest distressing answers be given.

After about 3 months of mainly telephone contact with the counselor, Elizabeth felt much less distressed and started planning a trip to France to visit her daughter, a scientist at INSERM. By this stage, Elizabeth was sleeping much better and had regained her appetite. She still cried rather easily, particularly at reminders of Gerhard, or when confronted by anything particularly senti-mental in nature. She still had some guilty ruminations, but these were not as prominent as they had been earlier. The counselor left the way open for Elizabeth to make contact with her again, if the need should arise.

Commentary on case study 2

Elizabeth experienced a grief reaction that was more severe than usual. Although speculative, it might be that she had had a somewhat ambivalent relationship with Gerhard, given her concerns about his fidelity earlier in their marriage. Or perhaps she had been sensitized to loss through her upbringing as a displaced person. However, the counselor attached to the hospice was able to identify that this was severe grief rather than complicated grief. This distinction was helpful in devising a management plan that relied mainly on telephone contact.

Telephone contact is a common method of follow-up provided by palliative care services (Mather, Good, Cavenagh, & Ravenscroft, 2008; Field, Reid, Payne, & Relf, 2004). It is suitable for use in both urban and rural settings. Many palliative care services send routine condolence cards that also offer counseling services to the bereaved. In this case study, the counselor conducted supportive work mainly by telephone because of Elizabeth's geographical isolation and initial safety concerns related to driving long distances on country roads.

The question has arisen whether emotional disclosure *on its own* facilitates recovery from bereavement-related distress. The available evidence suggests that it does not (Stroebe, Stroebe, Schut, Zech, & van den Bout, 2002).

Non-pharmacological interventions in bereavement

Over a long period, experienced clinicians have generally been confident that psychotherapeutic interventions make a difference in the management of pathologic grief (Parkes, 1980). However, it has proved surprisingly difficult to confirm this clinical impression in controlled trials. The strong tendency for grief symptoms to improve over time without treatment has meant that control participants often do almost as well as participants in active treatment arms. Treatment modalities that have been examined in controlled trials include psychodynamic psychotherapy (Raphael, 1977), peer support (Vachon, Lyall, Rogers, Freedman-Letofsky, & Freeman, 1980), guided mourning (Mawson, Marks, Ramm, & Stern, 1981), group therapy (Lieberman & Yalom, 1992), interpersonal therapy (Reynolds et al., 1999), complicated grief therapy (Shear, Frank, Houck, & Reynolds, 2005), family focused therapy (Kissane et al., 2006), and cognitive behavior therapy (De Groot et al., 2007). Many studies demonstrate improvements over time without significant differences between treatment arms. The available evidence for all types of psychotherapy in the context of bereavement is, at best, modest. Most studies have been conducted in middle-aged women volunteers and generalization beyond this group might be problematic. A recent meta-analysis of 61 studies (Currier, Neimeyer, & Berman, 2008) concluded that there was evidence of a small effect at post-treatment but no statistically significant benefit at follow-up. This review included 14 studies with non-random assignment to treatment condition and 16 unpublished dissertations. Thus, at present, psychotherapeutic interventions for pathologic grief cannot unequivocally be considered evidence-based treatment. Despite the absence of strong evidence, there obviously remains a place for the humane care of highly distressed individuals.

Medication use in bereavement

There is generally considered to be no indication for the use of psychotropic medication in the course of normal grief. The one exception might be the temporary use of a hypnotic drug for marked sleep disturbance. However, most bereaved spouses would require a hypnotic drug for only a few days. Despite this, many older people are prescribed benzodiazepines to assist in the management of distressing grief symptoms. Warner, Metcalfe, and King (2001) conducted a randomized controlled trial (RCT) of diazepam 2 mg (up to thrice daily) against placebo in 30 recently bereaved older people. At 6 months post-loss, there was no difference in grief symptoms on the Bereavement Phenomenology Questionnaire between the diazepam and placebo treatment arms. So it appears that diazepam does not alter the outcome of grief reactions.

Antidepressants may be indicated in some cases of bereavement complicated by major depressive disorder. Although there are several open-label uncontrolled studies with positive findings, there appears to be only one published RCT of antidepressant medication against placebo in older people with bereavement-related depression. In a 16-week study, 80 older people with bereavement complicated by major depression were randomized to nortriptyline alone, nortriptyline plus interpersonal psychotherapy, medication placebo plus interpersonal psychotherapy, or medication placebo alone (Reynolds et al., 1999). Nortriptyline was superior to placebo and the highest rate of completion was found in participants randomized to nortriptyline plus interpersonal psychotherapy. With four treatment groups, the cell size was inevitably rather small, limiting conclusions about the efficacy of interpersonal psychotherapy. At the time of writing, there was no RCT evidence for the treatment of bereavement complicated by generalized anxiety disorder with psychotropic medication in older people.

Antipsychotic drugs are not indicated for the hallucinatory experiences of bereavement as these are not caused by a psychotic disorder and will resolve over time with no treatment. Indeed, some bereaved people find the hallucinatory voice of their loved one comforting rather than disturbing.

At the time of writing there was no RCT evidence for the use of antipsychotic medication in this situation. The risks of using antipsychotic medication in the absence of evidence of efficacy are likely to outweigh the potential benefits.

Future issues

In the draft DSM-V (Diagnostic and Statistical Manual of Mental Disorders, fifth edition) diagnostic criteria for MDE, it is proposed that the bereavement exclusion criterion be deleted (American Psychiatric Association, 2010). At present, in DSM-IV-TR (Diagnostic and Statistical Manual of Mental Disorders, fourth edition, text revision), criterion E for the diagnosis of MDE states that, "The symptoms are not better accounted for by bereavement, that is, after the loss of a loved one, the symptoms persist for longer than 2 months or are characterized by marked functional impairment, morbid preoccupation with worthlessness, suicidal ideation, psychotic symptoms, or psychomotor retardation." However, the predominance of evidence now suggests that depressive episodes associated with bereavement are not significantly different to depressive episodes associated with other stressful antecedents (Zisook & Kendler, 2007; Zisook, Shear, & Kendler, 2007; Kendler, Myers, & Zisook, 2008; Kessing, Bukh, Bock, Vinberg, & Gether, 2009). Thus, it appears likely that those people suffering from depression as well as grief will finally be recognized by the dominant psychiatric nosology.

Conclusions

Working with the bereaved allows the clinician to enter into the lives of ordinary people when they are at their most vulnerable state. This privilege should be approached with care and maturity. As grief reactions are one of the inevitable consequences of healthy attachments, they should not normally be considered pathologic entities. When pathologic grief does occur, it should be treated appropriately. However, this is not quite as straightforward as one might wish and clinicians should ensure they do no harm. Despite a voluminous literature on bereavement, the evidentiary basis for both pharmacological and non-pharmacological interventions in older people with pathologic grief is still rather sparse. Much of the available research has been of limited rigor and most has been conducted on middle-aged women. Older people and men are seriously underrepresented in the scientific literature. Thus, there is great scope for further methodologically sound research in older bereaved persons.

Points for reflection

1. Consider the pathoplastic effect of premorbid personality on the expression of grief. How might obsessionality or histrionicity influence the presentation of bereavement phenomena?

2. How might the therapist's own past experience of grief affect their approach to the recently bereaved?

3. Consider cultural influences on mourning. How might cultural differences between the bereaved person and their therapist influence the interpretation of grief symptoms?

4. How should the therapist proceed when the evidentiary basis for intervention is inadequate?

Suggested reading

Bowlby, J. (1973). *Attachment and loss. Volume II: Separation, anxiety and anger*. London: The Hogarth Press and the Institute of Psychoanalysis.

Jacobs, S. (1993). *Pathologic grief: Maladaptation to loss*. Washington, DC: American Psychiatric Press.

Raphael, B. (1983). *The anatomy of bereavement*. New York, NY: Basic Books.

References

American Psychiatric Association (2010). *DSM-5 development. Mood disorders.* Available at: www.dsm5.org (accessed 16 October 2010).

Bonanno, G.A., Wortman, C.B., Lehman, D.R, Tweed, R.G., Haring, M., Sonnega, J., et al. (2002). Resilience to loss and chronic grief: A prospective study from preloss to 18-months post loss. *Journal of Personality and Social Psychology, 83*, 1150–1164.

Bowlby, J. (1969). *Attachment and loss, volume 1: Attachment.* London: The Hogarth Press.

Bowlby, J. (1973). *Attachment and loss, volume 2: Separation, anxiety and anger.* London: The Hogarth Press.

Bowlby, J. (1980). *Attachment and loss, volume 3: Loss: sadness and depression.* London: The Hogarth Press.

Bruce, M.L., Kim, K., Leaf, P.J., & Jacobs, S. (1990). Depressive episodes and dysphoria resulting from conjugal bereavement in a prospective community sample. *American Journal of Psychiatry, 147*, 608–611.

Byrne, G.J., & Raphael, B. (1994). A longitudinal study of bereavement phenomena in recently widowed elderly men. *Psychological Medicine, 24*, 411–421.

Byrne, G.J., & Raphael, B. (1999). Depressive symptoms and depressive episodes in recently widowed older men. *International Psychogeriatrics, 11*, 67–74.

Currier, J.M., Neimeyer, R.A., & Berman, J.S. (2008). The effectiveness of psychotherapeutic interventions for bereaved persons: A comprehensive quantitative review. *Psychological Bulletin 134*, 648–661.

De Groot, M., de Keijser, J., Neeleman, J., Kerkhof, A., Nolen, W., & Burger, H. (2007). Cognitive behaviour therapy to prevent complicated grief among relatives and spouses bereaved by suicide: Cluster randomised controlled trial. *British Medical Journal, 334*(7601), 994.

Field, D., Reid, D., Payne, S., & Relf, M. (2004). Survey of UK hospice and specialist palliative care adult bereavement services. *International Journal of Palliative Nursing, 10*, 569–576.

Holley, C.K., & Mast, B.T. (2009). The impact of anticipatory grief on caregiver burden in dementia caregivers. *Gerontologist, 49*, 388–396.

Kasper, S., Hajak, G., Wulff, K., Hoogendijk, W.J., Montejo, A.L., Smeraldi, E., et al. (2010). Efficacy of the novel antidepressant agomelatine on the circadian rest-activity cycle and depressive and anxiety symptoms in patients with major depressive disorder: A randomized, double-blind comparison with sertraline. *Journal of Clinical Psychiatry, 71*, 109–120.

Kendler, K.S., Myers, J., & Zisook, S. (2008). Does bereavement-related major depression differ from major depression associated with other stressful life events? *American Journal of Psychiatry, 165*, 1449–1455.

Kessing, L.V., Bukh, J.D., Bock, C., Vinberg, M., & Gether, U. (2009). Does bereavement-related first episode depression differ from other kinds of first depressions? *Social Psychiatry and Psychiatric Epidemiology*, Aug 20 [Epub ahead of print].

Kissane, D.W., McKenzie, M., Bloch, S., Moskowitz, C., McKenzie, D.P., & O'Neill, I. (2006). Family focused grief therapy: A randomized, controlled trial in palliative care and bereavement. *American Journal of Psychiatry, 163*, 1208–1218.

Kübler-Ross, E. (1969). *On death and dying.* New York, NY: Springer.

Li, G. (1995). The interaction effect of bereavement and sex on the risk of suicide in the elderly: An historical cohort study. *Social Science & Medicine, 40*, 825–828.

Lieberman, M.A., & Yalom, I. (1992). Brief group psychotherapy for the spousally bereaved: A controlled study. *International Journal of Group Psychotherapy, 42*, 117–132.

Mather, M.A., Good, P.D., Cavenagh, J.D., & Ravenscroft, P.J. (2008). Survey of bereavement support provided by Australian palliative care services. *Medical Journal of Australia, 188*, 228–230.

Mawson, D., Marks, I.M., Ramm, L., & Stern, R.S. (1981). Guided mourning for morbid grief: A controlled study. *British Journal of Psychiatry, 138*, 185–193.

Onrust, S.A., & Cuijpers, P. (2006). Mood and anxiety disorders in widowhood: A systematic review. *Aging and Mental Health, 10*, 327–334.

Ott, C.H., Lueger, R.J., Kelber, S.T., & Prigerson, H.G. (2007). Spousal bereavement in older adults: Common, resilient, and chronic grief with defining characteristics. *Journal of Nervous and Mental Disease, 195*, 332–341.

Parkes, C.M. (1980). Bereavement counselling: Does it work? *British Medical Journal, 281*(6236), 3–6.

Raphael, B. (1977). Preventive intervention with the recently bereaved. *Archives of General Psychiatry, 34*, 1450–1454.

Reynolds, C.F. 3rd, Miller, M.D., Pasternak, R.E., Frank, E., Perel, J.M., Cornes, C., et al. (1999). Treatment of bereavement-related major depressive episodes in later life: A controlled study of acute and continuation treatment with nortriptyline and interpersonal psychotherapy. *American Journal of Psychiatry, 156*, 202–208.

Sanders, S., Ott, C.H., Kelber, S.T., & Noonan, P. (2008). The experience of high levels of grief in caregivers of persons with Alzheimer's disease and related dementia. *Death Studies, 32*, 495–523.

Shear, K., Frank, E., Houck, P.R., & Reynolds, C.F. 3rd. (2005). Treatment of complicated grief: A randomized controlled trial. *JAMA, 293*, 2601–2608.

Silverman, G.K., Jacobs, S.C., Kasl, S.V., Shear, M.K., Maciejewski, P.K., Noaghiul, F.S., et al. (2000). Quality of life impairments associated with diagnostic criteria for traumatic grief. *Psychological Medicine, 30*, 857–862.

Schaefer, C., Quesenberry, C.P. Jr., & Wi, S. (1995). Mortality following conjugal bereavement and the effects of a shared environment. *American Journal of Epidemiology, 141*, 569–577.

Stroebe, M., Stroebe, W., Schut, H., Zech, E., & van den Bout, J. (2002). Does disclosure of emotions facilitate recovery from bereavement? Evidence from two prospective studies. *Journal of Consulting and Clinical Psychology, 70*, 169–178.

Turvey, C.L., Carney, C., Arndt, S., Wallace, R.B., & Herzog, R. (1999). Conjugal loss and syndromal depression in a sample of elders aged 70 years or older. *American Journal of Psychiatry, 156*, 1596–1601.

U.S. Census Bureau (2008). *Current population reports* (pp. 20–547).

Vachon, M.L., Lyall, W.A., Rogers, J., Freedman-Letofsky, K., & Freeman, S.J. (1980). A controlled study of self-help intervention for widows. *American Journal of Psychiatry, 137*, 1380–1384.

Warner, J., Metcalfe, C., & King, M. (2001). Evaluating the use of benzodiazepines following recent bereavement. *British Journal of Psychiatry, 178*, 36–41.

Zhang, B., Mitchell, S.L., Bambauer, K.Z., Jones, R., & Prigerson, H.G. (2008). Depressive symptom trajectories and associated risks among bereaved Alzheimer disease caregivers. *American Journal of Geriatric Psychiatry, 16*, 145–155.

Zisook, S., & Kendler, K.S. (2007). Is bereavement-related depression different than non-bereavement-related depression? *Psychological Medicine, 37*, 779–794.

Zisook, S., Shear, K., & Kendler, K.S. (2007). Validity of the bereavement exclusion criterion for the diagnosis of major depressive episode. *World Psychiatry, 6*, 102–107.

Zisook, S., Shuchter, S.R., Sledge, P., & Mulvihill, M. (1993). Aging and bereavement. *Journal of Geriatric Psychiatry and Neurology, 6*, 137–143.

Chapter 14

Effectively using cognitive behavioral therapy with the oldest-old: case examples and issues for consideration

Dolores Gallagher-Thompson
and Larry W. Thompson

Background: setting the context

Within the first half of this century (2005–2050), the number of people 80 years or older through-out the world will increase from 88 million to 402 million (United Nations, 2007). With this rise in the number of oldest-old individuals we can expect a concomitant increase in the number of depressive and other mental health disorders, as well as a marked increase in age-related severe chronic diseases (e.g. cancer, heart disease, stroke, severe arthritis, dementia, etc.), that are often accompanied by increased symptoms of depression. Thus, it is clear that many nations around the world can anticipate substantive increases in health and mental health problems among older adults during this time period. In particular, we can expect larger proportions of older individuals with depression, anxiety, and dementia, which will place an immense burden on the mental health resources of many countries.

Cognitive behavioral therapy (CBT), since its introduction more than 40 years ago, arguably has become one of the most predominant treatment programs used to treat depression and numerous other mental health disorders. By the year 2005, there were at least 16 published methodologically sound meta-analyses that reviewed more than 300 published outcome studies from many countries around the world that have evaluated the effects of CBT in the treatment of numerous psychiatric disorders (Butler et al., 2006). In general, these authors report that the efficacy of CBT for the treatment of depression and many other psychiatric disorders has been documented repeatedly over the past four decades in patients below 65 years of age.

A number of studies have also shown the efficacy of CBT in the treatment of older adults with a variety of mental health disorders (cf. Gallagher-Thompson, Steffen, & Thompson, 2008 for illustrations of work in this area). Of particular relevance for the present chapter is the effective-ness of CBT for the treatment of late-life depression and anxiety, which has been documented as well—even to the extent that CBT for late-life depression is now considered an "evidence-based treatment" for this disorder (Laidlaw, 2006; Laidlaw, Thompson, Dick-Siskin, & Gallagher-Thompson, 2003; Scogin, Welsh, Hanson, Stump, & Coates, 2005; Thompson & Gallagher, 1984; Thompson, Gallagher, & Breckenridge, 1987; Thompson, Coon, Gallagher-Thompson, Sommer, & Koin, 2001). However, virtually none of these published studies enrolled any substantive number of depressed older adults over the age of 80. Generally, the mean age was between 60 and 70 in these outpatient studies. Yet, as noted above, the fact that people are living longer all over the globe, and that depression is the "common cold" of mental health problems, means that practitioners will be seeing clients in their 80s and 90s for outpatient therapy before long. This leads to the question that we attempt to address in this chapter, namely, what data do we have that CBT can be effectively used to treat depression in these individuals? Since there are few clinical trials with this oldest-old age group, we have to draw on the base of "clinical experience" to provide at least a starting point for addressing this question.

What is cognitive behavioral therapy?

A major impetus in the emergence of CBT as an effective treatment modality has been the theoretical and empirical work of Aaron T. Beck and his colleagues (Beck, 1976; Beck, Rush, Shaw, & Emery, 1979). Referred to as cognitive therapy (CT), this treatment emphasizes the importance of identifying and modifying negative unhelpful thoughts that occur automatically, usually in response to negative stressful events or other negative thought constructions. The monitoring of daily activities and the creation of behavioral assignments for work outside therapy were also integral components of the therapy, but more often were employed in the service of collecting evidence for or against the validity of distorted or unhelpful thoughts, and/or to assist in the development of more helpful thought reconstructions. Continued refinement of the model over the years has called attention to the role of behaviors, *per se*, that often are implicated in the development and maintenance of depressive symptoms (Beck, 1987). As interest in CT increased among other researchers, the importance of behavioral functioning increased. Depending on the specific problem under consideration, modification of specific behaviors often received emphasis, which led eventually to the label of CBT. In fact, behavioral activation is often the starting point when treating older individuals with severe depression—and, as we shall illustrate in this chapter, it is often a very effective way to begin to work with the oldest-old.

Although a variety of CBT models are currently in use, our model is derived primarily from the work of Beck et al. (1979) and Lewinsohn, Hoberman, Teri, and Hautzinger (1985). This model emphasizes that depression results from the reciprocal interplay of cognitive, behavioral, emotional, and physiological changes in response to stressful events, which when left untended can lead to a downward negative spiral resulting in a clinical disorder of depression and anxiety. CBT for older depressed patients is time-limited and focuses on changing the negative thoughts and/or unhelpful behaviors as a means of interrupting this cyclical process before its accelerating intensity leads to a clinical dysfunctional state.

Patients learn specific cognitive and behavioral skills that can be used as tools to help them minimize their negative thinking and to employ more constructive behaviors, both of which can reduce symptoms of distress and improve emotional functioning. Of necessity, this is a highly structured approach in which therapists maintain an active and directive role in order to facilitate the acquisition of requisite skills. First and foremost among these is that patients must learn how to monitor their mood, thoughts, and activities during each day in order to identify antecedent and consequent events associated with a particular emotional or behavioral reaction. As patients begin to understand the relationships between events, thoughts, and behaviors, they then learn relevant cognitive or behavioral techniques required to address specific therapy goals.

The development of a collaborative relationship between therapist and patient is crucial to the success of this approach. It starts with attentive listening to patient's complaints, and then working together with him/her to develop potential therapy goals that can be addressed within the time-limit of therapy. The importance of practicing newly learned techniques outside of therapy sessions is emphasized, and compliance with this part of the therapy clearly increases the likelihood that the patient will show substantive improvement in his/her level of distress. Frequently, this will require a concerted effort and considerable patience to overcome barriers to compliance in addressing treatment goals. Therapists must attend to the idiosyncratic nature of patient's problems, his/her overall strengths and weaknesses in dealing with adverse events, and the need to tailor treatment strategies for each individual patient to maximize treatment gains. Although at first glance this therapy may appear as a conglomerate of specific "technical fixes" for particular problems that can be applied pretty much as a recipe is used to create a favorite dish, therapists quickly find that they must understand how each patient attributes meaning to events in his/her world and what the patient does to deal with the distress he/she experiences, in order to develop successful individualized interventions to maximize patient improvement, which is particularly the case when dealing with patients in the oldest age ranges.

Cognitive behavioral therapy with older adults

The "nuts and bolts" of how to do CBT with depressed older adults is well-described in Laidlaw et al. (2003). More recently, a detailed session-by-session protocol has been published in the Oxford University Press "Treatments that Work" series (Gallagher-Thompson & Thompson, 2010—Treatment Guide; Thompson, Dick-Siskin, Coon, Powers, & Gallagher-Thompson, 2010—Workbook). This is a three-phase program designed to be delivered over the course of 16–20 sessions, depending on the general capabilities of each patient. Key aspects of this program are described below. With patients who are frail, cognitively challenged, or are suffering from significant co-morbid health problems—which is typically the case with the oldest-old— additional sessions are usually needed for acceptable symptom reduction.

The first phase of the treatment, which is usually comprised of two to three sessions, focuses primarily on orienting and engaging the older patient in the therapy process. Psychotherapy is often a unique experience for older individuals; it requires a new way of thinking and acting as they learn the expectations and general procedures of this unique relationship. Target complaints that brought the person into treatment need to be explored, and one or two that are likely to be addressed successfully within the time-limited period of therapy need to be focused on, so that specific treatment goals can be formulated. Some time must be spent explaining the rationale of this approach, and how therapy will progress. Particularly if the patient has engaged in other psychotherapies it often is necessary to explain how this therapy is different. The patient needs to understand that this is a structured time-limited approach that will require him/her to be actively engaged in learning new skills and practicing these outside of session. The therapist needs to develop an empathic positive relationship with the patient that will engender the expectation of a positive outcome in therapy. Finally, additional history may be required to complete assessment and by the end of the third session or so the therapist should have developed a conceptual formulation of the patient's problems, issues, and initial plan for techniques required to address the patient's therapy goals. This formulation is likely to change as additional information about the patient's thinking process and behavior becomes available.

The next 8–12 sessions are used to help the patient learn appropriate skills to help him/her to achieve high priority treatment goals. The success of doing so typically increases patient's confidence in his/her ability to deal with similar complaints in the future. Available tools may involve learning how to modify thinking through the development of rational reconstructions, increase pleasurable behaviors, or decrease unpleasant life events through problem solving, modify the intensity of emotional states with relaxation or other behavioral techniques, and improve effective communication in situations where conflict resolution is needed. Not all available strategies are covered in this phase. The patient and therapist collaboratively decide on the techniques to be learned that will address therapy goals most effectively. As noted earlier, some form of behavioral activation is most often a starting point with patients in their 80s to help get them energized and involved in the therapy process.

In the final three to four sessions, the focus is on preparation for termination and on reviewing what was learned during treatment, in order to develop specific reminders to help the patient maintain the gains made in the therapy. Often this is a difficult period for older individuals, as the therapeutic relationship may be one of the few relationships they have to offset loneliness. It is often useful to space these session out to help the patients adjust to loss of the therapist and to try out some of the new skills while they still have a connection with the therapist. Development of a written "maintenance guide" to help the patient deal with future stressful situations is a key component of successful termination. It includes referrals of patients to community-based services when possible, to augment the gains made in therapy—for example, to increase socialization and decrease loneliness, one goal during therapy may have been to link the patient into the local senior center, with the aim being that regular attendance will continue after therapy ends.

Issues in providing cognitive behavioral therapy to the oldest-old

There are three major issues that complicate the implementation of the CBT protocol described above: (1) significant co-morbid health problems; (2) presence of some type of impairment in cognitive processing; and (3) the absence of a strong support network. When these are found in combination, as they frequently are in this age group, they present challenges to even the most well-trained CBT therapist. These issues will be illustrated with case examples and a description will be provided of the therapists' attempts to address them.

Co-morbid health conditions: Mary and John

"Mary" was a white widowed woman who was referred by her primary care physician for treatment of depression that she believed was associated with Mary's worsening physical health status. Mary began therapy at the age of 82 (about 3 years ago). At intake she was diagnosed as having major depressive disorder, recurrent, based on her history of several prior episodes during her adult life. There was no evidence of any form of cognitive impairment. She lived independently, drove to appointments, and was always well groomed and articulate in sessions. She had been trained as an elementary school teacher and after her three daughters were grown she went to work in that field. She retired at age 65 but retirement was not a positive thing for her: she missed her work life and soon had to provide significant care for her chronically ill husband at home. After his death (when she was 80) she realized how alone she was: she described being psychologically estranged from her daughters, although she had some contact with the grandchildren as they were growing up. At intake, she clearly was physically frail—she was significantly underweight, did not eat regular meals, had several different medical conditions that required frequent medical visits, regular laboratory testing, and often, changes in her medications that had untoward side effects. She was taking antidepressant medication as part of her regimen but said it had not helped her (although she continued to take it).

Initially, she was very receptive to the CBT approach and seemed eager to learn about how her thoughts and behaviors contributed to her "down" moods. She understood the model and was able to see how it applied to her. She readily engaged in the therapeutic relationship and agreed to do homework between sessions. Goals included developing relationships with persons her age (beginning with involvement in the local senior center) and repairing relationships with her adult daughters, if possible. Behavioral activation seemed to be an appropriate place to begin, and she was asked to complete an activity schedule on a weekly basis, as well as a questionnaire about potentially enjoyable activities that she could incorporate into her everyday life. However, it quickly became apparent that she was not able to keep appointments on a regular schedule: visits to her physician always took priority over therapy sessions. She was hospitalized several times during the course of the treatment as well (for medical emergencies), so that it took about 18 months to complete 20 sessions with her. The fact that there were so many interruptions in treatment made it difficult to maintain a consistent focus and as a result, progress was slow, and remission was not fully achieved. This is reflected in scores on the Beck Depression Inventory (BDI) II: she started at 35 at intake and got down to a score of 20 at the conclusion of therapy; although this is a significant improvement, it is still in the depressed range. However, Mary said her mood was "better, most days" and that she knew at least some things to do to maintain her mental health. On examination of the BDI, it was found that she scored high on virtually all of the somatic items—this may have been due to her health problems, and not indicative of depression *per se*. There was more improvement on the psychological items reflecting sadness, pessimism toward the future, and the like.

Over the 18 months, we did work on increasing her engagement in positive experiences with non-family members. She was able to establish friendly relationships with several neighbors; she took classes at a local adult school; and she attended the local senior center 2 days a week. Thus, the behavioral activation component of therapy was able to be implemented effectively. However, we were not able to progress to completing thought records or using other tools to examine her dysfunctional thinking with regard to her estranged relationships with her daughters. This was very difficult to implement due to the inconsistency of the sessions and the fact that she was reluc-tant to go into the matter in detail, fearing that she would, somehow, alienate them all the more. Therapy ended when Mary entered an assisted living facility, which was deemed medically neces-sary due to her declining health and gradual loss of ability to provide adequate self-care. Several follow-up phone calls were conducted after she moved into the facility: she indicated she was "making an adjustment" but felt badly that her daughters did not visit her. She expressed a desire to have "a supportive person to talk to" if possible, so the CBT therapist located a "friendly visitor" program in the community that provided periodic supportive contacts in the assisted living facility. At the last follow-up call, Mary reported that she was "doing all right" in the new setting and actually was relieved that there were people to help take care of her as her needs changed over time. This meant she would not have to rely on her daughters, who remained out of the picture as far as their mother was concerned.

Was this a successful outcome? Given the circumstances, the answer seems to be "Yes, but ..." On the one hand, Mary was able to obtain more pleasure from her daily life, despite her medical limitations, and was relatively more active than most women her age—at least for the time she was in CBT. On the other hand, the long-standing conflicts within her family were not addressed, and continued to bother her, as reflected in her depression score at the conclusion of therapy. It is also not clear whether she will be able to establish friendships in her new residence, and/or continue to engage in potentially pleasurable activities on a regular basis. It is possible that with-out regular therapy—even though it was quite intermittent—she will lose the reinforcement that the therapist provided and her depression will again increase. It is also possible that with contin-ued decline in her health and functional abilities, she may become significantly depressed again in the future.

The case of "John" indicates that a more complete course of CBT can be accomplished with an older gentleman who had significant medical problems (comparable to those of Mary) and whose adults sons were "there" to provide emotional support and to reinforce the aims and procedures of CBT.

John was 85 years old when he was referred for CBT by his primary care physician, who had referred other patients for CBT and found it effective in treating co-morbid depression. John was a highly educated, white, widowed man who had worked in several professional careers during his lifetime. He retired at the age of 70 but still remained active in the organizations and activities associated with several of these fields. He was very "computer literate" and was pleased to report that he read the NY Times online every day. His wife had died when he was 75; they had a wonderful marriage, by his report, and had raised two sons, both of whom lived in the area and with whom he was in regular contact. It was his wife's death that precipitated John's becoming depressed. He says that he'd been in that single episode of major depression since that time; he took medication for this but said it did not help much. At intake, there was no evidence of cognitive impairment but there was evidence of concomitant anxiety such that he had a secondary diagnosis of generalized anxiety disorder. He had severe heart disease and was in remission from prostate cancer. As with Mary, he had multiple and frequent medical appointments, laboratory testings, and changes in his medication to contend with. However, unlike Mary, he kept virtually all therapy appointments as scheduled, rarely canceling or asking to re-schedule because of competing medical appointments. This was notable considering that he was skeptical about therapy at the outset and did not believe it would help him—he came only on "doctor's orders" and said that he doubted he would complete more than three or four sessions. His skepticism was reflected in his direct questioning of the qualifications of the therapist (Dolores Gallagher-Thompson [DGT]) who was female and considerably younger than him: he studied the degrees and license on the office wall, and announced that he would "give it a try since you are a nice person and remind me of my wife."

Given his high level of education and his agile mind (along with the skeptical attitude noted), CBT was explained to him as an opportunity to "learn something new" about himself—specifically, to learn methods to manage his moods better so that he did not have to remain in therapy any longer than necessary. He was told that the therapist could help him use his life experience to deal with his current issues, and that we would not focus on "toilet training" or "how he felt about his mother when he was boy." These are comments he raised in the initial sessions that needed to be dealt with by education in the CBT approach. Finally, he agreed to a "trial run" of four sessions. John acknowledged periods of acute discomfort due to his anxiety attacks and was more comfortable starting with this than working on his depression. He understood that undue stress was not good for his heart problems and so, from a medical perspective, he was able to "buy in" to the therapy. Treatment, therefore, began with relaxation training which took about four sessions to complete. He utilized a combination of music, deep breathing, and what he called "refocusing" to reduce his perceived anxiety, and felt that he was successful in this effort. The completion of these four sessions coincided with the end of the "trial run" at which time he agreed to continue in CBT, and to work on his depression.

The next phase of therapy was difficult and required persistence and creativity on the part of the therapist. John was reluctant to examine the thoughts that apparently fueled his depression, namely that he did not provide adequate care for his wife before her death; that he was "nobody" without a job and an income; and that he was destined to be a "lonely old man" who would become more and more of a "burden" to his sons. He did not want to complete thought records, preferring to discuss examples verbally. However, without taking notes or having thought records to refer to, he often went over and over the same material, without any apparent progress. He claimed "you can't teach an old dog new tricks," that his mind was "made up" about these things and that the therapist should "stop arguing" with him about this. The usual CBT techniques of guided discovery and Socratic questioning were not effective with this patient because he went off on tangents and into philosophical discussions about the issues. There were only two methods that had success with him: (1) examining the evidence: he learned to make lists of evidence "for" and "against" his negative thoughts and was able to keep these lists in a notebook that he could add to between sessions and (2) assigning ratings of the degree to which he believed his negative thoughts before and after he examined the evidence. Over time, he was able both to reduce the intensity of his negative beliefs, and to reframe some of the more important ones, such as: "I believe that I did the best I could for my wife; I wish there would have been more to do but medical science had not advanced far enough so that I could help her more" and "I have some meaningful things to do with my time—it's not the same as working and earning a living, but I have my retirement funds so I really don't need the money. I can do more of what I like to do now." Achieving these changes took 26 sessions to accomplish.

To prepare for termination, John was asked if one or both of his sons (whose families he spent considerable time on weekends) could be asked to join for a few sessions, with the idea that if they understood their father's tendency to think so negatively about himself, and to become highly anxious over small things, perhaps they could learn to reinforce the adaptive coping strategies John had learned in therapy and thereby help him to avoid relapse. He liked that concept and selected his oldest son to come in; the son was eager to help, had been treated himself with CBT for depression secondary to a job loss, and quickly saw how the specific coping skills worked on would be useful to prevent relapse. The son attended four sessions together with his father and pointed out several ways that he could reinforce what John had learned. Two final sessions with John were spaced out, about 4–6 weeks apart, to determine how he would do without regular therapeutic contact and with the son's support. These went well; a final 6-month follow-up call revealed that John continues to do well and is not in need of further therapy. His BDI score had been 32 at intake and was 15 at termination. As with Mary, much of the score was due to high ratings on the somatic items. Although his health did not decline significantly over the course of therapy, he had persistent sleep, appetite, and fatigue problems that were quite troublesome to him.

Was this a successful outcome? Many clinicians would say "Yes . . . but" (but with fewer qualifications to the "yes") with this individual. Thirty-six sessions (spread out over a 2-year period) were required for a positive response; this is considerably more than the "standard" protocol. In addition, his BDI did not get down to the "normal" range, and although he made progress in reframing some of his persistent negative thoughts, others remained and probably will give him problems down the road (such as "being a burden" to his sons). Although one son willingly engaged in several sessions, John was reluctant to ask him to do anything specific. It is possible that over time, the son will get busy with his own family's demands again, spend less time with his father, and that source of positive reinforcement will diminish. If that is the case, then John's depression may worsen and he may again need professional assistance. It is also possible that a health crisis may exacerbate his condition: he may be the one needing care (vs. providing care to his beloved wife) and that kind of dependency will likely be very difficult for him to tolerate. It is the therapist's opinion that considerably more time (perhaps another year) would have been needed to delve into these issues, but this was not practical, given the constraints of insurance coverage and the fact that the original goals had been met to a reasonable degree. Therefore, termination was done by "mutual consent" although one could argue that more CBT would have been beneficial to this patient.

Contrasts between Mary and John

In the opinion of the authors, John had the more successful outcome, and this appears to be related to several factors: (1) his commitment to therapy, despite skepticism at the beginning; (2) his family's support (as evidenced by his oldest son's participation in several treatment sessions), and (3) his relatively stable health status—although he had serious health problems, he suffered no notable decline during the time he was in therapy. In contrast, Mary's decline in health and her several medical emergencies (with the concomitant scheduling problems and the frequent re-scheduling of sessions) made it much more difficult for her to participate fully in the therapy.

The lack of family support and the strained relationship with her daughters were significant factors in her continuing to be depressed, despite some very real gains in CBT. The move to an assisted living facility provided both opportunities and challenges to her mental health.

Points for reflection about Mary and John

1. How might the course of treatment with Mary been changed in a positive or negative way by more directly addressing her lower commitment to attend regular therapy sessions? Paradoxically, was it her easier acceptance of the benefits of therapy and greater faith in its benefits that allowed her to not see difficulties with missed sessions?

2. In all therapy cases, there is arguably a point of "diminishing returns." At what point in your own mind would you have felt comfortable terminating therapy with John?

The role of the family in cognitive behavioral therapy

In our experience with other patients aged 80 and above, the important role of the family cannot be overemphasized. Family support can greatly enhance the CBT process, whereas family criticism or dismissal of the therapy can prove to be quite damaging. Unfortunately, there is little written in the mainstream CBT literature about how to evaluate and/or involve family members in the treatment of depressed individuals of any age, so we are "learning by experience" and hope that sharing this experience will be of value to other practitioners and stimulate research in this area.

We recommend that inquiries be made about who is in the family, where they live, what the quality of these relationships is like, and what level of involvement the older patient has with each family member (or friend, or "significant other" if actual family is not available). This information is not likely to be covered in a standard intake and so time may need to be set aside in the first appointment to obtain it. It is also helpful to ask whom the elderly patient turns to for support and what kind of support (emotional, instrumental, financial) is provided by each person. Many older individuals will mention friends or neighbors (not family members), pets, and/or clergy as sources of support as well (or in lieu of) family members. We have treated many patients in their 80s and 90s who report that they are closer to their cats or dogs than to any people in their lives. At any rate, "family" may include any of the above. However, of greatest relevance here is finding out whom the older patient feels closest to, who they turn to for help and support, and who the patient lives with and spends leisure time with. It is these individuals who may be either a help or a hindrance to the therapy.

In our clinical work, we have found that a surprising number of older adults move out of their homes and familiar surroundings to be nearer to their adult children and grandchildren. However, the relationship they envisioned with these individuals often does not materialize, and depression ensues. In the most common case, the adult children are working outside the home, have their own friends and interests, and experience stress in their marriages and jobs, so may have little left over to give to their aging parents—particularly a parent with significant depression who may be difficult to be around. Past history is also important here: if the relationship was generally positive, the son or daughter may be more inclined to try to include their aging parent(s) in their lives, but if there was significant conflict and turmoil in the past, then it is unlikely the parent will be welcomed with open arms. A related issue is just how much involvement an older person can anticipate having in the lives of their grandchildren (or great grandchildren, as the case may be). He/she may be too frail to provide babysitting services or have so many health problems that it is not wise to be around active children or teenagers whose antics could precipitate a fall, or intensify the stress the older person experiences on a daily basis. In most healthy relationships a process of role negotiation occurs, to sort these things out and give the older person a place in the family. However, if relationships are strained, this may lead to numerous negative cognitions and increased negative mood.

In the best case scenario, the adult child is willing to help the aging parent and is supportive of the patient being in therapy. The adult child will also help to reinforce the messages and approaches used in CBT—as was illustrated in the case of John. Other examples include an older bipolar woman who came to live with her adult daughter following a mental collapse after the sudden death of her husband. The daughter had married late in life but still had children of her own, who were under 5 at the time the mother moved in. The patient Jane found that being with the children exacerbated her mood swings to such an extent that the daughter sought treatment for herself and her mother, to learn how to best handle the situation. They were seen together for 10 sessions of CBT focused on techniques for managing the situation. Jane's bipolar disorder generally was stable as a result of her medications but it became unstable when Jane spent too much time with the children which caused her daily schedule and routines to be disrupted. The daughter was willing to track her mother's responses carefully for a 2-week period to determine what triggered the mood swings. Once that information was available, the family was able to problem solve how, when, and under what conditions Jane could be with the children without experiencing significant mood fluctuations. An adjustment was also made to Jane's medication which helped to resolve the issue. In this case the daughter was very proactive in seeking treatment; she said she had done a lot of research on the Internet and learned that CBT was effective in the treatment of bipolar disorder, so she sought it out for herself and her mother (see Reiser et al., 2008, for more case examples of the effective use of CBT with older bipolar patients). Although this may not be a common occurrence, it does happen, and this example illustrates how the active involvement of the daughter improved the mother's response to a CBT treatment approach.

Other examples that can be shared are not as positive as this one. For instance, in several cases, with the patient's permission and encouragement, adult children were invited to participate in "family meetings" to discuss the impact of a particular co-morbid condition of the depressed parent (such as intense anxiety in certain situations). However, family members do not always see eye to eye on how to handle these matters (e.g. "give her another pill, there must be something for anxiety" without realizing the potentially negative side effects of common anti-anxiety medications) and that can only confuse or inflame the situation. We have learned that "family meetings" are best held only after the therapist has met with the family members individually and had the opportunity to inquire about where they stand on whatever the critical issues are that are to be discussed.

In one complex case, the issue arose as to whether or not the older depressed patient (a man in his 80s who occasionally got lost while outside his familiar area) should be allowed to continue driving. This is a common question that adult children raise, often out of concern for insurance rates and/or liability in the case of an accident, as well as genuine concern for the parent. For the older adult, particularly the depressed older adult, driving may be one of the few ways he/she can express independence and get out to do enjoyable activities with other people. If this privilege were taken away by the family (not a physician or the motor vehicles department) this could intensify both immediate and longer-term depression. However, this is an issue that can raise strong feelings on both sides. The case of Mr. Z illustrates this dilemma. This 92-year-old gentleman developed a depressive reaction to learning that his wife had full-blown Alzheimer's disease and could not longer be the partner that he cherished. Mr. Z's son wanted him to continue driving as long as possible, so that he could take Mrs. Z to the Alzheimer's day care center, and get out once a week to spend time with his "buddies" at the senior center, but Mr. Z's daughter wanted to put an end to the driving, saying that her father was "too depressed" to have this kind of responsibility. In this particular case, Mr. Z was also becoming concerned that he might be developing dementia and himself questioned if perhaps he should stop driving. He said that the criticism from his daughter was very disconcerting and made him doubt himself. This issue then became the focus of therapy. The therapist did not see any clear evidence of cognitive impairment in his responsiveness to CBT but to collect more conclusive evidence on this matter, the patient was referred to a neurologist, who found him normal. He was then referred to a neuropsychologist for more fine-grained evaluation. It was found that Mr. Z did have some short-term memory loss but this was regarded as within normal limits and not a cause for concern. His other test results were similar. In addition, his primary care physician had not diagnosed him as having any form of dementia. Therefore, once all the data had been collected (that entire process took about 3 months to complete), a family meeting was held to share the information and allay their fears. As predicted, the son was relieved but the daughter was not convinced. She thought it was just a "good idea" for a person of his age to stop driving. After considerable discussion of the pros and cons, with much tension during the meeting, the son offered a solution that seemed to assuage his sister and reassure his father: he agreed to purchase a GPS system for Mr. Z and teach him how to use it. This proved to be an excellent solution, and Mr. Z no longer got lost while driving. This positive outcome markedly improved his depression and reduced his anxiety. It should be noted here that the therapist learned from this experience (which could have turned out unsuccessfully had the daughter not modified her thinking during the meeting)—it may be preferable to work individually with distraught family members who could otherwise undermine the work to be done. If time and insurance coverage permit that to occur, we have learned from other patients as well that this is a good way to hear the concerns of family members and hopefully to provide them with psychoeducation about the issues. When there is a greater likelihood of consensus being achieved at the family meeting, then it can be very useful to have the meeting and thereby solidify the family's support for the patient.

Common barriers to participation in cognitive behavioral therapy

In our experience with very elderly patients, there are many potential barriers to consider and to try to overcome whenever possible, so that the individual can really engage in CBT. The most common is lack of reliable transportation to the therapy location. In the case of a 90-year-old depressed woman treated by the first author, for example, therapy was ended abruptly when the husband had a stroke and became very disabled and in need of considerable home care. Mrs. H was no longer able to come in for sessions since she did not drive and was too fearful to take public transportation or arrange for outreach type transportation services.

A second very common issue is family interference with treatment. A 95-year-old woman was "taken out" of therapy by her adult daughter who felt she should have electroconvulsive therapy (ECT) because she was "too depressed all the time." However, the daughter was unable to find any psychiatrist in the area willing to administer ECT to a woman of that age; despite this fact, she refused to bring her mother back for therapy appointments, telling the therapist by phone that it was a "waste of time" despite the therapist's efforts to encourage her to give CBT a chance. In other cases, the family members knew of another treatment that they thought should work and was less expensive or time-consuming, such as acupuncture, or herbal remedies, or they had seen a particular medication advertized on television and wanted that medication, and that *alone*, to treat their depressed relative.

A third issue that unfortunately is all too common is the presence of some kind of elder abuse—most frequently, verbal abuse and/or fiduciary abuse. For example, a case of fiduciary abuse became apparent in the course of CBT with an 85-year-old widowed patient who lived with her adult son. This necessitated involving adult protective services, who removed the patient from the home and placed her with her daughter who lived in another state and was not aware of the situation—this was a good outcome for the patient but it effectively terminated the therapy.

A fourth and final issue that can markedly interfere with effective engagement in CBT is the presence of mild-to-moderate cognitive impairment in the patient. For this reason, it is always recommended that a brief cognitive screening measure be routinely incorporated into the intake or first appointment (see Laidlaw et al., 2003 for fuller discussion of this issue). Although screening measures are far from perfect, they do give a quick idea as to whether or not further neurological and/or neuropsychological assessment may be needed. This issue is covered in detail in Chapter 2 in the therapist's guide (Gallagher-Thompson & Thompson, 2010) referred to earlier.

Cognitive behavioral therapy with cognitively impaired, depressed individuals

A detailed case example is now presented that will illustrate the challenges when doing effective CBT with patients with mild-to-moderate cognitive impairment. Jim is an 86-year-old widowed white male who was diagnosed by his primary care physician (about 6 months prior to starting CBT) as having "mild dementia." He was put on Aricept for its treatment. The physician also suspected depression was present, as Jim struggled to understand what was happening to him and to adjust to it, and referred him for therapy. The intake diagnosis was dysthymic disorder due to his history of having had a low-grade depression more or less continuously since his wife's death about 10 years prior to his coming for therapy. At the first session, Jim indicated that he did not have much education, did not understand about dementia, but was fearful that he would soon not be able to take care of himself. He lives independently and is able to get around on his own, though he reports having few interests or hobbies and said he had virtually no friends left. Most had predeceased him or were in nursing homes. He has three adult children in the area but they all have significant mental health problems and are in no condition to care of him, even in his present condition. His BDI was 20 at intake and his mental status screening measure showed mild-to-moderate cognitive impairment. For CBT this is a challenge since so much of the therapy depends on learning new information, being able to take a perspective on oneself, write things down for homework, and remember to do all of this on a regular basis. There are no empirical studies at this time indicating if CBT can be effective when deficits in these types of cognitive capabilities are present, and if so, what modifications are needed to enable the patient to derive at least some benefit from treatment.

CBT began with psychoeducation about dementia and the likely rate of progression, plus the fact that Aricept has been shown to slow this progression in several research studies. This was somewhat reassuring to him and he agreed to continue. Given Jim's lack of engagement in regular pleasant activities, and lack of socialization opportunities, behavioral activation was the first CBT component to be implemented. He was asked to keep an activity log for a week. He tried to complete it, but despite successful accomplishment in session, he brought it back just with X's marked in several of the blank spots on the form; nothing was written in the boxes (as he'd been instructed to do). The form was reviewed and re-assigned for homework, but the next week, it was still filled out incorrectly: this time there were comments in most of the boxes but not information on what activities he had engaged in during the time blocks. Jim said he could not remember the instructions and so just wrote whatever came to his mind. This indicated to the therapist that creativity would be needed to develop assignments, as well as simplified instructions and "memory aides," so that Jim could complete his home practice assignments. Following the suggestions contained in Coon, Thompson, and Gallagher-Thompson (2007) about adapting homework for cognitively impaired persons, a form was developed that contained a list of positive activities that Jim said he liked to engage in (such as preparing his own home cooked meals; watching sports on TV; and going to church on Sundays). Across the top were the days of the week. Jim was instructed to make an X or a check mark for the days when he did each of these things. This assignment he could complete successfully. When queried at the next session about the activities, his verbal report seemed to corroborate what was on the form. However, he often forgot to bring the completed form with him to the sessions; to deal with this problem, a brightly colored, labeled file folder was prepared for him and he was asked to keep all his therapy papers in it, and to put it by the front door of his apartment, to remind him to fill in the boxes each day and to remind him to bring it with him to the appointments. This worked well most the time. Subjective mood ratings on a 1–10 scale were used instead of more formal (and intimidating) questionnaires, to track progress. Over time his mood improved, and it was clearly associated with his doing (or not doing) the positive activities on his list. Given this strong association, which he clearly was able to see himself, this assignment was continued for 16 more sessions.

These sessions were held biweekly. On the "off week" the therapist called him to remind him of the homework assignment and also to remind him of the date and time of the next appointment. This proved very helpful after several appointments were a "no show" due to his having forgotten to check his calendar.

Some cognitive reframing was also accomplished with Jim when we decided (at about session 8) to spend some time in virtually every subsequent session discussing two issues that bothered him: (1) helping him to accept that he had done all he could for his adult children and reinforcing that he was not responsible for them anymore. These were beliefs that waxed and waned; they seemed to be associated with his Christian faith in that he was able to see that "God's will" was responsible for much of this and so it was not his fault that they had their own problems to deal with; (2) helping him plan ahead for the future when he would need more care in his everyday life. He was encouraged to work with a social worker to explore options for assisted living in the future, and he did so. Meanwhile, he was found to be eligible for in-home supportive services and the social worker arranged this for him, so that he had some assistance with medication management and other complex tasks in his daily life. This was empowering to some extent in that he saw that he was able to get some things done: he was persistent, followed through, and was able to achieve good outcomes. The final two (planned) sessions were spaced out so that they functioned as "booster sessions"—Jim reported that he taped the pleasant activities list to his refrigerator so that he would remember to do the things on the list. However, he also said that he thought he "should be writing down" when he did them (as he'd done in therapy) and was afraid he'd get out of the habit if he did not have continued appointments. Once approval was obtained to continue with him, he was put on a monthly maintenance schedule and that continues to the present time. He appears to be holding his own in terms of his depression while his dementia seems to have progressed somewhat since the start of therapy. His last BDI was 10 (however, it took him almost 30 minutes to complete the questionnaire) and his most recent mood rating was 7 (with 10 being "best ever").

Was this a successful outcome? Again, most would say "Yes, but ...." Jim's mood improved and he has learned several skills to compensate for his memory and learning deficits. He appears to be more "at peace" with his family situation and is clearly doing more everyday pleasant activities. However, he needs ongoing support and reinforcement to maintain these gains. Attempts are being made to find a community resource that can provide that for him, but to date, that has not been successful. It appears that he may continue on a "maintenance dose" of CBT for some time to come.

Jim's experience in CBT is quite typical of patients with some form of cognitive impairment. They need to learn strategies to compensate for their losses, and they need to use their strengths to remain engaged in life as much as possible. The absence of a supportive family or network of friends in Jim's case is not typical, however; in fact, most older adults with dementia are cared for by family members, in the home setting (National Alliance for Caregiving/AARP, 2009). Often, in the later stages, family members accompany the patient in for therapy. In many instances, CBT becomes more of a form of "couples" or "family" therapy so that the needs of the primary caregiver can also be addressed. Many dementia patients find it reassuring that their family member participates in therapeutic discussions, and they in turn learn ways to support the patient better in the home environment, and to manage their stress more effectively.

Points for reflection about Jim

1. Would the outcome likely have been better for Jim if he'd had family that could be counted on to help and support him as his cognitive decline increased over time? In what ways could family have been involved in the CBT, given their own mental health problems? As Jim's dementia progresses, are there other services (e.g. adult day care) that could be recommended, to help maintain his function? Is that part of the role of the CBT therapist in these cases— namely, to refer to social service and other community-based programs likely to be of assistance?

2. Does this case suggest that there might be some forms of cognitive processing skills that are more important than others, for adequate participation in CBT (such as problem-solving ability, and attention and concentration skills)? What are the clinical implications? For example, should all patients with known cognitive deficits be tested by a neuropsychologist, whenever possible, before initiating CBT, so that a fuller description of their cognitive strengths and weaknesses is available, for the therapist to use in treatment?

Summary and clinical recommendations

Although it is very true that CBT can be effective to treat moderate levels of depression in very old adult outpatients, as evidenced by the case examples presented here, CBT may require more sessions than is typical, and more creative problem solving on the therapist's part, to engage and retain these very old patients in treatment. Practical problems such as transportation and scheduling need to be dealt with on an individual basis, and the health status of the patient must be inquired about and adjusted for—particularly for those patients with significant medical co-morbidities. In addition, the role of the family (along with any part they will play in the therapy) needs to be assessed at the outset and re-assessed as therapy progresses. As well, the presence of mild-to-moderate cognitive impairment signals that therapy will take longer, move more slowly, and have many challenges along the way.

Taken together, these observations suggest that CBT should be used cautiously with patients over 80 who have significant health issues and/or mild-to-moderate cognitive impairment concomitant with their depression. We recommend that CBT be initiated on a trial basis and that four to six sessions be held to evaluate the extent to which it is likely to be responded to effectively by each particular patient with these characteristics.

In about one-third of patients referred to the authors for therapy, only one or two sessions took place, and then the patients discontinued on their own. Follow-up phone calls with patients who discontinued indicated reasons such as: they did not feel comfortable with the explanation provided of what CBT involved, or they did not feel they could make the commitment to come in for regular sessions over a sustained period of time, or they really felt they needed a different kind of help.

Others wanted only a "supportive listener" and not a true therapist. For example, both authors have had experience with patients who just want someone to talk to, and who do not want to do the work of CBT. This becomes apparent when trying to delineate goals, or when discussing the expectation that home practice will be done between sessions to foster learning and therapy gains. When patients say they don't have any goals except to "feel better" and despite one's best efforts, no specific goals can be set, or when patients say they simply will not be able to do any home practice assignments between sessions, these are therapeutic "red flags" that CBT is not likely to be successful and perhaps an alternative therapy should be considered. Those who are medically unstable are not likely to be able to fully participate in CBT (even if they want to) due to unexpected health declines, medication reactions, required tests, and frequent medical appointments. This is more likely to happen with increasing age, so unless the therapist can be extremely flexible with the timing (and location) of appointments, these are patients who perhaps should be referred for another form of therapy. On the other hand, a CBT approach with more limited goals may be appropriate and helpful to such patients—although full remission from the depressive episode may not be achieved due to the intermittent nature of the therapy contacts. Finally, in our experience, patients with extensive social work needs (housing options; how to get a financial benefit they feel they are entitled to, etc.) are usually not able to engage in CBT until these needs have been met. For those individuals, completing work with the social worker first may be necessary before CBT commences.

In conclusion, the CBT therapist who works with the oldest-old needs to recognize that at the very least, the following modifications to "standard" CBT will be needed with virtually every patient:

1. Linkages to community resources. Although some therapists might see this as falling into someone else's job duties (e.g. a social worker), we have found that making such referrals an integral part of your CBT enhances its effectiveness.

2. Scheduling phone call "check-ins" in between sessions. These reinforce home practice and provide encouragement and support. Calls can be relatively brief (5–10 minutes) and should remain focused. Patients are grateful for the follow-up and in our experience they do not abuse this privilege by trying to turn it into a mini-therapy session.

3. More sessions, extended over a longer period of time, seem to be the norm. It seems unrealistic to expect anyone but the most healthy, non-impaired patient to be able to complete the full course of CBT in 16 sessions over a 4-month period of time. Although length of therapy, and timing and frequency of sessions, are individual decisions made with each patient, it seems reasonable to plan for a longer treatment interval, and to recognize that sessions will probably need to be spaced out over time to enhance effectiveness.

4. Active involvement of the patient's support network whenever possible. Although this is not without its pitfalls, it can be of great value for maintenance of gains and relapse prevention.

5. Respect for, and knowledge about, the patients' medical condition, their medication regimens, and their functional limitations, are essential for CBT to succeed since these issues present realistic problems and limitations that have to be dealt with and/or that require adaptations to be made. Having the patient's permission to communicate with the primary physician, as well as specialty providers as needed, we believe to be a key component of the success of CBT.

6. Finally, the therapist's recognition that full remission may not occur in all cases; however, significant symptom reduction is possible, along with improved quality of life, for most very old patients who actively engage in CBT.

Acknowledgment

This work was partially supported by grant #RO1-MH37196 to LWT and grant #UO1-AG-13289 to DGT. The authors are grateful to Dr. Ken Laidlaw for his thoughtful comments on an earlier draft of this chapter.

References

Beck, A.T. (1976). *Cognitive therapy and the emotional disorders.* New York, NY: International Universities Press.

Beck, A.T. (1987). Cognitive models of depression. *Journal of Cognitive Psychotherapy: An International Quarterly, 1,* 5–37.

Beck, A.T., Rush, J., Shaw, B., & Emery, G. (1979). *Cognitive therapy of depression* (p. 425). New York, NY: Guilford Press.

Butler, A.C., Chapman, J.E., Forman, E.M., & Beck, A.T. (2006). The empirical status of cognitive-behavioral therapy: A review of meta-analyses. *Clinical Psychology Review, 26,* 17–31.

Coon, D.W., Thompson, L.W., & Gallagher-Thompson, D. (2007). Adapting homework for an older adult client with cognitive impairment. *Cognitive and Behavioral Practice, 14,* 252–260.

Gallagher-Thompson, D., & Thompson, L. (2010). *Treating late-life depression: A cognitive behavioral therapy approach—therapist guide.* Oxford: Oxford University Press.

Gallagher-Thompson, D., Steffen, A.M., & Thompson, L.W. (Eds.) (2008). *Handbook of behavioral and cognitive therapies with older adults.* New York, NY: Springer.

Laidlaw, K. (2006). Psychological treatment for depression and anxiety in older adults. In C.P. Freeman & M.J. Power (Eds.), *The handbook of evidence-based psychotherapy.* Chichester, West Sussex, UK: John Wiley & Sons.

Laidlaw, K., Thompson, L.W., Dick-Siskin, L., & Gallagher-Thompson, D. (2003). *Cognitive behaviour therapy with older people.* Chichester, West Sussex, UK: John Wiley & Sons.

Lewinsohn, P., Hoberman, H., Teri, L., & Hautzinger, M. (1985). An integrative theory of depression. In S. Reiss & R.R. Bootzin (Eds.), *Theoretical issues in behaviour therapy* (pp. 331–359). New York, NY: Academic Press.

National Alliance for Caregiving/AARP (2009). *Caregiving in the U.S.* Washington, DC: MetLife Foundation.

Reiser, R., Truong, D., Nguyen, T., Wachsmuth, W., Marquett, R., Feit, A., et al. (2008). Cognitive behavioral therapy for older adults with bipolar disorder. In D. Gallagher-Thompson, A. Steffen, & L.W. Thompson (Eds.), *Handbook of behavioral and cognitive therapies with older adults* (pp. 249–263). New York, NY: Springer.

Scogin, F., Welsh, D., Hanson, A., Stump, J., & Coates, A. (2005). Evidence-based psychotherapies for depression in older adults. *Clinical Psychology: Science and Practice, 12*(3), 222–237.

Thompson, L.W., & Gallagher, D. (1984). Efficacy of psychotherapy in the treatment of late-life depression. *Advances in Behavior Research and Therapy, 6,* 127–139.

Thompson, L.W., Gallagher, D., & Breckenridge, J.S. (1987). Comparative effectiveness of psychotherapies for depressed elders. *Journal of Consulting and Clinical Psychology, 55,* 385–390.

Thompson, L.W., Coon, D., Gallagher-Thompson, D., Sommer, B., & Koin, D. (2001). Comparison of desipramine and cognitive/behavioral therapy in the treatment of elderly outpatients with mild-to-moderate depression. *American Journal of Geriatric Psychiatry, 9,* 225–240.

Thompson, L.W., Dick-Siskin, L., Coon, D.W., Powers, D.V., & Gallagher-Thompson, D. (2010). *Treating late-life depression: A cognitive behavioral therapy approach—workbook.* Oxford: Oxford University Press.

United Nations (2007). *World population prospects: The 2006 revision.* New York, NY: Population Division, Department of Economic and Social Affairs.

Chapter 15

Values, validity, and ethical angst: assessment of mental capacity in older adults

Bret L. Hicken, Angela Plowhead, and William Gibson

Introduction

Mr. W is 79 years old and lives independently in his own home with his wife and two adult sons. A poor student as a child, he dropped out of school during the ninth grade. At the age of 16, he found a job at a local Army base where he worked as a general laborer and painter for 39 years until he took medical retirement at the age of 55. Now at 79, he has multiple chronic health problems and takes several medications prescribed by a primary care physician (PCP). However, Mr. W has a long history of poor adherence to medications, a frustration to his doctor who has consulted with several community agencies for help. Over the last 2 years, Adult Protective Services, the county health department, and a home health service have visited his home. All found his living conditions to be unsanitary and potentially unsafe and several questioned whether he should be managing his medications himself. The PCP requested an evaluation from a psychologist to determine whether Mr. W is "competent."

These consults are common for psychologists practicing in medical settings but similar questions may also occur in outpatient settings with a large proportion of geriatric patients. With aging populations in many Western countries, such questions about capacity among older adults will surely increase. In the United States, for instance, Alzheimer's dementia occurs in 6–10% in persons aged 65 and older and in 47% in those older than 85 (Kukull & Ganguli, 2000). With an anticipated 47% increase in the 85 and older population the next 50 years (United States Department of Veterans Affairs, 2003), we can anticipate a significant increase in the number of older persons with impaired capacity, which has the potential to affect health care delivery on a grand scale. Therefore, geropsychologists must be familiar with the principles of capacity evaluation in order to respond to questions about patient capacities.

Two terms are important to differentiate for the purposes of this chapter: capacity and competency. The terms may be used interchangeably in the literature; however, each has a distinct meaning with related implications for clinicians. In the United States, competency is a legal term, with incompetence being determined by a court of law (Barbas & Wilde, 2001; Kim, Karlawish, & Caine, 2002). Capacity, in contrast, refers to specific abilities to make decisions or act in a specific domain. Thus, "competency" is comprised of many individual skills or "capacities." This chapter concerns the evaluation of several individual mental capacities that are commonly evaluated by geropsychologists.

A multivariate concept

Grisso (1986, 2003) and later Moye (2000, 2003) described a conceptual framework outlining components common to all legal capacities:

- **Functional component** Activities that an individual can actually do on a daily basis including the knowledge, understanding, or beliefs necessary to act. This domain is broadly defined to include functional abilities (e.g. a formal assessment of one's ability to manage money or medications), behaviors (e.g. day-to-day observations of one's abilities), and cognitive skills (e.g. thinking, communicating, memory, judgment).

- **Causal component** Inferences that explain apparent deficits in an individual's functional abilities related to an area of capacity. Causal factors of incapacity may be permanent (e.g. traumatic brain injury) or temporary (e.g. delirium) and an explanation of such factors is essential to ensure that consequences of a judgment of incapacity are appropriately applied.

- **Interactive component** The interaction between functional abilities and the environment in which they are utilized. An absolute measure of ability is insufficient to determine incapacity. Rather, the context in which the person must function determines the abilities essential to the specific capacity in question.

- **Judgmental component** Expert decision regarding capacity based on an evaluation of the discrepancy between an individual's functional abilities and the context in which he or she operates. The evaluator determines whether any discrepancy is of sufficient magnitude to warrant a finding of incapacity.

- **Dispositional component** A determination of incapacity may deprive an individual of rights to make decisions. Thus, an evaluation of capacity must also consider dispositional consequences of a finding of incapacity.

Capacities commonly evaluated in older adults

This chapter focuses on four capacities that are commonly questioned in older adults: medical decision making, independent living, financial, and testamentary. We have labeled these abilities as "mental" capacities because they are predominantly cognitive in nature and their evaluation is concerned primarily with underlying thought processes as opposed to physical abilities. Certainly, physical disability can limit one's ability to function in some of these areas (e.g. a person with severe arthritis may have difficulty writing checks), but physical impairment is not as primary a criterion for incapacity as it might be for other capacities (e.g. driving).

- **Medical decision-making capacity** Four functional abilities are considered relevant to medical decision making (Appelbaum & Grisso, 1995). *Understanding* refers to the ability to comprehend and remember information about a treatment including risks, benefits, and expected outcomes. Patients demonstrate understanding by paraphrasing the information related to diagnosis and treatment (Wong, Clare, Gunn, & Holland, 1999). *Appreciation* is the ability to consider the diagnosis, treatment, and potential outcomes in the context of personal values and goals. *Reasoning* is the ability to use logical thought processes to compare and weigh treatment alternatives, benefits and risks, and the potential effects of treatments on functioning. Patients should be able to indicate major rational factors behind their decisions and the relative importance of those factors in the decision process. *Expressing a choice* refers to the ability to communicate a preference and maintain choice stability so that a choice can be acted upon (Grisso & Appelbaum, 1998).

- **Independent living capacity** The new American Bar Association/American Psychological Association (2008) handbook on capacity assessment in older adults notes that legal standards for capacity to live independently are not clearly defined. In the United States, state guardianship laws offer some guidance, typically citing at least one of four capacity "tests": (1) the presence of a disabling condition; (2) functional deficits limiting ability to meet needs to live independently; (3) cognitive problems; and (4) failure of less restrictive alternatives. Functionally, these tests may be evident in persons who are dependent on others for care but cannot delegate responsibility; make, communicate, or implement decisions; understand the risks and consequences of behavior; manage self or property; perform or obtain services; or protect self.

- **Financial capacity** Financial capacity is conceptualized as a broad continuum of activities associated with specific skills (Hebert & Marson, 2007). Griffith et al. (2003) proposed a model of financial capacity that includes nine domains: basic monetary skills, financial conceptual knowledge, cash transactions, checkbook management, bank statement management, financial judgment, bill payment, knowledge of assets/estate, and investment decision-making. Each general domain consists of specific underlying tasks required to demonstrate capacity in that area. For example, the "basic monetary skills" domain comprises several tasks including "counting coins/currency."

- **Testamentary capacity** The International Psychogeriatric Association recently published guidelines for expert evaluation of testamentary capacity. Based on English case law, the guidelines stipulate five general criteria: (1) understanding the act of making a will and its consequences; (2) understanding the extent of one's assets; (3) comprehending and appreciating the claims of those who might expect to benefit from the will, both those to be included and excluded; (4) understanding the impact of the distribution of the assets of the estate; and (5) the testator is free of any disorder of mind or delusions that influence the disposition of assets (Shulman, Peisah, Jacoby, Heinik, & Finkel, 2009). Testators only need to have testamentary capacity at the time the will is executed; they may lack testamentary capacity before and after the will is written. They do not need to demonstrate capacity to manage other affairs or financial activities (American Bar Association/American Psychological Association, 2008).

Complexity of capacity evaluation

The four cases that follow illustrate the complex nature of capacity evaluation. Except in cases of extreme and obvious impairment, persons with questionable capacity often have subtle and equivocal deficits that decline at different rates and are influenced by different contextual factors. Capacity is often unquestioned until a particular decision or goal conflicts with decisions or goals of others with a vested interest in a patient's well-being. The case of Mr. G, for instance, concerns the testamentary capacity of a man whose family members only questioned this ability after he decided to change his will to exclude family members from an expected inheritance.

It is common to question capacity in these situations and it is incumbent upon the evaluator to sort through the competing values and interests of different stakeholders to determine the "truth." Stakeholders include the patient, of course, but may also encompass other important entities including family members (both close and distant), friends, treatment providers, and health care systems. As many of the following cases demonstrate, these entities sometimes have values and goals that are in conflict. Ultimately, most questions about capacity emerge from a conflict of values, which must be understood to properly render a decision.

Physicians have difficulty assessing capacity and are often unprepared to evaluate cognitive issues in their patients (Marson, Ingram, Cody, & Harrell, 1995). Even clinicians experienced in assessment of capacity in older adults may disagree in their judgments (Marson, McInturff,

Hawkins, Bartolucci, & Harrell, 1997) suggesting that capacity evaluation is neither intuitive nor simple. The case of Mr. D presents an illustrative example of this challenge. Clinicians' own values, experiences, and training may have a significant impact on their judgments of capacity. To improve reliability, numerous instruments have been developed to assist evaluators to obtain more objective or standardized information about patients' capacities. The cases in this chapter utilize a variety of instruments, including vignette-based tools, skills, or functional tests, standardized question sets, and cognitive testing.

Finally, a finding of incapacity will typically encroach upon an individual's civil rights in order to protect that individual and other people. Furthermore, an incapacitated individual creates a new set of responsibilities for family, medical providers, and social institutions. Often, minor interventions can be introduced to maintain individual civil rights to some degree. Therefore, a determination of incapacity should also consider the implications of that finding on the patient and others. For example, in the case of Ms. P, a determination of incapacity resulted in specific plans for her children and her medical providers.

Case studies

Case study 1: Mr. W

As discussed in the introduction, Mr. W was referred for an evaluation of capacity after a long history of poor medication adherence. The evaluation, which took place in Mr. W's home, revealed an extensive psychiatric history that included a current prescription for medication to treat schizoaffective disorder. During the interview, Mr. W was dirty and unkempt but he was polite, pleasant, and cooperative. His speech was extremely circumstantial and tangential; his responses were often almost incoherent and he was very difficult to redirect. At times, his thought processes appeared delusional and illogical. For example, Mr. W believed that he was responsible for the recent deaths of some people because he had "prayed for snow."

Mr. W was able to report his medical diagnoses and current medications but his understanding of both of these was clearly limited. For example, he believed his antihypertensive medication was also a source of vitamins; he switched asthma inhalers to protect the ozone layer; his olanzapine helped his lungs; and he described schizophrenia as "something in the brain that grows." Mr. W had run out of olanzapine 2 weeks earlier but he expected to get a refill at his next psychiatry appointment, though he did not know if or when that appointment was scheduled. The only symptom he had experienced since stopping olanzapine was the "flu" and he did not feel like the medication was necessary anymore.

Mr. W was generally unconcerned about taking medication, believing that his physicians are merely worried that his non-adherence "messes up their record keeping." His medication bottles were all over his bed mixed with old bottles and garbage. The psychologist had him read the labels to explain the purpose of each medication. He picked up an apparently full bottle of olanzapine and said it was for his gastroesophageal reflux disease (GERD) but after reading the label several more times he realized that it was for schizophrenia. He explained that when the medication had arrived, he had thought it was for GERD so he had thrown it on the bed without looking at it.

Mr. W provided a tour of his home, which was extremely filthy with large floor areas that were rotted away and "repaired" with cloth and duct tape. He showed his living space, which was reduced to a third of the living room. The area around his bed was cluttered with empty boxes and trash. Mr. W remarked that he'd had an infestation of rats and mice, but that he had spread rat poison all over the floor, which cleared up the problem. He found 17 dead rats throughout the house. He then asked if it was ok to take rat poison in place of a blood thinner. He explained that a neighbor had told him that one of his antihypertensives was the same type of blood thinner used in rat poison so Mr. W wondered if he could save money by using that instead of buying medication. He said he did not know how much he would need to take, and further indicated that he was a little afraid to take it.

Mr. W completed the Repeatable Battery for the Assessment of Neuropsychological Status (RBANS), demonstrating deficits in learning/immediate memory (5th percentile), visuospatial/constructional (3rd percentile), language (30th percentile), attention (<1st percentile), and delayed recall (<1st percentile). This pattern of deficits coupled with his report in testing suggested an individual who was easily overwhelmed by data and who lacked the executive functions to filter and organize information effectively.

Regarding capacity for medical decision making, Mr. W's understanding of his medical conditions and treatments was marginal at best. He appeared confused about his diagnoses and the purpose of some of his medications. Mr. W could not acknowledge any risks to his current treatments nor was he able to describe many benefits. Mr. W was aware at some level of a risk to "alternative" treatments (rat poison as a blood thinner); however, he was not even prescribed anticoagulation therapy, which further supported the conclusion that Mr. W had a fundamental lack of understanding regarding his medical conditions. Significantly, his decisions regarding his medical care appeared to be guided at times by delusional reasoning. Considering the test data, his responses to interview questions, and his lack of insight into his deficits, the psychologist concluded that Mr. W lacked capacity for medical decision making.

Case reflection on Mr. W

♦ The data collected in the Mr. W's home were particularly informative in this assessment. Although clinic providers had some idea that cognitive problems might be affecting Mr. W's medication adherence, the home assessment revealed a more complete picture of the degree to which he was impaired.

♦ The apparent delusional nature of Mr. W's decision-making process was a particularly important piece of data in this evaluation because it signaled a second area of impairment, namely, in the reasoning domain.

♦ In this case, Mr. W had impairment in other areas that supported the finding of incapacity but it is not uncommon for a patient to be relatively intact in other areas and still be sufficiently delusional to warrant a finding of incapacity because decisions are not grounded in a rational process.

Case study 2: Ms. P

Ms. P was an 86-year-old female patient with several chronic medical problems who was referred by her PCP to home care for assistance with medication adherence because her Christian Scientist faith made her unfamiliar with taking medications. The PCP also reported that Ms. P's daughter was pressuring her to decline medication intervention consistent with her and her daughter's religious convictions. A psychologist first evaluated Ms. P when her home care nurse case manager became concerned about possible short-term memory impairment and poor social support. The early assessment concluded that Ms. P had possible mild Alzheimer's dementia based on difficulty encoding information, variability of performance across tasks in most domains, a tendency toward perseverative thinking, and poor awareness of her own deficits.

At that time, Ms. P appeared to have capacity to make medical decisions. However, she was unable to report her total monthly income and she devoted a significant amount of attention to worrying about her finances, making her capacity to handle financial matters suspect, though an evaluation was not done at that time. A social worker was able to assist the patient in obtaining complete financial information and the family became more involved with the patient's medical and financial management. As the patient's family became more acquainted with the severity of her medical diagnoses they became less resistant to her medical treatment.

Eleven months later, Ms. P began exhibiting increased perseveration, irritability, and difficulty finding her way home. Family and medical staff were concerned about her ability to safely live alone, particularly as Ms. P seemed to lack insight into her cognitive deficits. Ms. P declined psychological evaluation at that time. Two months later, however, Ms. P consented to a capacity evaluation after her family reported that she was refusing assistance with activities of daily living (ADLs) and instrumental activities of daily living (IADLs) and she had fallen victim to a telephone scam.

During this evaluation, Ms. P perseverated on her desire to remain in her home but also admitted having a difficult time managing her home. Throughout the interview, Ms. P complained that her family was neglectful and were unwilling to provide her the care that she wanted. She specifically complained that her daughter would not move in with her to provide care, even though her daughter had taken a leave of absence from work to be of more assistance to her mother. Ms. P continued to vehemently refuse to consider a higher level of care.

On the Independent Living Scales (ILS), Managing Money subtest, Ms. P could not recall her sources of income or her social security benefits. She also had difficulty describing how to avoid financial exploitation and why it is important to pay her bills. She could not describe the purpose of a will, and had difficulty completing a check register without considerable guidance. Her performance suggested a need for significant amount of assistance in managing her finances.

On Managing the Home and Transportation subtest of the ILS, Ms. P had moderate difficulty formulating a plan for dealing with home repairs or an electrical outage and even greater difficulty articulating how she would enact these plans, suggesting a disconnect between her abilities to plan and to execute. Though her score on this subtest suggested moderate to high functioning in this area, her difficulty explaining how she would execute her plans suggested that this score may have overestimated her actual abilities.

Ms. P's performance on the Health and Safety subtest of the ILS suggested very low functioning in this domain. She could not describe how she would handle several emergency or safety situations such as responding to heart attack symptoms, mitigating fall risk, maintaining home safety, or contacting emergency services. She could not describe any of her medical diagnoses stating "I used to ride a bicycle," when asked to describe changes in her medical condition. Ms. P knew she was prescribed six medications but did not know their indications. She did not know about alternative treatment options, the risks or benefits of treatment, or rational reasons for choosing one treatment over another.

The psychologist concluded that Ms. P did not have capacity to make medical and financial decisions or to live independently based on an inability to encode and recall information vital to making these decisions rationally. However, Ms. P did retain the ability to designate her own surrogate decision maker. In deference to her long-held values and ability to articulate her preferred living situation, despite her cognitive deficits, the treatment team and family developed a plan to increase assistance and supervision, to allow Ms. P to remain at home. A family meeting involving the patient, her treatment team, and her family produced a plan for an adult grandchild to move in with her and help with household chores. Her daughter assumed fiduciary responsibilities. Other family members committed to regular visit schedules with Ms. P.

Case reflection on Ms. P

◆ Ms. P's capacity was only questioned after she refused apparently reasonable treatments, which contradicted her doctors' wishes. Her wishes were consistent with her long-standing religious faith. Initially, the conflict in values created frustration for the treatment team and mistrust with Ms. P and her family. Compromise from the medical team and education about the severity of her conditions to the patient and family helped resolve the disagreement.

♦ Decisions about capacity were not forced as long as the patient remained safe and had significant oversight and assistance; once that changed and the situation became tenuous, a decision about capacity became necessary.

♦ With her advancing dementia, the team's understanding of her religious beliefs informed future treatment planning. Though she could no longer live independently, an understanding of and respect for her housing preferences allowed the team to coordinate with the family to develop a plan to help Ms. P remain safely in her home and maintain her dignity and self-identity as an independent adult.

Case study 3: Mr. D

Mr. D was a 71-year-old widower with a history of post-traumatic stress disorder (PTSD) and alcohol abuse in addition to numerous chronic medical conditions. He completed high school equivalency while in the military, owned a successful locksmith business for 30 years, and retired 15 years ago. He lived alone but two daughters provided some functional support as needed. Mr. D had a long history of alcohol use and until recently drank fairly heavily. However, 2 years ago he began to limit his consumption secondary to his declining physical health.

As part of a recent application for an increase in his Veterans Administration (VA) pension, he underwent an evaluation of his cognition and mental status. The psychiatrist's report noted that Mr. W had significant deficits in memory, attention, calculation, and abstract thinking. The psychiatrist concluded that Mr. D was not capable of "managing his affairs in his own best interest because of his significant medical problems, his cognitive disorder, and his alcohol dependence." One consequence of this determination was that, under U.S. law, Mr. D would now be prohibited from purchasing firearms. An avid gun collector, Mr. D appealed the determination and this evaluation was completed as part of his appeal.

At this evaluation, Mr. D's daughter verified all his responses to questions about his finances. He was able to identify multiple sources of income, payment amounts, monthly pay days, and the accounts to which his checks were deposited. He explained in detail how his disability payments were deducted from his Navy retirement and the tax advantages of VA disability. He was unsure of the type of bank account he had, but knew that checks could be written from it. He did not remember how much was in his account but suspected it was fairly low since he had just used some for Christmas gifts. His daughter reminded him that a pension check was deposited at the first of the month. He remembered his monthly mortgage payment. He did not know the value of his home, but estimated its worth based on the sale price from two homes recently sold in his neighborhood and his total square footage.

In terms of exploitation risk, Mr. D had not lent money or given excessive monetary gifts to anyone. He paid his granddaughter $6–8 per hour to clean his house each week. He had not had any money stolen recently, though he reported an incident 10 years ago when his niece stole money and possessions when she was cleaning the home. When he discovered the thefts, he fired the niece. Mr. D had a will with his daughter designated as executor and he was not currently involved in or planning any changes to his will.

Mr. D knew his monthly expenses. Historically, his wife managed their finances and after she died, his daughter began assisting with bill paying. He encouraged her to set up electronic bill payment to make it more convenient for her. He would collect all his bills as they came, which his daughter reviewed with him before making payments. She had access to all his accounts online and reviewed statements with him on a monthly basis. She also did his shopping because of his physical limitations, though he sometimes accompanied her in a wheelchair. His future financial plans mainly involved taking care of household and medical expenses. Mr. D said he might use some of his savings to help family members in the event of a life-threatening emergency. If his daughter were no longer able to assist with his finances, he would do it himself or ask his grand-daughter for help. He had a home computer he used for games and online shopping and he felt he could learn to pay his bills online, if necessary. The psychologist and Mr. D reviewed his tax statement together and he correctly explained his withholdings and deductions for that year. They also reviewed a bill for a recent purchase and Mr. D correctly identified the amount owed, sales tax, and the company to whom payment should be sent.

Mr. D also completed several hypothetical scenarios involving monetary transactions from the Revised Observed Tasks of Daily Living (OTDL-R) (Diehl, Willis, & Schaie, 1995). He was able to mentally calculate change for a lunch tab and enter debits and credits in a check register then correctly balance it after accounting for these transactions. He correctly wrote a check for a hypo-thetical bill for services, but had to be reminded to enter the dollar amount.

His overall performance on the RBANS fell in the Average range across all areas of cognition including learning/immediate memory, visuospatial/constructional, language, attention, and delayed recall. The psychologist concluded that his performance was consistent with his educa-tional and occupational background, suggesting he had not experienced much decline if any from his baseline cognitive abilities. His performance on testing and his responses to interview ques-tions suggested that Mr. D had the cognitive capacity to grasp basic financial concepts, conduct financial planning in his own behalf, detect situations with high exploitation risk, and manage his own finances, including any funds paid to him by the VA.

Case reflection on Mr. D

♦ Clearly Mr. D's performance at his first mental status examination was not indicative of his true abilities. More extensive cognitive testing and a practical examination related to financial capacity offered a more comprehensive view of his cognition.

♦ Mr. D's purchase of alcohol and guns with his pension, both of which were legal under U.S. law, could be indicative of poor judgment. However, there was no evidence that these purchases were the result of decisional impairment. Mr. D's purchases reflected personal values and the assessment suggested that he could use reasoned thought processes to make financial decisions.

Case study 4: Mr. G

Mr. G was an 86-year-old, widowed Caucasian veteran referred for psychological evaluation after his wife of 60 years died and he scored poorly on a cognitive screening measure. He had two chil-dren, a son living out of state and a daughter living locally. His daughter reported that he had a history of verbal abuse toward his wife, children, and other family which limited the amount of family support they were providing.

He denied a history of depression and said that he had been feeling and doing better lately, though he acknowledged feeling sad after his wife died. His appetite continued to be depressed but his weight was stable. Mr. G admitted that he was never good with names, but denied any decline in short-term memory and also denied any other cognitive complaints. His home health aide, who worked with him 5 days a week since his wife died, was present and agreed that his cognitive functioning had been stable and that his mood has improved.

On the Dementia Rating Scale-Second Edition (DRS-2) and clock drawing, Mr. G performed in the Average range on all tests except Initiation/Perseveration, where he scored in the low average range, primarily due to his performance on semantic fluency. The psychologist concluded that

Mr. G appeared to be generally cognitively intact, with some mild problems with verbal sequencing and processing speed. His poor performance on cognitive screening was more likely due to depression and bereavement which were resolving.

Several months later, the psychologist re-evaluated Mr. G at the request of his doctor and his daughter for decline in cognition and behavioral changes. Since the last evaluation, Mr. G had reportedly become increasingly close to his aide. They would sit on the couch and hold hands while watching television and Mr. G would put his arms around her and kiss her on the cheek and neck. According to the daughter, Mr. G also gave some of his wife's clothing and jewelry to his aide and gave her $100 for her birthday. However, when Mr. G eventually requested more affection from his aide (he asked her for a kiss), she reported this to her employer who removed her from the home. Mr. G became upset and blamed his daughter for the aide's departure.

During this same period, Mr. G's providers and his daughter observed changes in his sleep-wake cycle and possible delusional beliefs, specifically, that a stray cat lived in his basement and was having sex with his own cat. According to the daughter, Mr. G was also becoming more sexually preoccupied and was attempting to discuss his sex life with his late wife with his daughter. He also had several falls in the last few months without loss of consciousness, although his daughter reported she had found him confused and disoriented after one fall. His daughter also voiced concern over his decision to forgo additional treatment for prostate cancer. He continued to be demanding and verbally abusive to his children, especially his daughter, whom he would call for help and then berate for not taking good care of him.

At the second evaluation, Mr. G was initially gracious and cooperative but he became irritated as he was asked about his relationship with his aide. He perseverated on her absence and frequently asked for help getting her back. As Mr. G described it, "they took my little maid away." Though he initially said he did not know why she left, he later admitted it was because of their "relationship." He confirmed reports about their physical contact and stated that she did not mind his advances. He denied any other touching beyond that already reported and denied wanting any further relationship with her. He eventually admitted to giving her gifts and saw nothing wrong with this. He attributed her removal from his home to the "guards" who "thought I was molesting her." He said that his aide always told him she would "be there until the end."

Mr. G explained his refusal of additional treatment for prostate cancer by citing his advanced age and saying that did not want to "pay that doctor any more money." He acknowledged that his death may be hastened by this decision, "Yes, I might die, but we all have to die, most people my age do." Mr. G also admitted that his relationship with his daughter was "not too good," that he was angry at her for leaving her first husband, and compared her to a prostitute. He said his daughter only visits about once per week and is not affectionate with him.

He admitted to daily sadness, mostly about the loss of his aide, but denied tearfulness. Although he also denied suicidal ideation, he admitted that his physical decline has made him feel "ready to go" so that he could be reunited with his late wife. He reported variable appetite but without significant weight change. He said his sleep was "pretty good." He denied any changes in memory. He admitted to three recent falls but denied any head injury.

Mr. G again completed the DRS-2 and the Hopemont Capacity Assessment Interview (HCAI) (Edelstein, 1999). He remembered the DRS-2 from before and even recalled some of the test items. At one point he remarked that he would probably perform better on testing if it would help him get his aide back. On the DRS-2, Mr. G exhibited significant declines in processing speed and flexibility, orientation, and short-term memory. On the health care decision-making portion of the HCAI, Mr. G had difficulty articulating an understanding of the concept of risk, but could adequately articulate his understanding of benefit and choice. On the hypothetical scenarios presented in the test, he could explain the risks and benefits of the hypothetical treatment choice and understood reasons for treatment choices that differed from his own. The psychologist concluded that Mr. G had experienced a cognitive decline since the first testing with multiple potential etiologies including possible mild head injuries from falls, declining mood, neurological involvement from advancing prostate cancer, and continued cerebrovascular changes. However, the psychologist determined that Mr. G's capacity to make medical decisions remained intact as long as the options were clearly explained.

Three months later, Mr. G was seen again for an assessment of financial and testamentary capacity. During this time, Mr. G had decided to change his will to bequeath his estate to his former aide and exclude his children entirely from any inheritance. At this evaluation, Mr. G soon became angry, defensive, and hostile when questioned about his relationships with the aide and his daughter. Mr. G reiterated both his desire to have his aide care for him again and his suspicion that his daughter was responsible for her removal. He refused to believe that the aide asked to be reassigned herself, saying that her supervisor had told him that his daughter had written a letter calling the aide a thief. He minimized any inappropriate behavior on his part, saying he did not know it was wrong. He said he believed his late wife sent him the aide.

When questioned about his financial assets, he reported a value from a recent home appraisal. He accused his daughter of stealing the $40,000 he had in savings, opening his mail, and taking his money. He confirmed his desire to leave his estate to his aide, explaining that she is a "fine young woman" who treated him better than his children. He did not want either of his children to inherit any of his estate because of his anger over the aide's removal from his home. He also wanted to exclude his son from his will "because he's in with my daughter."

On the ILS, his strongest performance came on the subscale measuring orientation and memory. He performed very poorly on all other subscales and the Problem Solving and Performance/Information factors. Of most relevance to this evaluation, he performed very poorly on the Managing Money scale. Moreover, Mr. G demonstrated slightly better knowledge than problem solving, suggesting that even if he could answer a question about a particular issue related to his daily life, he may well be unable to work with this information in a practical way.

The psychologist concluded that Mr. G did not have full financial capacity. Although he could participate in decisions about how his resources were used, he lacked the skills and understanding to manage his money soundly. The evaluation suggested that Mr. G was susceptible to financial exploitation. Fortunately, his daughter was already his financial power of attorney, and seemed to be managing his money properly. In contrast, the psychologist determined that Mr. G still enjoyed basic medical decision-making capacity. He was able to describe the purpose for and the use of his emergency alert device, and he was able to describe the circumstances under which he would go to the hospital emergently. Furthermore, he was able to articulate consistent, coherent, and defensible reasons for his medical decisions.

With regards to testamentary capacity, Mr. G appeared to have a general understanding of his assets that his children were his "natural heirs." He also understood the purpose of a will. However, his perseveration and odd ideas about his former aide and his suspiciousness about his daughter's motivations raised questions about the rationality of his decision making. State case law stipulated that the presence of an "insane delusion" negates testamentary capacity if that delusion directly affects the person's disposition of his or her assets. This seemed to be the case with Mr. G as his persistent and irrational beliefs about his relationship with his aide bordered on the delusional. His desire to change his will based on these beliefs rose to the level of "insane delusion," and thus suggested that he lacked testamentary capacity.

Case reflection on Mr. G

♦ Consistent with progressive dementia, Mr. G experienced a progressive decline in capacity, though not all capacities declined at the same rate. Though he lacked testamentary capacity, he still retained medical decision-making capacity, which illustrates the multifactorial nature of capacity and supports the idea that capacities are somewhat individual, though interrelated, constructs.

- ◆ The testing data offered supplemental information about Mr. G's abilities and deficits. Although one of Mr. G's ILS scores suggested impaired medical decision-making capacity, the evaluator's conclusion was based on a synthesis of all the evidences.

Discussion

Normal aging is associated with a decline in certain fluid cognitive abilities (e.g. mental flexibility, processing speed, and complex attention) (Anstey & Low, 2004) and sensory changes (e.g. vision and hearing) that may reduce a person's capacity to function as he/she once did. Even in the absence of any known disease affecting cognition, an individual may lose capacity for certain functions. For example, it is common for many older persons to stop driving due to visual deficits, physical weakness, or poor mobility. Although they remain intact cognitively, they nevertheless lack capacity for this skill because they can no longer perform some components essential to that activity. Among the individuals described in these case examples, all had experienced physical and mental declines that affected their capacity to perform different activities. Ms. P, for instance, could no longer drive or clean her house due to limited physical mobility and Mr. G's daughter was already paying his bills due to his cognitive deficits.

It should be noted, however, that specific capacities are individual, albeit interrelated, abilities that may decline at different rates. Thus, an individual may lose one capacity, such as the ability to safely drive a car, but retain other capacities such as the ability to make medical decisions, as was evident with Mr. G and Mr. D. Both men had experienced declines in capacity that prompted a formal psychological evaluation. Mr. G's evaluation concluded that he lacked capacity to manage his money in his own best interest or to make out a will. For those capacities, surrogates were identified to act in his behalf. However, Mr. G still retained basic medical decision-making capacity and was, therefore, able to continue making his own choices about his health care, including whether to forgo further treatment for prostate cancer.

However, even when cognitive deficits are documented, individuals may still retain their mental capacities. Early research on evaluation of medical decision-making capacity found that physicians commonly based their estimations of patient capacity entirely upon brief tests of mental status, such as three-word recall, and subjective impressions (Fitten & Waite, 1990; Grisso, 1986). However, it is not unusual for a patient to perform poorly on a MiniCog, Mini-Mental State Examination (MMSE), or even more extensive cognitive tests but still be able to make medical decisions or manage finances. For this reason, a determination of capacity must be based on more information than MMSE alone. The evaluation must be specific to the capacity in question with assessment derived from accepted criteria. When legal standards are not available, the clinician should consult with legal experts. Mr. D's situation highlights the danger of basing a determination of incapacity on brief tests of cognition. The initial evaluation was incomplete and the determination of incapacity was based on inadequate data. A more comprehensive examination of cognition that was also specific to Mr. D's financial abilities clearly showed that this capacity remained intact.

Diagnosis and capacity

These cases also highlight how other psychiatric conditions may affect capacity. Just as cognitive disorders like Alzheimer's disease may raise questions about capacity, psychiatric diagnoses like schizophrenia may also impact cognition and eventually impair capacity. Nevertheless, a psychiatric diagnosis by itself is not prima facie evidence of incapacity and patients may still retain mental capacities despite psychiatric impairment. For instance, multiple studies have found that individuals with schizophrenia (Grisso & Appelbaum, 1995; Moye et al., 2008) or major depressive disorder (Appelbaum, Grisso, Frank, O'Donnell, & Kupfer, 1999) can retain capacity for medical decision making even while they have active psychiatric symptoms.

A capacity evaluation will always be better informed when based on accepted criteria that underlie a given capacity rather than focusing on a specific diagnosis. For example, while Mr. W's diagnosis of schizoaffective disorder prompted the evaluator to assess more carefully for psychotic symptoms, especially delusional beliefs, the diagnosis was not a relevant factor in determining whether he had medical decision-making capacity. Rather, the finding of incapacity was based on his performance on cognitive testing, his answers to specific medical questions, and especially the apparent delusional thought process underlying his decisions.

Basing a determination of capacity solely on the presence or absence of any diagnosis may lead to incorrect assumptions about an individual's capacities. Mr. D's diagnosis of PTSD and history of chronic alcohol dependence were important factors at his first capacity evaluation, which resulted in a questionable determination of incapacity. As revealed by the second evaluation, however, these diagnoses had minimal influence on his ability to manage his finances, despite his having active PTSD symptoms that were not adequately treated. By building the evaluation around accepted standards for financial capacity, the evaluator minimized the influence of these psychiatric diagnoses on the outcome, resulting in a more complete and defensible determination.

The specific deficits that underlie incapacity often differ even in persons with similar diagnoses, again supporting the importance of a comprehensive evaluation based on accepted capacity criteria. For persons with Alzheimer's disease, for example, the cognitive deficit underlying incapacity is often impaired short-term memory, which limits acquisition and retention of information. Such was the case with Ms. P whose capacities were challenged in the context of declining memory. With Mr. G, however, the delusional beliefs that influenced some of his decisions were important evidence in determining lack of testamentary capacity. In his case, the incapacity determination was based on legal standards which stipulated that decisions about a will should be the result of a reasoned, logical process. Indeed, though Mr. G knew the purpose of a will, his assets, and his natural heirs, an evaluation focused solely on these "understanding" elements of decision-making may have discounted the influence of delusional beliefs on his decision to change the will. Basing the evaluation on legal criteria shifted focus away from the diagnosis and individual deficits, allowing the psychologist to consider these delusional beliefs along with all the other data to form a conclusion about testamentary capacity.

An individual's psychiatric or cognitive diagnosis is important when explaining causal factors that may be contributing to incapacity. Some causal factors like severe depression or delirium may resolve over time. For example, a person may lack capacity while in the midst of a delirium, but capacity may be restored once symptoms resolve. In contrast, patients with Alzheimer's disease, an irreversible form of dementia, are unlikely to ever regain capacities once lost. In both instances, knowing these diagnoses allows the evaluator to express an opinion regarding the permanence of incapacity—either to ensure civil rights are eventually restored or to avoid raising false hopes of improvement and to ensure the safety of the patient and others.

Values and goals

These cases illustrate the impact of values and goals in any capacity evaluation. All cases of questionable capacity essentially involve the conflict between two or more value systems. It is paramount that the evaluator be aware of these underlying demands because strongly held values may influence decision-making in both automatic and conscious or rational ways. Karel, Gurrera, Hicken, and Moye (in press) noted that values come into play at multiple levels. That is, besides the patient's own values, the interests of family, providers, the health care system, and society as a whole all influence how capacity is determined, how incapacitated persons are treated, and whether capacity is even questioned in the first place.

Even in the context of significant cognitive deficits, a person may still be able to articulate his/her values and make decisions consistent with individual preferences. Indeed, a decision based on a personal value system may be perfectly rational even when it falls outside accepted standards of practice (Moye, 2007). Therefore, an assessment of capacity should also capture an individual's underlying values and goals (Moye & Braun, 2007). The Assessment of the Capacity to Consent to Treatment (ACCT) model actually incorporates an assessment of values within an evaluation tool. As with earlier models, ACCT stipulates the four legal standards of medical decision-making capacity. However, the model also emphasizes the role of individual values in decision-making and suggests that assessing a decision's consistency with underlying values and goals is a critical part of capacity evaluation (Moye et al., 2008).

The importance of understanding a patient's system of values was evident in Ms. P's case. Her refusal of reasonable medical treatments in light of suspected cognitive impairment raised questions about her capacity to consent. However, her refusals were consistent with her lifelong religious beliefs. As a practicing Christian Scientist before she became cognitively impaired, her providers were correct in considering whether her non-adherence reflected underlying beliefs despite her cognitive impairment. Similarly, the importance she placed on remaining in her home informed the team and family as they developed a plan to address her incapacity. However, two additional value systems were also involved in this case. Consistent with the medical model, Ms. P's PCPs were prescribing and encouraging her to accept treatment that would prolong her life and reduce her symptoms. Also, when Ms. P began to consider accepting some of these treatment recommendations, her daughter began exerting pressure consistent with her own religious beliefs. Her daughter's pressure to adhere to these beliefs created additional tension among competing values, which prompted the capacity evaluation.

Another set of values can also influence a capacity evaluation in important ways. The "impartial" evaluator's own values will affect interpretation of the interview and test data, the weight given to certain pieces of data, and even the types of questions asked during the evaluation (Karel et al., in press). In Mr. D's case, for example, two evaluators reached discrepant opinions about his ability to manage his VA pension. The two evaluators' own beliefs about mental illness and its influence on capacity, alcohol use, gun control, the relative value of cognitive assessment, and even their beliefs about their own expertise, likely influenced their approach to their evaluations. The second evaluator had a personal relationship with Mr. D as his therapist for about a year while the first evaluator did not. Although their underlying values are not known, surely the second evaluator's relationship with the patient (and a probable desire for the patient to remain independent) influenced that assessment. Likewise, the VA system's expectation that pension funds be used wisely may have influenced the conclusion in the first evaluation. Thus, in addition to assessing a patient's values, clinicians must also be aware of the potential influence of their own values, experiences, and biases and those of other interested parties (e.g. family, other providers, etc.).

Reliability and validity

Mr. D's case also illustrates another challenging aspect of capacity evaluation, namely the reliability and validity of capacity determinations across clinicians. Marson et al. (1997) were among the first to empirically demonstrate that clinical determinations about capacity can vary significantly, even among experienced clinicians. Indeed, in one study, he found that a group of five physicians agreed only 56% of the time when evaluating medical decision-making capacity in a group of patients with mild Alzheimer's disease. Moreover, significant variability existed across physician judgments. Although one physician concluded that 90% of the patients evaluated lacked capacity, another physician determined that none of them was incapacitated. These physicians were neurologists, geriatricians, and psychiatrists, who, presumably, had expertise in evaluation of mental capacities.

The two evaluations of Mr. D's capacity offered two opposite conclusions about his ability to manage his own finances. The first evaluator, a psychiatrist, concluded that the patient "shows significant cognitive problems on MMSE including decreased memory functions, decreased attention, decreased calculation, and decreased abstractive ability," which led him to conclude that the patient lacked capacity to manage his VA pension. This evaluation included several brief tests of cognition including serial 7s, digit span, three-word list memory, backward spelling, historical memory, and proverbs.

The second evaluator, a clinical psychologist, concluded that Mr. D had "Average cognitive abilities across most areas of functioning" and retained the "cognitive capacity to grasp basic financial concepts, conduct financial planning in his own behalf, and detect situations with high exploitation risk." The second evaluation included cognitive testing using an instrument with age-appropriate norms and an assessment of Mr. D's financial knowledge and ability to manage money. Thus, in addition to the potential impact of clinicians' values as mentioned above, clearly their assessment strategies had a major impact on the evaluation outcome.

Measurement tools

To improve reliability and validity, clinicians may use a variety of assessment tools to assist in the clinical evaluation of capacity. In addition to clinical interview, the cases above utilized formal capacity assessment instruments and collateral data to inform the evaluation. All the cases used cognitive testing which, alone, is typically insufficient to permit a determination about capacity. However, cognitive tests are useful for quantifying underlying cognitive deficits that may impact a particular mental capacity. Most evaluations of capacity should include general measures of cognition and measures specific to a particular capacity. However, the value of each method is dictated by several factors including the type of capacity(ies) under question, the significance of the decision being made (Dunn, Nowrangi, Palmer, Jeste, & Saks, 2006), the patient's tolerance of formal testing, suspected need for guardianship, facility policy, and the laws of the particular region or country.

As demonstrated with Mr. W, a patient's capacity may be determined through the use of a thorough and targeted clinical interview and assessment of cognitive functioning. The remaining cases involved the use of various measurement instruments designed specifically for assessing different capacities in conjunction with clinical interviews, cognitive testing, collateral data, medical records reviews, and direct observation. The weighty and life-altering consequences of capacity evaluations dictate that clinicians must be thorough and creative in gathering all pertinent information. For example, if an assessment of capacity for independent living cannot be conducted in a patient's home, family members could video or photograph the home to provide some information about these living conditions.

Many measurement tools have been developed over the last three decades for objectively assessing various domains of mental capacity (Table 15.1), including the OTDL-R, the ILS, and the HCAI, which were used in the last three cases. These instruments do not provide a cut-off score below which a person is said to lack capacity. Rather, they provide an organized method of collecting

Table 15.1 Measurement tools for evaluation of mental capacities

Measurement tool	Type of capacity*			Method		
	Medical	Independent living	Financial	Vignette	Semi- or structured interview	Performance-based
Adult Functional Adaptive Behavior Scale (AFABS): *Informant-based 14-item assessment of adaptive functioning.*	X	X	X		X	
Aid to Capacity Evaluation (ACE): *Interview with questions based on patient's actual medical decision.*	X				X	
Assessment of Capacity to Consent to Treatment (ACCT): *Standardized interview that includes assessment of patient values in addition to legal standards.*	X			X	X	
Capacity Assessment Tool (CAT): *Assesses six abilities as patients choose between two actual treatment options.*	X				X	
Capacity to Consent to Treatment Interview (CCTI): *Based on two clinical vignettes presented in verbal and written formats.*	X			X	X	
Cognitive Competency Test (CCT): *Hypothetical vignettes are presented throughout; the financial subscale has a performance element.*	X	X	X	X	X	
Competency Interview Schedule (CIS): *15-item assessment initially developed for consent to ECT.*	X				X	
Decision Assessment Measure: *Hypothetical vignette to assess understanding, reasoning, understanding a choice, and retention of information based on legal standards of capacity in England and Wales.*	X			X		

(Continued)

Table 15.1 (continued) Measurement tools for evaluation of mental capacities

Measurement tool	Type of capacity*			Method		
	Medical	Independent living	Financial	Vignette	Semi- or structured interview	Performance-based
Decision-Making Instrument for Guardianship (DIG): *Standardized vignettes with information on administration and scoring for use in guardianship decisions.*	X		X	X		
Direct Assessment of Functional Status (DAFS): *Assesses ADLs and IADLs required for independent living in patients with dementia.*		X			X	X
Financial Capacity Instrument (FCI): *Information provided for administration and scoring.*			X		X	X
Hopemont Capacity Assessment Interview (HCAI): *Two sections with standardized instructions.*	X		X	X	X	
Independent Living Scales (ILS): *Standardized test of six scales measuring capability of caring for self and property.*	X	X	X	X		X
MacArthur Competence Assessment Tool-Treatment (MACCAT-T): *Questions are based on the patient's actual medical condition.*	X				X	
Multidimensional Functional Assessment Questionnaire (MFAQ): *Developed for use with an older population. Assesses ADLs, IADLs, and utilization of services.*		X			X	X
Philadelphia Geriatric Center Multilevel Assessment Inventory (MAI): *Developed to determine need for services and placement in an older population. Three versions available based on length (165, 38, and 24 items).*		X			X	

Table 15.1 (continued) Measurement tools for evaluation of mental capacities

Measurement tool	Type of capacity*			Method		
	Medical	Independent living	Financial	Vignette	Semi- or structured interview	Performance-based
Revised Observed Tasks of Daily Living (OTDL-R): *Performance-based test of everyday problem solving that evaluates nine functional abilities.*	X	X	X			X

*There are currently no standardized tools to assess testamentary capacity (Shulman et al., 2009).

Source: Adapted from American Bar Association/American Psychological Association (2008). *Assessment of older adults with diminished capacity: A handbook for psychologists.* Washington, DC: American Bar Association Commission on Law and Aging/American Psychological Association.

data about the component skills important to different capacities to inform, not supersede, the provider's clinical judgment about a patient's abilities (Moye & Marson, 2007). With Mr. G, for example, the psychologist's use of all the data available led to a different conclusion about capacity than what was evident from scores on the ILS, a measure used for evaluating several different capacities including medical decision making. His scores on the ILS Health and Safety subscale suggested he could not safely make important medical decisions. However, the psychologist's opinion differed from this interpretation based on the patient's report that highlighted his understanding and appreciation of his medical decisions, his consistency in expressing a choice, and his ability to provide sound reasoning for his decisions.

Disposition with incapacity

Finally, capacity evaluations must balance the need to foster the safety of patients and others against the need to maintain patient independence. A poorly done capacity assessment could either deprive someone of civil rights to which they are legally entitled, as in the case of Mr. D, or deny an incapacitated person and others protection from potential harm. It is vitally important, therefore, that clinicians who evaluate capacity understand the potential consequences of their decision for the patient, concerned others, and society. Clinicians must not overstate their assessment by offering conclusions about capacities that were not evaluated. As discussed earlier, capacities decline at different rates; a patient may not fully appreciate the nuances of a financial contract, but may retain the ability to balance a checking account. In the cases above, recognizing that patients retained some capacities allowed clinicians to develop a plan for retaining patients' independence consistent with their values and abilities while securing assistance for areas of incapacity.

Information gathered during the evaluation can be used to capitalize on the patient's cognitive strengths and further facilitate areas in which they maintain capacity. In developing a plan, it is important to consider the patient's consistently held values, the environment in which the patient will be living, and possible support from collaterals. For example, if a plan assumes that the patient will be moved to a higher level of care, but the proxy decision maker refuses based on the patient's strong resistance, the plan will be ineffective. Having a firm grasp of available resources is integral to developing a successful plan. Family conferences or involvement of the support network to determine the realities of accessible resources can be the determining factor in whether a dispositional plan will succeed.

The disposition should also consider whether a patient's capacity may be fully or partially restored. As noted earlier, lost capacity may be restored when temporary conditions that affect cognition are resolved or adequately treated. In geropsychology settings, conditions affecting capacity are often chronic and/or progressive (e.g. Alzheimer's dementia), so restoring capacity is unlikely. But in some patients, even in some older patients, restoration of capacity is possible. A delirium may clear after an infection is treated or psychosis may abate with psychotropic medication, which may restore patients' capacity in some areas. Clinicians must account for conditions affecting the patient's cognitive and psychological functioning in the dispositional plan and be prepared to conduct follow-up assessments where indicated to update the clinical data regarding the patient's capacity in various areas.

Summary and conclusion

The evaluation of mental capacities can be challenging—the process is neither simple nor necessarily intuitive. Mental capacity is a multivariate concept rather than a single, unitary construct and capacities can be permanently or temporarily affected by a variety of circumstances, including psychiatric conditions. A capacity evaluation could also potentially infringe on patients' civil rights, obligating family, providers, or society to act in a patient's behalf to prevent harm, which can result in some ethical angst on the part of the evaluator. The case scenarios above suggest several points that clinicians should consider to facilitate evaluating mental capacities:

◆ What accepted legal or clinical criteria for this mental capacity can inform the evaluation process? Capacity evaluation should be grounded in an underlying model. In doing so, the clinician minimizes the risk that the capacity determination will be based solely on particularly salient features about a patient (e.g. short-term memory deficits, dementia diagnosis, etc.). Instead, the evaluation will account for multiple relevant factors that should all be considered prior to making a determination. Using standard criteria also provides some legal protection to the clinician. In the absence of accepted standards, the clinician should obtain legal counsel prior to conducting an evaluation.

◆ What values and beliefs are at play in this case? The clinician should find out patients' preferences and how their decisions are being influenced by the goals of family, friends, and providers. Perhaps most importantly, clinicians must be aware of their own biases and then take steps to minimize their impact on the evaluation.

◆ In what ways can the evaluation be supplemented in order to improve the reliability and validity of the outcome? Capacity-specific measures and tests of cognition can provide more objective data about abilities but clinicians may also obtain data from other sources including caregivers and clinicians. At times, an in-home evaluation may be helpful, particularly with questions about capacity for independent living. Clinicians should bear in mind, however, that no single test or piece of evidence can typically be relied upon to make a determination regarding a mental capacity.

◆ Finally, what are the consequences of a capacity determination, positive or negative? Are the deficits observed in an interview permanent or might abilities be restored through medication or improved health? Addressing these questions will help to maintain patients' dignity and to the extent possible, their agency to act in their own behalf.

References

American Bar Association/American Psychological Association (2008). *Assessment of older adults with diminished capacity: A handbook for psychologists.* Washington, DC: American Bar Association Commission on Law and Aging/American Psychological Association.

Anstey, K.J., & Low, L.F. (2004). Normal cognitive changes in aging. *Australian Family Physician, 33*(10), 783–787.

Appelbaum, P.S., & Grisso, T. (1995). The MacArthur Treatment Competence Study. I. Mental illness and competence to consent to treatment. *Law and Human Behavior, 19*(2), 105–126.

Appelbaum, P.S., Grisso, T., Frank, E., O'Donnell, S., & Kupfer, D.J. (1999). Competence of depressed patients for consent to research. *American Journal of Psychiatry, 156*(9), 1380–1384.

Barbas, N.R., & Wilde, E.A. (2001). Competency issues in dementia: Medical decision making, driving, and independent living. *Journal of Geriatric Psychiatry and Neurology, 14*(4), 199–212.

Diehl, M., Willis, S.L., & Schaie, K.W. (1995). Everyday problem solving in older adults: Observational assessment and cognitive correlates. *Psychology and Aging, 10*(3), 478–491.

Dunn, L.B., Nowrangi, M.A., Palmer, B.W., Jeste, D.V., & Saks, E.R. (2006). Assessing decisional capacity for clinical research or treatment: A review of instruments. *American Journal of Psychiatry, 163*(8), 1323–1334.

Edelstein, B. (1999). *Hopemont capacity assessment interview manual and scoring guide.* Morgantown, WV: West Virginia University.

Fitten, L.J., & Waite, M.S. (1990). Impact of medical hospitalization on treatment decision-making capacity in the elderly. *Archives of Internal Medicine, 150*(8), 1717–1721.

Griffith, H.R., Belue, K., Sicola, A., Krzywanski, S., Zamrini, E., Harrell, L., et al. (2003). Impaired financial abilities in mild cognitive impairment: A direct assessment approach. *Neurology, 60*(3), 449–457.

Grisso, T. (1986). *Evaluating competencies: Forensic assessments and instruments.* New York, NY: Plenum Press.

Grisso, T. (2003). Legally relevant assessments for legal competencies. In T. Grisso (Ed.), *Evaluating competencies: Forensic assessments and instruments* (pp. 21–39). New York, NY: Plenum Press.

Grisso, T., & Appelbaum, P. (1995). MacArthur Treatment Competence Study. *Journal of the American Psychiatric Nurses Association, 1*(4), 125–127.

Grisso, T., & Appelbaum, P.S. (1998). *Assessing competence to consent to treatment: A guide for physicians and other health professionals.* New York, NY: Oxford University Press.

Hebert, K.R., & Marson, D. (2007). Assessment of financial capacity in older adults with dementia. In S. Qualls & M.A. Smyer (Eds.), *Changes in decision-making capacity in older adults* (pp. 237–270). Hoboken, NJ: John Wiley & Sons.

Karel, M.J., Moye, J., Hicken, B., & Gurrera, R.J. (in press). Reasoning in medical consent capacity: The consideratio of values. *The Journal of Clinical Ethics, 21*(1).

Kim, S.Y.H., Karlawish, J.H.T., & Caine, E.D. (2002). Current state of research on decision-making competence of cognitively impaired elderly persons. *American Journal of Geriatric Psychiatry, 10*(2), 151–165.

Kukull, W.A., & Ganguli, M. (2000). Epidemiology of dementia: Concepts and overview. *Neurology Clinics, 18*(4), 923–950.

Marson, D.C., Ingram, K.K., Cody, H.A., & Harrell, L.E. (1995). Assessing the competency of patients with Alzheimer's disease under different legal standards. A prototype instrument. *Archives of Neurology, 52*(10), 949–954.

Marson, D.C., McInturff, B., Hawkins, L., Bartolucci, A., & Harrell, L.E. (1997). Consistency of physician judgments of capacity to consent in mild Alzheimer's disease. *Journal of the American Geriatrics Society, 45*(4), 453–457.

Moye, J. (2000). Mr. Franks refuses surgery. Cognition and values in competency determination in complex cases. *Journal of Aging Studies, 14*(4), 385–401.

Moye, J. (2003). Guardianship and conservatorship. In T. Grisso (Ed.), *Evaluating competencies: Forensic assessments and instruments*. Second edition (pp. 309–389). New York, NY: Plenum Press.

Moye, J. (2007). Clinical frameworks for capacity assessments. In S. Qualls & M.A. Smyer (Eds.), *Changes in decision-making capacity in older adults*. Hoboken, NJ: John Wiley & Sons.

Moye, J., & Braun, M. (2007). Assessment of medical consent capacity and independent living. In S. Qualls & M.A. Smyer (Eds.), *Changes in decision-making capacity in older adults*. Hoboken, NJ: John Wiley & Sons.

Moye, J., & Marson, D.C. (2007). Assessment of decision-making capacity in older adults: An emerging area of practice and research. *The Journals of Gerontology Series B: Psychological Sciences and Social Sciences*, 62(1), P3–P11.

Moye, J., Karel, M.J., Edelstein, B., Hicken, B., Armesto, J.C., & Gurrera, R.J. (2008). Assessment of capacity to consent to treatment: Challenges, the 'ACCT' approach, future directions. *Clinical Gerontologist*, 31(3), 37–66.

Shulman, K.I., Peisah, C., Jacoby, R., Heinik, J., & Finkel, S. (2009). Contemporaneous assessment of testamentary capacity. *International Psychogeriatrics*, 21(3), 433–439.

United States Department of Veterans Affairs (2003). *State summary*. Washington, DC: United States Department of Veterans Affairs.

Wong, J.G., Clare, I.C.H., Gunn, M.J., & Holland, A.J. (1999). Capacity to make health care decisions: Its importance in clinical practice. *Psychological Medicine*, 29(2), 437–446.

Chapter 16

Clinical geropsychology practice in long-term care facilities

Anne Margriet Pot and Bernadette Willemse

Introduction

Long-term care facilities (LTCFs) are focused on providing a normal life for older adults with a wide variety of complex problems. Much of what is described in this book is also feasible for residents in LTCFs. However, clinical geropsychologists working with residents in LTCFs will be confronted with questions that are typical, although not exclusive, for this specific target group. Four of these questions will be discussed in this chapter:

1. How to improve the quality of life of residents with dementia?

2. How to diagnose depression in residents with co-morbidity?

3. How to assess residents' mental capacity?

4. How to prevent or treat residents' problems via mobilizing their care and social support system—so-called mediators—for example, nursing staff and family members?

Each of these questions will be discussed separately, prefaced with a case that is exemplary. For each case, the role of the geropsychologist will be explicitly described. Before going into the cases, some background about Dutch nursing home care in general, and group living home care specifically, will be provided.

Nursing home care in the Netherlands

Around 6% of people aged 65 years and older live in a LTCF in the Netherlands, for the most part in homes for the aged; approximately 2% live in nursing homes. The traditional nursing homes resemble a hospital, with long corridors and bedrooms for six people who had to share a bathroom. Although there was a time when older adults could move to a home for the aged when they were 70 years of age and healthy, nowadays only people with severe somatic and/or psychogeriatric problems, mostly older adults with a mean age above 80, who need intensive and complex care are referred to LTCFs.

For placement in a LTCF, a referral from the Dutch Center for Referral in Care (CIZ) is needed. There are 10 so-called care-load packages available, ranging from sheltered living with support to protected stay with intensive (nursing) care. These packages also include short stays, for example for older adults who broke their hip or have had a stroke and who need rehabilitation, and people who need intensive palliative care. The referral may be viewed as a ticket for admission to home care. With such a ticket, people can choose a living arrangement where the care they need is provided.

The care-load packages, including nursing home care, are paid by the Exceptional Medical Expenses Law or AWBZ (all Dutch citizens in paid employment pay an AWBZ premium of 15%

of their income). People who receive nursing home care must pay their own contribution as well depending on their income, composition of the household, and the duration of their stay. The Dutch government encourages substitution here, or in other words, the replacement of expensive care (intramural care) by cheaper care (community care). This is due to financial considerations, but also is based on the idea that it is important to take the preferences of older adults into account. Older adults mostly prefer to stay at home as long as possible.

In the Netherlands, LTCFs provide multidisciplinary (MD) care, by addressing residents' complex problems in a MD care-plan. MD care is based on the assumption that the collaboration of different disciplines leads to a higher quality of care as compared to the sum of their separate efforts. Joint goals are set for the problems of the individual resident and one shared language is used to describe problems, goals, and actions. Therefore, nursing homes employ MD teams, including specialists in old age medicine, geropsychologists, occupational therapists, speech therapists, physiotherapists, psychomotor therapists, and others. The exact composition varies between homes. Most nursing homes made specialists in old age medicine responsible for the MD care-plan. To guarantee the quality of care, the care has to fulfill the Dutch norms for responsible care. These norms can be summarized as effective, efficient, safe, and client-oriented care, adapted to the needs of the client.

Over the past decade, nursing home care for people with dementia has changed drastically in the Netherlands. Several types of living arrangements for people with dementia where nursing home care is provided have been developed. In particular, the development of the concept of group living home care for people with dementia has received much attention. Currently, several types of nursing home care arrangements for people with dementia exist, including: (1) traditional large-scale nursing homes; (2) nursing home wards in homes for the aged; (3) large nursing homes where group living home care is provided; (4) group living homes nearby the main care facility; and (5) stand-alone group living homes in the community.

In the next section, the development of group living home care, the ideals of this type of care, and the role of MD teams and geropsychologists in particular, will be discussed in greater detail.

Group living home care[1]

In the 1980s, the need for starting small-scale group living home care for people with dementia was felt. At that time, large-scale institutions for people with mental retardation or psychiatric disorders had already been the subject of discussion for several years. These institutes were increasingly seen as inhuman and dehumanizing, stimulating dependency. Critics emphasized the importance of human care, where clients have more privacy and autonomy, the right to self-determination, and a normal life. The first Dutch group living home care for people with dementia dates back to 1981. Equivalent living arrangements followed at the end of the 1980s after visits to Sweden—where the development of group living homes had started—and a Dutch national reported stimulating group living home care. Since then, the number of group living home care arrangements in the Netherlands has rapidly increased.

Over the years, there have been many studies about the outcomes of group living home care as compared to modern traditional nursing home care in the Netherlands. Results show a varied picture. Group living home care has some beneficial effects on its residents, but recently build nursing homes—having bedrooms for one or two persons—perform well too. Six months after admission, residents of group living homes needed less help with Activities of Daily Living and were more socially engaged as compared to people in nursing homes. No differences were found

---

[1] This section is based on Depla and te Boekhorst (2007).

in behavioral problems or cognitive status between the groups. Residents of group living homes had greater aesthetics and had more activities to keep them engaged. Less physical restraints were used in group living settings, but no differences were found in the use of psychotropic drugs (te Boekhorst, Depla, de Lange, Pot, & Eefsting, 2009).

In addition, group living home care seemed to be associated with less burnout and less job dissatisfaction in nursing staff (te Boekhorst et al., 2008). With regard to family caregivers of the residents, no differences in perceived burden or health were found 6 months after admission. In both settings, burden and health of family caregivers were improved. The only differences found showed that family caregivers were more satisfied with essential aspects of the care in the group living home situations. They perceived the staff in these homes as less rushed with care tasks, while displaying more respect for the world as experienced by the residents. They also had the impression that the staff showed more interest in the life history of the residents (te Boekhorst, Pot, Depla, Smit, de Lange, Eefsting, 2008).

Ideals of group living home care

We carried out a concept-mapping exercise to clarify what Dutch pioneers of small-scale group living home care for people with dementia thought were the most crucial features in such settings (te Boekhorst, Depla, de Lange, Pot, & Eefsting, 2007). Six clusters of features could be distinguished. The first and most important cluster found can be summarized as "Residents for better for worse." The pioneers of this type of care argued that in an ideal group living home care, residents stay until their death. That means no referral to another facility when the disease is progressing or behavioral problems are increasing. This is different from the situation in Sweden, where group living homes are meant as an intermediary type of facility. However, in the Netherlands as well, some group living homes do not always fulfill this ideal, in contrast to what the pioneers would advocate.

The second cluster of features that could be distinguished is "daily life is organized analogous to that of a normal household." Residents must have the rights and duties that they would in a normal household. For example, they must be able to go outside safely and by themselves. The feature most often mentioned in this cluster was "cooking takes place in the group living home." Thus, dinner is not prepared in a huge kitchen by professional cooks as in hospital-like nursing homes.

The third cluster encompassed residents' right to be their own boss in their own home and their own life. They have freedom of choice. Examples included: choosing your own hairdresser and not simply be sent to the one in a care facility. But it also means the right to quarrel with other residents or to choose whether you do or do not want your name at the front door. The most important feature mentioned was that residents may get up, go to the toilet, or go to sleep whenever they want.

The fourth cluster showed that the staff need to be part of the household. This includes staff not wearing a uniform, but also that the group living home care must have a vision that puts the residents' needs at the forefront.

A fifth cluster is that residents form a group together. Residents live as a family, where their family members are welcome and may join in for dinner, help provide care, and stay overnight. Thus, visiting hours are not in line with the ideals of group living home care.

The last cluster, namely that people live in an archetypal house, was viewed as the least important. However, there is still a debate in the Netherlands whether stand-alone group living homes are preferred above smaller units within the walls of large-scale institutes. Some pioneers argue that an archetypal home is an essential feature. As one states: "This is not because you live with a small number of people together in a home *per se*, but it is a necessary condition to run a normal household. With six you can sit around a table, but with more people one table is not enough.

An archetypal house stands for a common environment, familiar stimuli of daily life, and clarity" (Depla & te Boekhorst, 2007).

In conclusion, to provide group living home care, care needs to move from a hospital model to a person-centered model, and from institute dictated care to individual, human care.

Organization of care and the role of geropsychologists

Providing group living home care does not mean that nursing staff is less needed or can be replaced by housewives. In contrast, in Dutch group living homes more nursing staff are in charge and a higher percentage of these staff have a relatively high educational level. Thus, in that sense group living home care is more expensive; however, professional cooks, cleaners, and other such services are not or only rarely required.

The question arises as to whether small-scale care can be sustained with the greying of the population and the increasing tightness in the labor market. Recruitment and maintenance of nursing staff in group living homes might be easier, because they have higher job satisfaction and less burnout in comparison to their colleagues in newly built nursing homes. This is partially explained by the staff having greater control; they can do their job in accordance with their own insights into what is best. They also feel less job demands. They feel they have more time for the residents and for providing care, maybe because there are less strict rules and regulations and the focus is more on residents' wishes and needs rather than on tasks that need to be performed. A third reason for more job satisfaction and less burnout is that staff believe they receive more support from co-workers. High levels of control mean sharing responsibility for the residents with just a few colleagues. It seems likely that interactions with these colleagues will revolve around the residents and thus increase social support.

In group living homes, the role of the MD team is not different from the role of such a team in traditional nursing homes. MD teams need to support the nursing staff and take responsibility for the care of the residents. Because of the change from a hospital model to a living one's life model, MD teams will operate at a greater distance from the residents. As a consequence, psychologists and other members of the MD team are increasingly dependent on the "eyes and ears" of the nursing staff. Therefore, a regular screening of the residents with regard to biological, psychological, and social aspects increases in importance. Another difference in the role of geropsychologists in group living homes as compared to traditional nursing homes is related to the emphasis on individual, person-centered care. In group living homes, psychologists are more focused on improving the well-being of the residents instead of treatment or prevention of problems. Because of the emphasis on well-being instead of problems or diseases, some group living homes made the geropsychologist responsible for the MD care-plan.

Person-centered care

In Dutch group living homes person-centered care is provided, which means that care is provided in a way that creates a daily life as normal as possible for a specific resident. In person-centered care, there is much attention paid to the individuality of the residents. There is continuous attention to what fits best for the individual: how does someone respond to his/her environment and what does it mean for the way in which we approach that person? Person-centered care is characterized by the following principles (de Lange, 2005; Woods, 1995):

- No discussion about the truth, in the sense of absolute orientation to reality, but instead communications showing respect for the dignity of a person with dementia and his or her unique experience of reality
- Looking for possibilities, in spite of limitations

- Emphasizing identity and the life cycle
- Attention to individual needs and wishes
- Consideration of the individuals' need for either autonomy or dependence

Nursing staff in homes for people with dementia are trained in several ways to provide person-centered care. Examples are reality orientation, validation, reminiscence, and "snoezelen." These types of care focus on coping with cognitive deterioration, coping with the past, or stimulating the expression of feelings or senses (de Lange, 2007).

There is a growing emphasis on the implementation and enhancement of person-centered care in living arrangements for people with dementia in the Netherlands. Geropsychologists are often involved in the decision to change the care policy from a more task-oriented approach into a person-centered approach, especially but not exclusively in group living homes. In addition, geropsychologists teach and coach the nursing staff in person-centered care. This is an important—indirect—role for the improvement of residents' quality of life, since the educational level of the nursing staff is rather low due to the absence of registered nurses in Dutch nursing homes. Meetings with the nursing staff and a geropsychologist are organized to reflect on the way they care for the residents.

Improving quality of life in dementia[2]

Maria, 83 years old with a diagnosis of Alzheimer's disease, recently moved to a group living home for people with dementia. Maria is the mother of two daughters and is someone who is very loyal to her family and does not ask much for herself. Her family is very important to her. She never worked; she was at home with the children and took care of the household. She likes working in the garden and cooking very much. She is a very active woman and almost never sits down. Maria seems to feel at home in the group living home and helps out in the household as much as she can. Sometimes the nursing staff have to remind her to sit down for a minute and drink a cup of tea herself. She folds the laundry, does the dishes, and helps the nursing staff to prepare dinner. She especially likes to help residents in the group living home who are less independent and need help. For example, there is a resident who is not able to talk anymore and eat herself. Maria helps her very carefully. Maria does not go to activities that are organized outside the group living home very often. She prefers to stay at home and help out in the household chores.

To illustrate the role of the geropsychologist in the Dutch nursing home care, we will discuss the care process after Maria's admission to a group living home care.

Multidisciplinary meetings

In order to keep Maria's quality of life as high as possible, an important question after admission is: What are her preferences and needs?

In all Dutch living arrangements for people with dementia, every resident has to be discussed a few weeks after admission as well as reviewed on an ongoing and regular basis, at least twice a year, in MD meetings. On wards where people with dementia are living, usually the geropsychologist joins these meetings. In addition, the MD team typically consists of a member of the nursing staff, the nursing home physician, and paramedics, depending on the needs of the resident. The role of geropsychologists in these MD meetings is threefold. First, they bring their expertise in the psychological functioning of older adults in general and older adults with neurological progressive diseases in particular, as well as their expertise in person-centered approaches

---

[2] This section is based on Gerritsen and Steverink (2007).

with people with dementia. Second, they can help to clarify the needs of the residents based on the information that other disciplines bring to the table, because of their communication skills and analytic approach. Finally, their analytic approach and methodological skills can help to evaluate the outcomes of the care or interventions.

Care-life plan

The care-life plan is a first tool to assess the needs of the residents, developed by the Netherlands branch organization (Actiz) of homes for the aged, nursing homes, and home care. A couple of years ago, the quality of care in nursing homes was regularly, and negatively, in the news. Therefore, norms for responsible care have been developed. Actiz states that residents' care plans not only need to be focused on medical care and nursing, but also on their living environment and well-being and developed within the care-life plan. This plan takes the following aspects into account:

◆ Mental well-being

◆ Physical well-being and health

◆ Daily scheduling according to the resident's own interest and maintenance of social contact and participation

◆ Housing and living circumstances

The central question in this plan is how the resident wants to live. The starting points are the preferences, questions, needs, and goals of the resident which are obtained during an interview with the person with dementia and a family member. In the care-life plan, how the resident wants to live and what support from the MD team (nursing staff and other disciplines) the resident can depend on is described. This plan is continuously changing and always focused on the best match with the (changing) needs of the resident.

To illustrate the functioning of the care-life plan, we describe one care question of Maria's plan concerning her daily schedule and the maintenance of social contact and participation for her. Her needs are formulated as follows: "Maria is a very active woman and likes to help other people and in the household. She likes to get compliments for her help and likes to feel useful. Sometimes she does not take time to rest." The goal is: "Maria feels useful and appreciated and has a balance between activity and rest."

Actions formulated for this goal are:

◆ Maria gets out of her room and is stimulated to help out with activities in the household such as doing the dishes, preparing dinner, and folding laundry.

◆ Maria helps other residents with things they need help with such as pushing their wheelchair, eating, and drinking.

◆ Maria takes care of the plants in the garden.

◆ Maria is reminded to take a break and sit down at least to drink coffee in the morning, to rest for 1 hour after lunch, and to drink tea in the afternoon.

When Maria and her plan are discussed in the MD meeting after 6 months, the nursing staff point out that Maria gets somewhat less careful when she is helping other residents with eating. The nursing staff is sometimes worried that a co-resident will choke on his or her food. The psychologist asks how they deal with it. They explain that they sometimes warn Maria to be careful or try to take over the task. When the psychologist asks how Maria reacts, one of the staff members says that Maria gets irritated or sad. The daughter of Maria, who is also present during the MD meetings, adds that she recognizes that the cognitive problems of her mother are increasing. She feels her mother is deteriorating and gets upset when she is not able to do the things she normally likes to do like helping other people.

Assessing quality of life: the Qualidem

Apart from the care-life plan, some nursing homes and group living homes in the Netherlands also use the Qualidem. The instrument is rated by professional caregivers and scored by a psychologist. The scale includes nine subscales: care relationship, positive and negative affect, self-esteem, restless behavior, social relations, social isolation, feeling at home, and having something to do (Ettema et al., 2006). This tool is used to obtain a picture of the way in which the resident is functioning well and what are points of concern where quality of care can be improved. Furthermore, the Qualidem is used to evaluate outcomes of care and treatment. In the group living home where Maria lives, they also use this instrument.

The Qualidem of Maria confirms what the nursing staff describe in the MD meeting. The psychologist explains that in comparison to 6 months ago, Maria is crying more and has a lower positive affect. Additionally, she has less frequently something to do and seems to have fewer social relationships and is more socially isolated. Finally, it seems that the care relationship between the nursing staff and Maria is diminished. It seems that the changing situation of Maria has had a great impact on her.

Meeting to discuss how best to cope with residents

The psychologist suggests making an appointment with the nursing staff to generate a plan for how to let Maria participate and feel useful in spite of her deteriorating cognition. This plan will be included in the care-life plan of Maria and will be evaluated in a MD meeting after 1 month. In the meeting on how to best cope with residents, first residents' problems are analyzed and alternative ways to cope with the resident are formulated. In the case of Maria, the following strategies are put forward: changing the place of the nursing staff and Maria at the table, asking her to lay the table, to fill the glasses, and to cut the meat for residents who need help.

In addition, the nursing staff wish to know how to stop Maria helping others without making her upset. Because feeling appreciated is very important to Maria, the psychologist suggests thanking Maria for her assistance and asking her to help with another task. They decide to try this new approach for a period of 2 weeks. If it works well they will continue. The psychologist writes the plan down and asks the nursing staff to report the results of the new approach after every meal. They will write down whether Maria wanted to help other residents with eating, whether they tried to stop her, and if so, how she responded and what the effect was of asking her to do something else.

After 2 weeks the new approach is evaluated. It seems that it is difficult to make sure that Maria does not help residents. She starts immediately when they sit down for dinner. The nursing staff does report that thanking her and asking to do someone else is an effective strategy to prevent her from getting upset. The new care approach is made definite in Maria's care-life plan and she will be discussed in a MD meeting in another 6 months.

The diagnosis of depression with overlapping somatic co-morbidity[3]

Monica is 82 years old and just has had a stroke in the left hemisphere. After a short stay in hospital, she is referred to a nursing home for revalidation. She has a significant loss in the strength of her right arm and leg and mild dysarthria. She has a chronic renal insufficiency for which she needs dialysis on a regular basis.

---

[3] This section is based on Pot and Falck (2002).

In the first month of her stay in the nursing home, Monica does her exercises faithfully. She wants to do as much as she can independently. She comes to the gym alone at the agreed-upon time. Nevertheless, the strength of her arms and legs is improving slowly. As a result she will not be able to return home, in contrast to her expectations.

In the MD meeting 6 weeks after admission, the physiotherapist mentions that Monica seems to be declining. She often forgets to come to the gym and she complains about fatigue. In addition, the nurse reports that she is confused in the mornings and wants to stay in bed. She does not sleep well, even though the physician had already prescribed temazepam (Normison). She does not eat well anymore and has lost seven pounds. The nurse also mentions that Monica feels tired and does not show any interest in things. Monica has told her that she is not able to stand and walk, because she is too tired. She also exclaimed: "And now, I am also having Alzheimer's disease," referring to her forgetfulness. Monica is heartily sick of it. Some professionals who attend the MD meeting say they can understand, because of her advanced age, the difficulties she has, in combination with not being able to go home soon.

Is Monica depressed? Does she have the first signs of Alzheimer's disease? And if so, what to do? The geropsychologist is asked for diagnosis and advice.

Factors hampering recognition of depression

Depression is highly prevalent among older people with co-morbid disorders like diabetes, rheumatism, cancer, stroke, or other cardiovascular problems (Bierman, Comijs, Depla, ten Have, & Pot, 2007). Prevalence of depression in residents with stroke ranges from 20% to 60%, with an estimated mean of about one-third. There is little agreement on causal mechanisms, risk factors, and consequences of depression in people who have had a stroke. These residents show a minor improvement in rehabilitation programs in comparison to non-depressed stroke patients (Lenzi, Altieri, Maestrini, 2008). The effectiveness of psychological interventions for people who have had a stroke and subsequently develop depression is still unclear (Hacket et al., 2008).

It is difficult to diagnose a depressive disorder in the presence of a co-morbidity like a stroke, for several reasons. First, there is symptom overlap. The fatigue of Monica may be a symptom of depression, but may also be a symptom of having had a stroke. There is no gold standard for diagnosing depression in stroke patients. In addition, older adults may mention physical problems more than mental problems or may attribute symptoms to a physical illness (attribution bias) rather than a psychological cause. Monica attributes her fatigue and loss of interest to the stroke she had, but this is not necessarily the case. Another reason for difficulties in recognition of depression is that older people may be less used to discussing mental health problems. Finally, there may be factors related to health care professionals' impeding diagnosis of depression. Apart from lacking expertise, they may think depression is related to getting older ("agism") or living in a nursing home ("nursing home-ism") or they do not want to stigmatize the person. However, if an existing depressive disorder is not detected, there will be no treatment. In cases where the diagnosis is not clear, a treatment trial is often recommended.

Screening for depression

If the geropsychologist is not sure whether or not Monica has depression, a screening instrument might be used to establish depressive symptoms. For geropsychologists in Dutch nursing homes, the preferred instrument is the Geriatric Depression Scale (GDS; Yesavage et al., 1983). For residents like Monica, the GDS has a few advantages in comparison to other depression screens. The items of the GDS have a straightforward response format (yes/no) and are therefore easier for frail people with limited energy or people with some cognitive problems like concentration deficits to answer. Furthermore, the items do not contain depressive symptoms, such as sleeping problems, which can also be related to other disorders. The sensitivity and specificity are good and the validity is guaranteed for people with absent to moderate memory problems (reflected by a score on the Mini-Mental State Examination of 15 or higher) (Gerety et al., 1994; Jongenelis et al., 2005). There are different versions of the GDS with varying numbers of items. The original version contains 30 items, but in Dutch nursing home care we often use the eight-item version, in which items are removed that are less appropriate for residents in nursing homes (Jongenelis et al., 2007). The GDS can also be used to measure the effect of an intervention (Smalbrugge, Jongenelis, Pot, Beekman, & Eefsting, 2008). Because the questions are often presented orally, preferably a psychologist will be involved to improve the validity of the answers.

Weighing symptoms

Self-evidently, screening for depressive symptoms is not the same as diagnosing a depressive disorder. To establish a depressive disorder, the symptoms of depression have to be weighted. The complexity of this weighing process becomes apparent in the case of Monica. Apart from the core symptoms of depression—lack of interest or pleasure—she has several symptoms that might stem from a variety of different causes. For example, fatigue and loss of energy may be due to Monica's stroke, renal insufficiency, medication, or sleeping problems. Her sleeping problems may be the result of a restless roommate. Her fatigue and sleeping problems may simply be a consequence of her age. Her bad appetite and related loss of weight might be due to difficulties with swallowing as a result of her stroke, but environmental factors may also play a role. Her symptoms might also be attributed to grief, since she cannot go home in contrast to her wishes and expectations. This is especially hard for her as she has always been an independent woman and cannot accept that she needs help from others.

Diagnosing depressive disorders in residents like Monica are complex puzzles. Because of what has been discussed, it will be difficult or even impossible to decide whether Monica has a depressive disorder, even after more research regarding her symptoms. However, treatment will not be different *per se*, because a high level of depressive symptoms is often related to significant suffering as well (Smalbrugge et al., 2006). It is clear that Monica suffers, as demonstrated by her desperate exclamation that she also thinks she has Alzheimer's disease.

Treatment trial

If questions remain, trial of a treatment is the only way to judge whether or not depression has been the right diagnosis and this was the right treatment. Possible treatments to trial include not only pharmacological, but also psychological, interventions. Which one will be administered will be determined by the preference of the patient.

In the case of Monica, psychological treatment was advised as a first step, in light of potential side effects of antidepressants. After a few sessions in which the slowing of her rehabilitation, and the consequences and the related difficulties of this for her were discussed, the symptoms of depression started to disappear.

Assessment of mental capacity[4]

Jacob, 85 years old and living in a nursing home, needs to decide whether or not he wants hip surgery. This is a complex decision, because the surgery is not without danger in light of

[4] This section is based on Diesfeldt and Teunisse (2007).

his frailty. Furthermore, there is a 50% chance that the surgery will not be successful. However, if he decides that he does not want surgery, the pain he has will continue. The specialist in old age medicine has tried to ask Jacob what he wanted. However, his answer was unclear, probably due to cognitive problems.

Clients' rights and psychologists' duties

In the MD meeting the question arises as to what to do. Geropsychologists may play an important role in these kind of sitiuations. Different questions arise: What kind of problems does Jacob have with his cognition? Do we need to do a (neuro)psychological evaluation? And if so, how to introduce such an assessment? May we ask his children for their opinion? And what if Jacob does not want us to get into contact with them? The question behind all these questions is: Does Jacob retain the mental capacity to make the decision about his hip surgery?

In the Netherlands, people—including those living in a LTCF—have the right to self-determination or the free choice of one's own acts without external compulsion. Advanced age is no reason to decide that Jacob no longer has the capacity to decide whether or not he wants the surgery. The same holds for having Alzheimer's disease or a related disorder. The mental capacity required to make specific decisions or take specific actions vary with the nature and complexity of the decision. Therefore, mental capacity must always be judged in relation to a specific decision or action. In other words, mental capacity is not a categorical concept. As long as there are no serious doubts or clear signs of the opposite, people have the right to self-determination, including nursing home residents.

There are also laws in the Netherlands stating that residents of nursing homes or homes for the aged need to agree with assessment or treatment, after they have been informed in a way they can understand. Clinical health care professionals like physicians and psychologists need to decide whether or not they think the client has the mental capacity to decide on a specific treatment. In the case of Jacob, the specialist in old age medicine had doubts and asked the geropsychologist to assess whether Jacob is able to decide for himself about the surgery. Before starting the assessment, geropsychologists need to realize that there must be a good reason to do so. In this case, it is clear that the decision whether or not to have surgery is complex and will have far-reaching consequences for the client.

First of all, geropsychologists must take the mental capacity of clients into account in their own clinical practice. Their role may also be to advise other disciplines with regard to the mental capacity of clients. If it turns out, after assessment, that a client like Jacob does not have the mental capacity to make a decision on treatment, a legal representative can be consulted. If there is no legal representative, than the following people can be consulted in order of importance: an official delegate; the partner or husband/wife; or a close family member (parent, child, brother, sister). Since Jacob has no legal representative, delegate, or partner, his children would be the ones to ask about their father's preferences in case he now lacks the mental capacity to decide. Note that this is NOT the same as asking what the preference of the children would be.

Assessment: role of geropsychologist

To assess whether Jacob has the mental capacity to decide whether or not he wants hip surgery, the geropsychologist makes an appointment to speak with him. She summarizes his situation concisely. Recognizing his cognitive difficulties, she uses simple words, repeats information, and asks questions to confirm that he understands the information. Easy, written information is presented to support her verbal description of the situation.

In addition, the geropsychologist asks questions to check if Jacob understands the problem, can tell what the consequences of a positive and negative decision would be, and which arguments he has to chose for one or the other. He has to show insight in the nature of the decision and the options available.

The preliminary conclusion drawn based on his answers is that he lacks the mental capacity to make this complex decision. To be sure, the geropsychologist did a neuropsychological examination to get some insight into his skills crucial for making an informed decision (e.g. memory and executive functions like planning and problem solving). His cognitive skills were sufficient for decisions with calculable consequences; however, for more complex decisions such as whether or not wanting hip surgery might have immense consequences for his life, his cognitive functioning was too limited.

Based on all the information gathered, the geropsychologist draws the conclusion that Jacob was no longer mentally capable of making the decision for the hip surgery himself. Therefore, his children were asked what to do, and they made it clear that their father would not have wanted the hip surgery.

Mediator-facilitated therapy[5]

Henk, 75 years old with a diagnosis of frontotemporal dementia, is living in a modern large-scale nursing home. In the last few months, it has become increasingly difficult to communicate with him. He resides on a ward with 30 other people with a dementia diagnosis. There are two living rooms were they can stay during the day. At the moment, he increasingly gets into conflicts with other residents and reacts in an agitated or aggressive manner when the nursing staff assist him in the morning. The nursing staff find it very difficult to deal with Henk's behavior.

Why is Henk so agitated and sometimes even aggressive to nursing staff and other residents? How could staff members cope with his behavior? The geropsychologist is consulted and he starts mediation therapy. Mediation therapy in this context means that we treat the problems of a client via key people, such as nurses or family members, also called mediators. The geropsychologist treats the client indirectly, by advising the mediators how to cope with the client. Because the same behavior of clients can have different causes and triggers, a functional analysis and holistic theory is essential. One of the aims of this type of therapy is to decrease challenging behavior.

Analyzing challenging behavior: the ABC model

In a meeting focused on analyzing the aggressive behavior of Henk, one of the nurses reports that the other day Henk was sitting in the living room in the afternoon. Some residents had a family member visiting them. Henk suddenly stood up and yelled to the husband of another resident and showed him his fist. This situation frightened other residents and shocked the nurse. She took Henk's arm and tried to take Henk with her to another room, to explain that he scared the co-residents. Henk reacted aggressively and tried to hit her. The other nurses recognize this situation and confirm that they also find it difficult to deal with his behavior, because of its unexpected and unpredictable nature. Some, but not all, staff members have the experience that Henk is also angry and tries to hit them while they help him with washing and dressing in the morning.

The nursing staff decides to start with analyzing the aggressive behavior of Henk in the living room because of its broad negative impact. It had a negative impact on several other residents,

---

5 This section is based on Hamer (2007).

their families, and the staff members themselves. The reactions of the people around him will make Henk feel unpleasant as well.

The ABC model offers a structured way to analyze the behavior of Henk. The letters ABC stand for Antecedents, Behavior, and Consequences.

A. Describe the Antecedents:

    a. What might be the matter with the client?

    b. What happens around the client?

    c. Did something change lately?

B. Describe the Behavior:

    a. What does the resident do?

    b. Where does it happen?

    c. For how long?

    d. How often and how serious is it?

    e. For whom is it a problem?

C. Describe the Consequences:

    a. How does the behavior continue when nobody responds?

    b. How do staff members and others respond to the behavior?

    c. What are the consequences for the resident?

In the case of Henk, the functional analysis looks as follows:

A. Antecedents:

- Hearing loss
- Problems understanding people
- Problems to make himself clear
- Tiredness in the afternoon
- Lot of noise when family members are visiting
- No control over his behavior

B. Behavior:

- Yelling
- Showing fist
- (trying to) slap

C. Consequences:

- Getting annoyed, but stays in the living room
- Nurses tell him to stop, that he may not do what he has done
- Co-residents and visitors react scared
- Grasping his arm to remove him

The holistic theory is as follows:

Henk is a 75-year-old man with frontotemporal dementia. He used to read a lot and was very interested in politics and liked to discuss this subject with individual friends. He did not like to be in a group. In situations with new people he was always ill at ease. Since the frontotemporal dementia started, he is not able to respond in social situations as normal people would. He makes inappropriate comments. Currently, it appears that his speech and understanding are decreasing and that communication is becoming more difficult. When he lived at home, in the afternoons he withdrew himself and sat in his study in a reclining chair and read a book, watched the TV, or listened to classical music. When he came to the nursing home, the nursing staff tried to let him rest in bed for an hour in the afternoon. He came out of his bed very quickly. From that time on Henk does not rest during the afternoon. In contrast, he stays in a room where visitors make a lot of noise. He gets more and more annoyed and agitated until his limit is reached and he starts to yell. The physical contact and the warnings of the nursing staff threaten him.

Behavioral therapy

Behavioral therapy assumes that behavior is learned by experience, triggered by internal and external stimuli (antecedents), and reinforced by its consequences. The assumption is that in the same way, alternative behavior can be learned. The geropsychologist helps the nursing staff to formulate alternative, desirable behaviors and to formulate antecedents and consequences that might stimulate the new behaviors. In this case, the following goal is formulated: "Henk does not get aggressive with other people in the living room." It is important to choose a realistic goal that can be achieved. It is preferable to start relatively small and to formulate a new goal when the first one is achieved instead of formulating a larger goal at the start. To formulate a plan, a fixed set of questions is being used in mediator-facilitated therapy in Dutch nursing homes. The desired behavior and the antecedents and consequences are described below:

- New behavior
  - Henk does not get aggressive with other people in the living room.
- New antecedents
  - His hearing loss, his problems understanding people, problems making himself clear, his tiredness in the afternoon, and the lack of control over his behavior are taken into account.
  - He is offered a pleasant quiet place several times during the day with the music he likes and a reclining chair.
- New consequences:
  - No warnings
  - Support what you say with body language
  - No physical contact when he gets angry
  - When he gets very agitated or aggressive, react by asking the people in the living room who are sitting at his table to go with you. Do not try to take Henk with you (e.g. by grasping his arm). Let him be for a while.
  - Go to him when he has calmed down and ask if he is feeling better. Do not talk about the incident, he might not remember or understand.

In the next meeting 4 weeks later the intervention for Henk is evaluated by the nursing staff and the psychologist. The result of this intervention is that the behavior did not reappear.

Conclusion

The aim of this chapter was twofold. First, we described nursing home care in the Netherlands, especially the change from traditional hospital-like care to person-centered care and the general role of geropsychologists in the nursing home setting. In addition, we described four typical cases in different nursing home settings to illustrate the role of geropsychologists. A few conclusions can be drawn based on what has been discussed. Geropsychologists have different roles in the Dutch nursing home care system. Their role as clinical practitioner includes the more traditional tasks such as (neuro)psychological assessment and treatment of mental health problems, but prevention and improvement of quality of life of the residents is increasingly part of this role. The same holds for their role as a coach of the care system around the residents, and especially the nursing staff. This broad expertise of geropsychologists, much broader than doing (neuro) psychological assessments alone, make them an essential partner in the care for nursing home residents. We did not discuss the other roles geropsychologists may also have: as a manager or as a scientific researcher in such a facility. The last one is especially important to improve the evidence-based practice of geropsychology and to improve the strength of the discipline to enhance and optimize the quality of life of nursing home residents.

Key readings

Unfortunately, most of the literature we referred to concerning the role of geropsychologists in long-term care is part of the Dutch Manual of Geropsychology and currently is not available in English. The literature concerning group living home care is available in English. The references by our research group (e.g. te Boekhorst et al.) are listed in the section "References." Furthermore, we are working on a large-scale study in 140 Dutch living arrangements for people with dementia: the Living Arrangements for people with Dementia study (LAD study). In the next few years the results of this study will be published.

Points of reflection

Changes in nursing home care from hospital-like care to person-centered care challenges practitioners to:

a. Reflect on the situations where geropsychologists could be involved in nursing home care, for example, structured evaluation of residents' different life domains on a regular basis.

b. Attend to improvements in quality of life before treatment of mental health problems.

c. Place a stronger emphasis on the role of a coach within the care system, especially with nursing staff.

References

Bierman, H., Comijs, M., Depla, M.F., ten Have, M., & Pot, A.M. (2007). Psychische problemen en GGZ-gebruik bij ouderen met lichamelijke aandoeningen [Psychological problems and mental health care use by older asdults with physical problems]. In A.M. Pot, M.F. Depla, & M. ten Have (Eds.), *Monitor geestelijke gezondheidszorg ouderen. Rapportage 2006 [Monitor mental health care older adults. Report 2006]* (pp. 32–37). Utrecht, The Netherlands: Trimbos-instituut.

Depla, M.F., & te Boekhorst, S. (Eds.) (2007). *Kleinschalig wonen voor mensen met dementie: Doen of laten? [Group living home care for people with dementia: Do or do not?]* (pp. 58–61). Utrecht, The Netherlands: Trimbos-instituut/EMGO-VUmc.

de Lange, J. (2005). Belevingsgerichte zorg bij mensen met dementie [Person-centered care for people with dementia]. In A. Schene (Ed.), *Jaarboek voor psychiatrie en psychotherapie [Yearbook for psychiatry and psychotherapy] 2005–2006* (pp. 218–229). Houten: Bohn Stafleu van Loghum.

de Lange, J. (2007). Persoonsgerichte benaderingswijzen bij dementie [Person-centered approaches in dementia]. In A.M. Pot, Y. Kuin, & M. Vink (Eds.), *Handboek ouderenpsychologie [Manual geropsychology]*. Utrecht, The Netherlands: De Tijdstroom.

Diesfeldt, H., & Teunisse, S. (2007). Wilsbekwaamheid [Mental capacity]. In A.M. Pot, Y. Kuin, & M. Vink (Eds.), *Handboek ouderenpsychologie [Manual geropsychology]*. Utrecht, The Netherlands: De Tijdstroom.

Ettema, T.P., Dröes, R–M., de Lange, J., Mellenbergh, G.J., & Ribbe, M.W. (2006). QUALIDEM: development and evaluation of a dementia specific quality of life instrument—validation. *International Journal of Geriatric Psychiatry, 5*, 424–430.

Gerety, M.B., Williams, J.W., Mulrow, C.D., Cornell, J.E., Kadri, A.A., Roosenberg, J., et al. (1994). Performance of case-finding tools for depression in the nursing-home. *Journal of the American Geriatrics Society, 42*, 1103–1109.

Gerritsen, D., & Steverink, N. (2007). Kwaliteit van leven [Quality of life]. In A.M. Pot, Y. Kuin, & M. Vink (Eds.), *Handboek ouderenpsychologie [Manual geropsychology]*. Utrecht, The Netherlands: De Tijdstroom.

Hacket, M.L., Anderson, C.S., House, A., & Xia, J. (2008). Interventions for treating depression after stroke. *Cochrane Database Systematic Review, 8*, CD003437.

Hamer, T. (2007). Gedragstherapie en mediatieve behandeling [Behavior therapy and mediative treatment]. In A.M. Pot, Y. Kuin, & M. Vink (Eds.), *Handboek ouderenpsychologie [Manual geropsychology]*. Utrecht, The Netherlands: De Tijdstroom.

Jongenelis, K., Pot, A.M., Eisses, A.M.H., Gerritsen, D.L., Derksen, M., Beekman, A.T.F., et al. (2005). Diagnostic accuracy of the original 30-item and shortened versions of the Geriatric Depression Scale in nursing home patients. *International Journal of Geriatric Psychiatry, 20*, 1067–1074.

Jongenelis, K., Gerritsen, D.L., Pot, A.M., Beekman, A.T., Eisses, A.M., Kluiter, H., et al. (2007). Construction and validation of a patient- and user-friendly nursing home version of the Geriatric Depression Scale. *International Journal of Geriatric Psychiatry, 22*, 837–842.

Lenzi, G.L., Altieri, M., & Maestrini, I. (2008). Post-stroke depression. *Revue Neurologique, 164*, 837–840.

Pot, A.M., & Falck, R. (2002). Diagnostiek van depressie: Instrumenten en aandachtspunten. [Diagnosis of depression: Instruments and points of attention]. In M.T. Vink, B.G. Deelman, & R.P. Falck (Eds.), *Senioren en CVA: Veranderingen in cognitie, emoties en gedrag.* [Seniors and stroke: Changes in cognition, emotion and behavior]. Houten/Diegem: Bohn Stafleu Van Loghum.

Smalbrugge, M., Pot, A.M., Jongenelis, L., Gundy, C.M., Beekman, A.T., & Eefsting, J.A. (2006). The impact of depression and anxiety on well being, disability and use of health care services in nursing home patients. *International Journal of Geriatric Psychiatry, 21*, 325–332.

Smalbrugge, M., Jongenelis, L., Pot, A.M., Beekman, A.T., & Eefsting, J.A. (2008). Screening for depression and assessing change in severity of depression. Is the Geriatric Depression Scale (30-, 15- and 8-item versions) useful for both purposes in nursing home patients? *Aging & Mental Health, 12*, 244–248.

te Boekhorst, S., Depla, M.F., de Lange, J., Pot, A.M., & Eefsting, J.A. (2007). Kleinschaligheid in de zorg voor ouderen met dementie: Een begripsverheldering. [Small-scale group living for elderly with dementia: A clarification]. *Tijdschrift voor Gerontologie en Geriatrie, 38*, 17–26.

te Boekhorst, S., Depla, M.F., de Lange, J., Pot, A.M., & Eefsting, J.A. (2009). The effects of group living homes on older people with dementia: A comparison with traditional nursing home care. *International Journal of Geriatric Psychiatry, 24*, 970–978.

te Boekhorst, S., Pot, A.M., Depla, M.F, Smit, D., de Lange, J., & Eefsting, J.A. (2008). Group living homes for older people with dementia: The effects on psychological distress of informal caregivers. *Aging & Mental Health, 12*, 761–768.

te Boekhorst, S., Willemse, B., Depla, M.F., Eefsting, J.A., & Pot, A.M. (2008). Working in group living homes for older people with dementia: The effects on job satisfaction and burnout and the role of job characteristics. *International Psychogeriatrics, 20*, 927–940.

Woods, B. (1995). The beginnings of a new culture in care. In T. Kitwood & S. Benson (Eds.), *The new culture of dementia care* (pp. 19–23). London: Hawker Publications.

Yesavage, J.A., Brink, T.L., Rose, T.L., Lum, O., Huang, V., Adey, M., et al. (1983). Development and validation of a geriatric depression screening scale: A preliminary report. *Journal of Psychiatric Research, 17*, 37–49.

Chapter 17

Suicide in later life

Helen Chiu, Sandra Chan, and Joshua Tsoh

Introduction

Suicide is a tragic end to an individual's life and public health crisis for the global community. In 2002, an estimated 877,000 lives were lost worldwide through suicide, representing 1.5% of the global burden of disease or more than 20 million years of healthy life lost through premature death/disability (World Health Organization [WHO], 2003). The United Nations (UN) estimates that by 2020, the population over 60 years of age will reach 1 billion, with 70% residing in developing countries (United Nations Population Division/DESA, 2009). Older adults, as the fastest growing population segment worldwide, are at greater risk for suicide than any other age group (Stevens et al., 1999; WHO, 1999). With the suicide death toll expected to climb in this high-risk age group in a rapidly aging population, calls to translate research findings into effective prevention and postvention strategies become all the more compelling. The design of effective suicide prevention strategies hinges on the identification of specific and quantifiable risk factors in epidemiological, cohort, and retrospective case-control psychological autopsy (PA) studies. As suicide is a multidetermined tragic outcome, further research is needed to define more precisely the interactions among emotional, physical, and social factors that determine risk for suicide in older adults. To provide a foundation for the case vignettes on later life attempted and completed suicide presented in this chapter, we begin with a broad overview of the correlates/risk factors for suicide and findings related to the application of prevention and postvention strategies in later life.

Epidemiology

Completed suicide

Among countries that provide statistics on suicide, nearly all report that suicide rates rise progressively with age, with the highest rates occurring among men aged 75 and over (Pearson & Conwell, 1995). There is wide cross-national variation in older adult suicide rates (Shah, Bhat, McKenzie, & Koen, 2007). In general, they are the lowest in Caribbean, Central American, and Arabic countries, and the highest in central and eastern European, some Asian, and some western European countries. Suicide rates are higher among men compared to women for both the 65–74 and 75+ age bands; however, suicide rates are higher in the latter age band compared to the former one for both women and men. In most Western countries, the ratio of male to female suicide rates is approximately 3:1, but in many Asian countries, the ratio is lower (Chiu, Chan, & Lam, 2001).

Attempted suicide and suicidal ideation

There is a dearth of epidemiological data on attempted suicide, especially in later life, as there is no systematic surveillance mechanism in even the most developed countries. As with suicidal ideation, attempted suicide is far less frequent in later life than among younger age groups

(Moscicki, 1997). In adolescence, the ratio of attempted to completed suicide is estimated to be 200:1 (Langley & Bayatti, 1984), while that of the general population ranges from 8:1 to 33:1 (Paykel, Myers, Lindenthal, & Tanner, 1974). There are approximately four attempts for each completed suicide in later life (Parkin & Stengel, 1965). Older people often have greater determination to die and use more lethal methods compared to other age groups (Conwell, 2001; Lawrence, Almeida, Hulse, Jablensky, & Holman, 2000), but they are driven by the same spectrum of risk factors including depression, ill health, and solitary living arrangements (De Leo & Scocco, 2000; Tsoh et al., 2005).

Older adults are less likely to endorse suicidal ideation than are younger subjects (Duberstein et al., 1999; Gallo, Anthony, & Muthen, 1994). Estimates of the prevalence of suicidal ideation vary widely across community, primary care, and tertiary care settings, ranging from less than 1% to over 20%. The frequency is higher among women, those with mental disorders (depression and dementia in particular), and those with a history of chronic physical disorders (Conwell, Duberstein, & Caine, 2002).

Risk factors for suicide in older adults

Risk factors for late-life suicide can be grouped into four general domains: mental health, physical health, social factors, and access to lethal means. Risk factors are often identified through prospective follow-ups of high-risk samples and retrospective case-control PA research. A prospective follow-up study of a high-risk group is often limited by a low base rate of suicide and lack of statistical power to demonstrate the effect size of the putative risk factors. PA is the term used to describe the method by which information about decedents is gathered retrospectively from relatives, friends, caregivers, others familiar with the decedents, and relevant records (Hawton et al., 1998). Limitations inherent in the PA approach are its retrospective nature and the potential for reporting bias.

Mental health

The presence of any axis I disorder is significantly associated with an elevated risk for suicide in older adults (Conwell et al., 2002). Depressive disorders stand out as significant predictors. Recurrent major depressive disorder is associated with the greatest relative risk, although single episode major depression, dysthymia, and minor depression are also significant predictors of completed suicide. Primary psychotic illness (e.g. schizophrenia, schizoaffective disorder, and delusional disorder), personality disorders, anxiety disorders, and alcohol and other substance use disorders appear to play a relatively small role in suicide among older adults compared to younger age groups. A PA study reported that depressive disorders associated with older adult suicide are often of a single episode and moderate severity, which suggests that older persons are likely to respond to standard therapies, especially when mood problems are not complicated by co-morbidities such as alcohol and other substance use disorders. Despite the prevalence of dementia in old age, it is infrequently diagnosed in completed suicide using the PA method (Conwell et al., 1996).

Prior history of suicide attempts is a statistically significant risk factor for suicide (Beautrais, 2002; Conwell et al., 2000). Chiu et al. (2004) found that almost one-third of older suicide decedents in a Chinese community had a history of a suicide attempt, and that over 30% of these attempts had occurred within 1 week prior to the completed suicide, which indicates the clinical significance of a prior suicide attempt in risk assessment.

Studies of the personality traits of late-life suicide completers are often uncontrolled ones. Harwood, Hawton, Hope, and Jacoby (2001) assessed the personality domain using a categorical approach and found no significant difference in the prevalence of personality disorder diagnosis between late-life suicide cases and controls. Duberstein, Conwell, and Caine (1994) examined personality traits using standardized measures in a case-control sample of suicide in older adults aged 50 years and over, and found that a high level of neuroticism and lower scores on the openness to experience factor on the NEO Personality Inventory distinguished suicide decedents from age- and gender-matched controls. The relationship of these traits to depressive disorders and their potential role as moderators of other putative risk factors for late-life suicide remain to be examined in future studies.

Physical health

Harris and Barraclough (1994) calculated standardized mortality ratios for suicide for more than 60 medical disorders and treatments including HIV/AIDS, Huntington's disease, multiple sclerosis, peptic ulcer, renal disease, spinal cord injury, and systemic lupus erythematosis. These disease/treatment entities are more characteristic of suicides among middle aged or young old than among old old adults. Case-control studies investigating risk for suicide associated with physical illness in older adults provide mixed results (Conwell et al., 2002). Some find that physical illness and the presence of a current serious physical condition significantly distinguish suicides from controls in analyses that do not control for the presence of depressive symptoms or syndromes. Others find that serious physical illness in any organ category is associated with suicide in men; however, these associations become insignificant when controlling for mood disorders. The foregoing studies indicate that physical illness and functional impairment may be associated with late-life suicide, but that the association is partly mediated through their relationship with affective disorders.

Social factors

Stressful life events are often implicated as antecedents to suicide attempts and completed suicide in older adults. The specific types of life events related to suicide in later life differ from those of younger suicide victims. For instance, interpersonal discord, financial and job problems, and legal difficulties are more typical of suicides in young and middle adulthood, whereas physical illness, loneliness, and social isolation are more typical of those in later life (Heikkinen & Lonnqvist, 1995; Carney, Rich, Burke, & Fowler, 1994). The apparent association between stressful life events and completed suicide may be mediated through other risk factors for suicide, such as depression. A case-control PA study that examined specific stressors in cases and controls found that financial/relationship problems distinguished the groups but that the associations became insignificant when controlling for other risk factors (such as depression). Further research is required to uncover the mediating effects of variables such as depression on the relationship between life events and suicide in later life.

Research findings on the role of social support and living situation in late-life suicide tend to be more consistent across uncontrolled and controlled studies. Studies comparing the living situation of suicide victims using census data find that older decedents are more likely than other older adults in the community to have lived alone, which suggests that social isolation and loneliness play a role in late-life suicide (e.g. Barraclough, 1971). Miller (1978) reported that controls were significantly more likely than suicides to have had a confidante. In a case-control study conducted in New Zealand, a low level of social interaction was found to be an independent risk factor for suicide even after adjusting for physical and mental health variables (Beautrais, 2002). However, case-control PA studies of late-life suicide conducted in an urban part of China showed that living alone was not an independent risk factor for completed suicide (Chiu et al., 2004; Tsoh et al., 2005). Given the inconsistent results across different sociocultural settings, the potential moderating role played by various cultural and social factors warrants further investigation.

Access to lethal means

Older adults tend to use more immediately lethal methods for suicide than do younger age groups, indicating that the former are more determined than the latter in their efforts to die. The prevalence of different means of suicide varies with the availability of means across diverse socio-cultural settings. For instance, about 70% of older adult suicides in the United States are committed with a firearm. The predominant use of firearms for suicide is unique to the United States, where civilian possession of firearms at home is lawful in most states. In a study of all medical examiner-certified suicides in New York City from 1990 to 1998, Abrams et al. (2005) compared the suicide methods used by older and younger adults, and examined associations between age and suicide method and place of occurrence. They found that individuals aged 65 and older were significantly more likely to use a fall from a height compared to those who were younger. It is debated whether access to lethal means is itself a risk factor for suicide or simply influences the prevalence of the preferred means of suicide. In contrast to findings about adolescent suicide (Brent et al., 1993), an earlier case-control PA study of late-life suicide found no difference between male suicides and controls in the proportion that owned a firearm (Miller, 1978). However, Conwell, Duberstein, Conner, Eberly, and colleagues (2002) found that the odds for suicide increased twofold with the presence of a gun in the home of older adults. Although method substitution might arguably obscure a change in overall suicide rates when access to lethal means changes in a community, means restriction has the potential to lower overall suicide rates where the method in question is common, with examples of success reported following firearm restriction in Canada and Washington, DC, in the United States, and domestic gas detoxification in Switzerland and England (Mann et al., 2005).

Other putative factors

Neurobiological theories

The body of literature on the neurobiological basis of suicidal behavior indicates the possible role of the serotonergic, noradrenergic, and neuroendocrine systems (Mann, 1998). Some studies find that age-related effects on serotonergic and other monoamine systems are more pronounced in men, while the findings of lower cerebrospinal fluid (CSF) levels of 5-hydroxyindoleacetic acid (5-HIAA) in older depressed patients who attempted suicide compared with older depressed controls suggest that the model may apply in later life as well (Mann & Stoff, 1997; Jones et al., 1990). A review of twin studies of death by suicide revealed that among 129 identical twin pairs, when one twin died by suicide, it was 17 times more likely that the other twin would die by suicide, whereas the risk was only two times higher among 270 non-identical twins (Roy, Rylander, & Sarchiapone, 1997). The genetic basis of suicide is also supported by adoption studies, which show that the rate of suicide among the biological relatives of adoptees is higher than that among the adoptive families (Shulsinger, Kety, Rosenthal, & Wender, 1979). Mann, Waternaux, Hass, and Malone (1999) found that individuals with impulsive/aggressive behavior and a tendency to experience suicidal ideation under stress were more likely to act on their suicidal feelings than persons without such behavior, and proposed that genetic predisposition is a biological vulnerability factor in a stress-diathesis model.

Neuropsychological studies show impaired executive function in non-demented late-life suicide attempters (King et al., 2000; Keilp et al., 2001). Ahearn et al. (2001) examined the MRI (magnetic resonance imaging) images of older depressives and found that those with a lifetime history of suicide attempts had significantly more subcortical gray matter hyperintensities and a trend toward more periventricular white matter hyperintensities compared to carefully matched depressives with no previous attempts. In a community case-control study of older adults aged 50 and over, clinical cerebrovascular risk factors were significantly higher among suicide decedents than among community-dwelling age- and gender-matched comparison subjects after adjusting for age, sex, depression diagnosis, and functional status (Chan, Lyness, & Conwell, 2007). Taken together, these findings suggest that late-life suicide is associated with disrupted neural pathways that play essential roles in impulse control, mood regulation, and cognition. We do not know enough of the direct neurochemical correlates of these clinical, functional, and neuroanatomical findings or whether they represent early subsyndromal presentations of vascular or other degenerative pathology. Despite the rapidly developing body of scientific literature in this area, the neurobiology of suicide in later life remains at the theoretical level without direct application to prevention strategies.

Psychological theories

Although the association between mental illness and suicide is clear, the majority of those with mental illness do not die by suicide. Various psychological theories have been proposed to bridge the gap between mental illness and suicide to better our understanding of suicidal people in clinical encounters. Schneidman (2004) posited that suicides have a common purpose, that is, to try to escape from unendurable psychological pain ("psychache"). The common emotion in suicide is hopelessness-helplessness, while the perceptual state is usually constricted ("tunnel vision"). Schneidman stated that suicidal individuals are typically ambivalent about dying and that this ambivalence can continue right up until the moment of death. For instance, it is not uncommon that an individual will call a hotline or ambulance after self-harming, and this scenario is often misinterpreted to indicate that the suicide attempt is "not so serious," which can induce negative feelings, disregard, and distrust among aftercare helping professionals attending to these situations.

Cognitive behavioral theories have made major contributions to the understanding of suicide. Based on empirical evidence, Beck, Steer, Kavocs, and Garrison (1985) argued that hopelessness is a risk factor for suicide. In a study of 207 patients hospitalized for suicidal ideation, only hopelessness predicted suicide deaths in the decade following a suicide attempt. Researchers have sought to uncover cognitive variables that may constitute the core components of suicidality or explain the compulsion to commit suicide. One line of research has focused on "over-general memory," in which suicidal persons tend to remember events in their personal history not in specific detail but rather in general terms, colored by their affect and cognitive appraisal of life (hopelessness). Cognitive behavioral theories of suicide have translated into psychological intervention approaches to chronic suicidality in younger age groups. For example, randomized controlled trials show that Linehan's dialectical behavioral therapy is effective in reducing suicidality in people suffering from borderline personality disorder (Linehan, 1993). A variety of psychotherapies, including interpersonal therapy (IPT), cognitive behavioral therapy (CBT), problem-solving therapy, and psychodynamic psychotherapies, have also been found to be effective in the acute treatment of older depressed outpatients (Niederehe, 1994). However, there is no direct evidence of the efficacy of IPT (either on its own or in combination with other treatment modalities for late-life depression) in reducing completed suicide in later life.

Prevention and postvention

Suicide prevention strategies usually adopt a multifaceted or multilayered approach with particular attention to mental health, but a systematic review of these strategies fails to find consistent evidence of their efficacy because of heterogeneity in study methodology and populations (Mann et al., 2005). Often the programs evaluated are not specifically targeted to older adults. Public health approaches such as gatekeeper programs focus on community or organizational gatekeepers, whose contact with potentially vulnerable populations enables referral for at-risk individuals to appropriate assessment and treatment facilities. The beneficial effect of such programs in lowering suicide rates has been demonstrated in well-defined high-risk communities such as the U.S. Air Force (Knox, Litts, Talcott, Feig, & Caine, 2003). However, the use of the same approach among less well-defined target populations in communities with lower base rates of suicide does not yield clear-cut benefits (Isaac et al., 2009). A number of ecological studies have found an association between increased antidepressant use and fewer completed suicides based on national registry and population statistics, which indicates that antidepressant prescription (used as a proxy of depression) reduces risk for completed suicide at a population level (Henriksson & Isacsson, 2006; Bramness, Walby, & Tverdal, 2007). Such an association was also observed among older adults in an Australian study, in which the association was found to be in the opposite direction among adolescents (Hall et al., 2003).

Aftercare for late-life suicide attempters may be a potentially useful means of suicide prevention (or postvention) as there is a significant overlap between the risk factor profile of suicide attempters and that of suicides in late life; however, there is not yet sufficient evidence of its efficacy. Aftercare programs for suicide attempters, including telecare, issuance of an emergency contact card, intensive psychosocial follow-up, and video education plus family therapy, show mixed results, and often no difference is found between standard aftercare and intervention groups in the rate of re-attempt and re-emerging suicidal ideation (Cedereke, Monti, & Ojehagen, 2002; Allard, Marshall, & Plante, 1992; Motto & Bostrom, 2001; Morgan, Jones, & Owen, 1993; Carter, Clover, Whyte, Dawson, & D'Este, 2005). Alexopoulos et al. (2009) found that up to three-quarters of older adults who died by suicide were seen by their primary care provider in their last month of life, and up to one-third in their last week. Primary care thus represents an important platform for launching prevention interventions for older adults. Among the different intervention strategies employed, physician education in depression recognition and treatment and collaborative care at the primary care level have been found to be effective in lowering suicide rates across diverse sociocultural settings and different age groups (Mann et al., 2005).

The National Institute of Mental Health (NIMH)-sponsored multisite PROSPECT (Prevention of Suicide in Primary Care Elderly Collaborative Trial) study in the United States specifically targeted the geriatric population (Alexopoulos et al., 2009). The goal of this study was to determine whether, as hypothesized, the placement of non-physician depression health specialists in primary care practices would have a favorable impact on rates of depression, hopelessness, and suicidal ideation in primary care patients with major depression, dysthymic disorder, or persistent minor depression. Practices were randomly assigned to either an intervention arm or a treatment as usual (TAU) arm. A total of 20 practices participated. Patients in the intervention practices received acute, continuation, and maintenance treatment (medication, interpersonal psychotherapy) provided by depression care managers who collaborated with primary care physicians in the detection, algorithm-based treatment, and outcome assessment of depressed patients over 24 months of care. The primary outcome measures that were assessed every 4 months for 2 years were measures of depressive symptoms, hopelessness, and suicidal ideation/intent/behavior. The results show a significantly greater decline in suicidal ideation among patients in the intervention group compared to those in the TAU group. Improved outcome was associated with a greater likelihood of receiving antidepressants and/or psychotherapy (IPT) in patients with major depression. Despite the promising results, it is difficult to anticipate what impact PROSPECT intervention would have on late-life suicidal behavior (attempted suicide and completed suicide) at a population level because suicide attempts and completed suicide are rare events. Also, the study lacks statistical power to demonstrate the magnitude of change in occurrence (if any) in the study sample. Studies conducted in Gotland, Sweden and Padua, Italy show that the effectiveness of community-based suicide prevention for older people is specific to women (Rutz, von Knorring, Pihlgren, Rihmer, & Wálinder, 1995; De Leo, Dello Buono, & Dwyer, 2002; Rutz, von Knorring, & Wálinder, 1989). Recent studies of community-based interventions in rural Japan also find that older women are more receptive to suicide prevention programs (Oyama, Fujita, Goto, Shibuya, & Sakashita, 2006; Oyama et al., 2005).

Barriers to suicide prevention

Psychological autopsy in older adults shows that the deceased are more determined in their suicidal acts, which are well planned, and issue fewer explicit warnings of suicidal intent compared to other age groups (Conwell et al., 1998). Intervention in the crisis or perisuicidal state might be less effective among older adults than among younger people, making it all the more important to implement early detection strategies to identify at-risk individuals and primary prevention programs. Uncapher and Arean (2000) reported that despite the established association between suicide and late-life depression in older adults, California physicians expressed reluctance to treat older adults with suicidal ideation. Duberstein et al. (1999) found that depression in older adults is difficult to detect because they are less likely to endorse depressed mood and suicidal ideation compared with younger people. Underreporting of depressive symptoms could lead to underdetection and low treatment rates of depression in older adults. In a PA study conducted among Hong Kong Chinese, Chiu et al. (2004) reported a low rate of psychiatric service utilization (less than 40%) among suicide victims, although 86% of them were found to have a psychiatric disorder shortly before their death.

Case studies and comments

Case study 1

Mr. A is a 60-year-old retired security guard living with his wife and children. His relatives described him as emotionally stable. Two years ago he was diagnosed with early-stage lung cancer and underwent bilateral upper lobectomy. Although there was no sign of tumor relapse, the patient became increasingly depressed because of the marked decrease in his tolerance of physical exertion, which forced him to retire from his job. More recently, he could not handle even basic house tasks, and developed a sense of uselessness. He also worried that he would soon exhaust his savings and become a burden to the family. He became increasingly anxious and inattentive, and experienced difficulty concentrating on simple daily tasks. He had difficulty maintaining sleep at night and was incapable of experiencing pleasure. He had on one occasion gone on a ferry alone and planned to throw himself into the sea, but lacked the courage to do so. He kept his suicidal thoughts to himself. His wife thought he was worrying too much, and brought him to a doctor. He was given mianserin as treatment but experienced limited improvement in his mood and sleep symptoms. He began to secretly stockpile the prescribed antidepressant pills. On the morning of the day of admission, he went to a forest and overdosed with 80 tablets of the medication, with a strong intent to die. However, he experienced intense nausea after taking the drug, and vomited a few times. Eventually he returned home, told his wife what had happened, and was brought to hospital for further treatment. He was diagnosed with a severe form of major depression by the attending consultation-liaison psychiatrist.

Case study 2

Ms. B is a 78-year-old widowed housewife. She had been living alone since her husband died from a heart attack 5 years ago, but showed no clear signs of pathological grief after her husband's death.

She was capable of performing household chores and self-care, and was visited weekly by her daughters. A year ago, she started to complain of intense, dull, and deep-seated toothache around the left molar area. Tooth extraction was performed; however, Ms. B complained that the pain persisted. Repeated examination by a dentist did not reveal specific local pathologies. The pain occurred almost daily. Ms. B experienced downswings in mood, weeping spells, insomnia at night, loss of appetite, and a drop in weight. More recently, she occasionally heard voices telling her that she had an incurable disease. Feeling desperate and hopeless, she intended to jump from her flat, but was afraid to carry out the act. She spotted a bottle of insecticide in her kitchen and drank half of it, leaving no suicide note. She passed out. Her daughter could not reach her by phone that evening, so she went to her mother's home and found her mother unconscious. The patient was admitted to the intensive care unit for treatment. She was reviewed and diagnosed to have severe major depressive disorder with psychotic features by the consultation-liaison psychiatrist after she was medically stabilized.

Case study 3

Mr. C, aged 64, is a retired driving school instructor. He lives with his family and is usually a fairly optimistic person. He occasionally quarrels with his wife over his smoking habit, but otherwise has stable relationships with his family members. For 3 months, he experienced inexplicable symptoms of anergia, lack of interest, and a feeling of mental dullness and downswings in mood with no clear precipitants. He had intermittent sleep and early morning wakening despite the general tiredness. He was prescribed hypnotics by general practitioners (GPs) whom he visited, but did not experience symptom alleviation. After yet another sleepless night, he felt upset. He took 40–50 sleeping pills together with red wine and passed out. His wife found him and he was brought to hospital for treatment. He told his attending psychiatrist that he was not sure whether he wanted to kill himself or drug himself into oblivion—he was just frustrated by his inability to sleep and somatic symptoms, and did not know why he had lapsed into this state. He was depressed and agreed to stay in the psychiatric ward for treatment. It was noticed a few days after his admission that he had a cough and hemoptysis. A chest X-ray revealed a thickened bronchial tree in the right lower lobe, and bronchoscopy and biopsy eventually confirmed local squamous cell carcinoma.

Comments

These three cases concern an older patient who made a suicide attempt against a background of late-onset depression (LOD). In contrast to younger suicide attempters, the overwhelming majority of suicidal older adults suffer from major depression, and other psychiatric diagnoses are relatively uncommon (Hawton & Fagg, 1990; Pierce, 1987; Frierson, 1991; Nowers, 1993; Draper, 1994; Takahashi et al., 1995; Beautrais, 2002; Tsoh et al., 2005). Depressive symptoms often escape detection by relatives because older adults tend to underreport, minimize, or fail to endorse their affective symptoms (Lyness et al., 1995; Duberstein et al., 1999). In Chinese and other ethnic groups, there is also a tendency toward somatization of such symptoms (Kleinman, 2004).

More importantly, symptoms of depression are likely to be overlooked because of significant physical discomfort/disease, as in cases 1 and 2, where the focus of the physician/dentist and relatives was on chest discomfort/toothache, respectively. The persistent strong toothache in case 2 might not necessarily have been a somatized depressive symptom but rather the result of undiagnosed trigeminal neuralgia, which resulted in significant distress. That the patient lived alone might have added to the risk for suicide in the midst of persistent stress and undiagnosed depression (Heikkinen & Lonnqvist, 1995).

The suicide attempts in cases 1 and 2 were serious and carried out with great resolve, which is typical of suicidal behavior in late life (Conwell et al., 1998). They might be better conceptualized as failed suicides; unfortunately, the underlying depression of the patients evaded detection by their doctors and relatives.

Although major life events or other stressors often precede or perpetuate depression in older adults, in patients with LOD without a clear precipitant—as in case 3—one should bear in mind that there are several potentially lethal diseases (including neoplasms and endocrine or metabolic disorders) that have depressive or depressive-like symptomatology as their only early manifestations, in which case there is often a lack of full cognitive quality of depression. Rather, the patient may feel indifferent, apathetic, or fatigued (Fountoulakis et al., 2003). It is possible that the patient in case 3 suffered from paraneoplastic syndrome accompanying lung cancer, which presented as depression. Other organic causes for the clinician to work up for LOD with no clear psychosocial causes would include silent cerebrovascular lesions (vascular depression) (Alexopoulos et al., 1997) and early dementia (Brommelhoff, 2009).

Case study 4

Mr. D is a 66-year-old married man who presented with a 1-year history of depression, lack of emotional reactivity, social withdrawal, and rumination about headache and other somatic discomforts. He had retired from his lifelong job as a teacher about 2 years ago but there were no initial signs of maladjustment to his post-retirement lifestyle.

The father of two sons, Mr. D was described as a mild-mannered, introverted person. A lifetime review showed that he had been mentally stable and sound until this presentation. No particular psychosocial precipitants were found on examination.

Mr. D was diagnosed with major depression but showed a limited response to two first-line antidepressants, each of which was tried over a few weeks. He became more and more irritable, reclusive, and preoccupied with headache. His wife was stressed by caregiving, as her suggestions that he go outdoors for a walk or do other activities were often met with vehement rejections and arguments. Her relatives also misinterpreted the patient's behavioral changes as symptomatic of marital strife, which resulted in much self-blame by Mr. D's wife. A brain computed tomography (CT) was arranged because of the persistent complaint of headache and relative treatment refractoriness, but there was no abnormal finding. The attending psychiatrist planned to prescribe another antidepressant, but on the evening before his scheduled follow-up, the patient impulsively attempted to jump from his balcony after another heated quarrel with his wife, claiming that the latter was not being "understanding" about his difficulties. He was prevented from jumping by his son, brought to hospital, and stayed for a fortnight's treatment. He responded favorably to venlafaxine but a few months later was hospitalized again for features of hypomania. His diagnosis was revised to bipolar affective disorder, and he was put on a mood stabilizer and discharged to a psychogeriatric day unit after initial stabilization for further monitoring of his condition.

Although Mr. D appeared more stable in mood, his wife found him emotionally indifferent and uncaring. On multidisciplinary assessment of his case, his wife was found to have adjustment disorder and given supportive counseling. On the other hand, signs of frontal dysfunction, namely, difficulty handling abstract concepts and verbal fluency (which were not on par with his general cognitive performance) were noted in the patient on routine cognitive profiling. Mr. D was referred to have a SPECT (single photon emission computed tomography) brain scan, which revealed bilateral moderate frontal hypoperfusion, which is characteristic of the frontal variant of frontotemporal dementia (FTD). The wife's counselor noted that there was less self-blame and some signs of relief on the wife's part with the discovery that her husband's condition, although not reversible, was primarily "organic" in nature and not the result of a lack of understanding or concern on her part.

Comments

The relationship between dementia and suicidal behavior is unclear. It was stated in the introduction of this chapter that a number of PA studies have found that dementia is not commonly associated with suicide, while early studies of mental disorders and suicide mortality suggest that dementia is among the few categories of mental illnesses associated with a lesser risk of suicide (Harris & Barraclough, 1997).

Although most PA studies do not show that dementia is a risk factor for late-life suicide, because of the proxy nature of PA interviews, they might be unable to identify early cognitive impairment. At the neuropathological level, Rubio et al. (2001) found that older suicide completers more frequently had severe Alzheimer's disease pathology than had age-matched controls in a post-mortem study. The relationship between dementia and affective disorders is strong and multifaceted (Lichtenberg, Ross, Millis, & Manning, 1995; Cummings, 1989). Suicidal ideations in demented persons have been attributed to co-morbid depression (Draper, MacCuspie-Moore, & Brodaty, 1998). Recent case-control studies of older suicide attempters find that dementia is an independent predictor of self-harming acts, controlling for depression and other mental disorders (Tsoh et al., 2005). Depressed older adults who attempt suicide can be distinguished from their non-depressed counterparts by their poorer executive functioning on neuropsychological profiling (Dombrovski et al., 2008; King et al., 2000), which indicates that they might be less capable of problem solving in times of stress. A recent nationwide longitudinal study in Denmark of persons aged 50 and over found that in both men and women, the diagnosis of dementia upon hospitalization was associated with a significantly elevated risk of completed suicide (especially in the first few years after the diagnosis was made) in the 10-year study period. The relative risk reached 8–10 times greater among those aged 50–69 years compared with those without the diagnosis, and the effect on suicide risk remained robust after controlling for depression (Erlangsen, Zarit, & Conwell, 2008).

The abovementioned study findings underscore the importance of identifying depressive features and suicidal tendency in older adults with cognitive impairment (and vice versa), and the need for careful monitoring during their respective courses of illness.

Similar to Mr. C in case 3, the patient in case 4 presented with LOD coupled with suicidal features, but without clear psychosocial precipitants. Careful examination of the patient's cognitive profile revealed executive dysfunction, which prompted a SPECT brain scan that confirmed features compatible with FTD. The findings in this case echo those of a study investigating the relationship between frontal dysfunction and elevated risk for suicidal behavior (King et al., 2000; Keilp et al., 2001). The formal diagnosis of FTD is often delayed among its many sufferers because in the early phase, its symptoms often mimic the features of affective or other mental disorders, and CT brain scans are often normal until a fairly late stage of the disease.

One of the debates in geriatric medicine in the past decade is whether LOD might be a prodrome in addition to being a risk factor for dementia. This notion is supported by the evidence from two earlier population studies (Berger, Fratiglioni, Forsell, Winblad, & Backman, 1999; Chen, Ganguli, Mulsant, & DeKosky, 1999) and a recent population-based twin study in Sweden (Brommelhoff, 2009). Interested readers may refer to a systematic review of the related literature by Schweitzer, Tuckwell, O'Brien, and Ames (2002). Again, mental health professionals should be aware of this link when they encounter patients with LOD who lacks clear psychosocial etiological factors.

Case study 5

Mr. E was a 72-year-old widower who had had chronic obstructive pulmonary disease (COPD) for more than two decades. He was described as being a strong and stubborn person by his children, who visited him infrequently. In the past year, his physical condition had appeared to decline, and he had been in and out of hospital a few times for COPD exacerbation. In between episodes, he experienced shortness of breath on walking and handling household chores. He started worrying about self-care. On a visit to his respiratory specialist clinic, the physician discussed long-term oxygen therapy and home care options with him. An appointment was booked for him to be seen again in 2 weeks' time for follow-up. Mr. E perceived that he had finally come to the stage where he would need to bring an oxygen cylinder with him wherever he went, and felt dejected about this. Two days later, he was found to have died from jumping from a height.

Case study 6

Ms. F was a 71-year-old widow who lived with her son's family. She had a history of osteoporosis, chronic back pain, hypertension, ischemic heart disease, and anxiety neurosis, and was receiving treatment from a GP. She had also been under chronic stress because of family conflict but had been ambivalent about moving out and living alone because of her health problems. Her son usually tried to intervene after she had arguments with her daughter-in-law.

Nine months ago, Ms. F was admitted to hospital after suddenly collapsing in the street. A brain MRI revealed stroke in the cerebellar and brainstem regions. She showed mild dysarthria after regaining consciousness, but made a gradual recovery and was discharged from hospital afterward. She was still ambulatory, but after discharge, she experienced intense episodes of dizziness throughout the day, which rendered her home-bound. She felt quite dispirited by her perceived functional loss and bothersome somatic symptoms. One night, after a dizzy spell, she became very upset and took about 40 tablets from a stock of medications for her cardiovascular condition. She was taken to hospital after her son noted that she had lost consciousness. She was resuscitated and medically stabilized. Ms. F was seen by a psychiatrist on a consultation-liaison basis and diagnosed to have depression. She was started on an antidepressant, which she tolerated well. Her somatic symptoms also appeared to improve on treatment by her physician. She was later sent to a convalescent hospital for 3 months' rehabilitative care. Her attending physician there was not aware that she had attempted suicide and did not refer her for further psychiatric care during her stay or upon her discharge, despite the recommendation by the psychiatrist at the acute hospital. A few months after her discharge, Ms. F was re-admitted to the acute hospital after another drug overdose, but this time she could not be revived. She left a suicide note stating that she wanted to escape from her "painful world."

Comments

A few case-control retrospective studies have examined the relationship between common physical illnesses (and their symptoms) and suicide in older age groups. A case-control PA study conducted in Sweden by Waern et al. (2002) revealed that visual impairment, neurological disorders, and malignant disease were associated with elevated risk for suicide. A Canadian study reported that COPD, congestive heart failure, and seizure disorder were the main correlates, and that their effect was cumulative (Juurlink, Herrmann, Szalai, Kopp, & Redelmeier, 2004). Studies conducted in Hong Kong by Chiu et al. (2004) and Tsoh et al. (2005) demonstrated that among older adults, COPD, arthritis, bone fracture, and malignancy were independently associated with completed suicide, and that stroke, bone fracture, arthritis, and malignancy were independently related to attempted suicide. A 10-year prospective multisite study conducted in the United States found that musculoskeletal disorders, in the form of bone fractures, were associated with suicide in those of advanced age (Turvey et al., 2002).

The patient in case 5 suffered from moderate to severe COPD. Because of his personality and interpersonal problems, he had difficulty in recruiting help when he experienced functional decline and the worsening of distressful physical symptoms, which affected his activities of daily living. It has been reported that loner status is among the strongest predictors for depression in COPD, in addition to disease severity (van Manen et al., 2002). In addition, patients with chronic COPD often have hypoxic brain damage, generally in the frontal lobe and hippocampus (Borson et al., 2008; Hynninen, Breitve, Wiborg, Pallesen, & Nordhus, 2005). Persons with frontal lobe damage are often impulsive and have diminished ability to resolve problems related to life change or crisis. All of these factors might have increased Mr. E's risk for suicide. Although he had attended the COPD clinic just prior to his suicide, the focus of his consultation was likely to have been on his physical condition. Routine screening for depression, anxiety, and suicidal symptoms in patients with moderate to severe COPD is indicated to reduce suicide risk in this group of patients that have a greater risk for self-harm.

The person in case 6 also had an array of risk factors for suicide, including several incapacitating physical disorders, chronic family discord, and history of a suicide attempt. Chronic family discord has been demonstrated to be a key life event that predicts suicide in later life (Rubenowitz, Waern, Wilhelmson, & Allebeck, 2001; Duberstein, Conwell, Conner, Eberly, & Caine, 2004; Tsoh et al., 2005). Attempted suicide, however, is probably the most important predictor of completed suicide (Beautrais, 2002; Conwell et al., 2000; Chiu et al., 2004). In case 6, the aforementioned service gap (which has since been closed with a specialized team on suicide prevention) might have contributed to Ms. F's completed suicide. The foregoing cases highlight the importance of structured and seamless postvention service whereby patients at high risk for suicide receive regular and intensive follow-up.

Case study 7

Ms. G was a 69-year-old Chinese woman who lived with her husband and her son's family. She portrayed herself as extroverted but anxiety prone and a perfectionist. She was financially well-off and looked younger than her age, but described herself as having been despondent for decades because of the repeated extramarital affairs of her husband, an allegation that was confirmed by her children. She occasionally had insomnia, and obtained hypnotics from GPs. She often had rows with her husband and had a history of repeated drug overdose after fighting with him. She had been diagnosed with idiopathic Parkinson's disease (PD) 5 years ago, and the symptoms had progressed more quickly in the past 2 years. She suffered from bradykinesia, tremor, dyskinesia, and postural instability. These symptoms did not improve much with drug management, even after an expensive operation to place an implant for deep brain stimulation (DBS) a year prior to her suicide. She overdosed on about 20 hypnotic tablets shortly after being discharged from hospital, after learning about another alleged affair of her husband while she was hospitalized. She was admitted to hospital and attended by a psychiatrist. She claimed that she was feeling unhappy because of the recent act of infidelity of her husband, and said that she had come to terms with it and felt well again. She played down her distress due to her neurological illness, and even apologized about her tremors during the interview, saying that they were "unsightly." Despite her attempt to minimize her mental distress, Ms. G was diagnosed with recurrent depressive disorder. In-patient psychiatric treatment was recommended but she discharged herself from hospital against medical advice. She also did not attend follow-up regularly as recommended. She was re-admitted to hospital after ingesting half a bottle of Dettol (a disinfectant) in front of her husband following a heated argument about another affair. Her daughter said that prior to this incident Ms. G had been quite depressed after receiving a phone call from her gynecologist 2 days previously, notifying her of an abnormal pap smear. Despite resuscitation efforts, Ms. G eventually died of acute pancreatitis (a complication of disinfectant ingestion).

Comments

We have discussed the effects of untreated depression, chronic familial discord, specific chronic physical illnesses, functional impairment, and repeated suicide attempts as factors that increase suicide risk in late age. All of these factors were present in case 7. However, unlike the former cases, the depressive illness and history of suicide attempts of the patient had started well before she entered old age. In addition, she had not chosen particularly violent methods in her past suicide attempts; however, we are not sure whether this can be translated into decreased suicide intent. Among Chinese people, suicidal acts are often seen as a socially sanctioned means of protest and escape from interpersonal conflict or other situations that may involve loss of face, with or without serious depressive disorder (Ji, Kleinman, & Becker, 2001; Phillips et al., 2002). We are also uncertain whether the woman's choice to ingest disinfectant instead of sleeping pills in front of her husband, who was alleged to be having an affair, carried symbolic meaning, as the incident took place shortly after she discovered that she might have cervical cancer, a kind of malignancy that can be sexually transmitted, or reflected greater intent and determination.

It is also worthwhile to consider Ms. G's treatment-resistant PD. Depression is estimated to occur in up to 40% of PD patients. Female gender and early age at onset of PD are risk factors, and depressed patients with PD also have greater frontal lobe dysfunction (Cummings, 1992), which might negatively impinge on their problem-solving ability.

The past decade has seen the more widespread use of DBS for the treatment of refractory cases of PD, a technique that has met with generally encouraging results. However, recently there have been numerous reports of patients killing themselves after DBS was performed, even when the operation was successful (Burkhard et al., 2004; Soulas et al., 2008; Voon et al., 2008). Although the causes of suicide are multifactorial, a specific effect of DBS on cognitive processes is suspected to be related to elevated risk for postoperative suicide (Voon et al., 2008).

A past history of depression, highly impulsive behavior, and past suicide attempt(s) in a candidate for DBS are now contraindications for the operation. Unfortunately, these side effects of DBS were not well known at the time Ms. G received the operation (in 2001).

Case study 8

Mr. H was a 62-year-old mechanical engineer newly presented to a psychogeriatric day unit. He had mild hypertension and diabetes mellitus (DM) but was otherwise healthy. He described his relationship with his wife as close but that with his only daughter as emotionally distant. He was a conscientious person. He had been emotionally stable until his wife suffered from a traumatic fracture dislocation of the thoracic spine in a serious road traffic accident 6 years ago. As a result of this accident, his wife suffered from paraplegia, sphincter dysfunction, and neuralgia in the lower limbs, which greatly upset her. She was diagnosed with depression. Disheartened by the lack of physical improvement after the first 6 months of rehabilitation, she refused further treatment and stayed at home. Mr. H felt torn by the conflict between his caregiving responsibility for his wife (despite the presence of a home helper), which was driven by his conscientious nature, and the bitter remarks of his wife when he was not at home, and his working life (he had financial fears as the cost of his wife's care was high). He became easily worried and anxious and had difficulty initiating and maintaining sleep at night, although he was not overtly depressed. He was attended by a psychiatrist who diagnosed adjustment disorder, and experienced sustained symptomatic relief after a short course of low-dose antidepressants and hypnotics.

Two year later, Mr. H developed mild but worsening weakness in his right foot. Initially thought to be a manifestation of DM neuropathy by his internist, weakness emerged in his other limbs months later, coupled with mild muscular fasciculation and spasticity, and he fell easily when walking. A comprehensive neurological evaluation was performed and he was eventually diagnosed with amyotrophic lateral sclerosis (ALS). The patient did not appear to be very shocked upon hearing of the negative outcome of the disease from his neurologist. He was apparently more bothered by his worsening gait, which eventually forced him into an early, unplanned retirement. He refused treatment with riluzole, which is costly (around USD 100 per month) and non-curative. He spent more hours caring for his wife and encouraging her with positive remarks. His physical condition continued to decline, but he coped with symptoms with assistance from the home helper. He and his wife continued to receive support and monitoring by their psychiatrists and community nurses.

A year after his original diagnosis, Mr. H experienced a major emotional episode when he found that he could not hold his wife in his arms to comfort her as usual, as his upper limbs had become too weak. He explained to his attending psychiatrist that he felt that his life had been deprived of meaning. He perceived that his role as a caring husband had been eroded, and that his further decline in health due to ALS would only add to the emotional burden of his wife. He admitted to having fairly strong suicidal wishes after the episode, saying, "The time has come to close the chapter, before it is overdue." He asked whether euthanasia was possible under certain circumstances. However, although Mr. H had suicide ideation and a sense of futility, careful examination revealed that there were insufficient features to substantiate a diagnosis of major depression. He and his relatives refused his hospitalization for psychiatric treatment. After a lengthy discussion, he agreed to be admitted to a psychogeriatric day unit; however, his wife was adamant in her refusal to join him.

Mr. H agreed to pass on some of the caring work for his wife to another home helper. Additional community nursing support was provided and his daughter and home helpers were trained to monitor the emotional condition and suicidal tendency of both the patient and his wife. He also received care from a physician on a consultation-liaison basis for his physical condition.

Mr. H experienced some improvement upon receiving multidisciplinary rehabilitation at the day unit. He became less anxious as he no longer needed to tend to every request made by his wife, felt that his daily routines were more structured with the mental and physical rehabilitative training, and spent less time ruminating on his situation. He was also able to sleep after an adjustment was made in the dosage of his antidepressant.

Mr. H never displayed overt depressive symptoms or emotional reactivity. Efforts to improve relations between the daughter and the couple met with some success. Mr. H felt that his daughter (who viewed Mr. H to be a "stubborn father") had become more empathetic and mature, and was glad to hear her promise that his wife would not be sent to a residential home after he died.

With guidance from his neurologist, Mr. H made an advance directive concerning the refusal of intubation for artificial ventilation, percutaneous endoscopic gastrostomy (PEG) nutritional support, and resuscitation. The patient respectfully declined resources for spiritual support. He was also unwilling to consider joining an ALS support group or to receive community palliative care.

Psychotherapy addressed Mr. H's existential despair, and attempted to reframe his views on his physical and interpersonal situation and new psychological bonding. Repeated assessments at the ambulatory unit revealed that he had a less absolutist stance on suicide. He was ambivalent about living an increasingly dependent life and admitted he would still opt for an early exit "in a controlled and graceful fashion should such be available"; however, when the focus was placed on the present situation, he was content with the continual support for his changing physical and psychological and interpersonal needs as his bodily functioning deteriorated. Mr. H received day rehabilitation services for 9 more months until he was admitted to the Department of Internal Medicine for repeated bouts of sepsis, to which he eventually succumbed peacefully.

Comments

Engaging and caring for persons with terminal medical conditions who display suicidal tendencies or make requests for hastened deaths are among the most onerous yet important tasks for mental health professionals. Issues arising in the psychological, medical, and legal domains and consideration for the patient's own values and belief system converge in the clinical management of individual cases. Macroscopically, powerful debates on the bioethical dilemma involved (autonomy, medical beneficence, non-abandonment, and non-malevolence) are ongoing, and might challenge and reshape societal attitudes toward suicide at large, especially for patients with incurable conditions like terminal cancer, ALS/motor neurone disease (MND), or Huntington's chorea.

Central to the arguments to relax prohibitions against measures to usher in hastened deaths for these cases are the principles of respect for autonomy and the importance of rationality (Clarke, 1999). Most people would agree that in the presence of a psychiatric disorder, the person's capacity to make a rational choice about his/her life might be eroded. Indeed, according to a systematic review, major depression is diagnosed in up to 58% of terminally ill cancer patients who have a significant desire for death (Chochinov & Wilson, 1995). It also occurs in about 25% patients with ALS (Ganzini, Goy, & Dobscha, 2008). Screening for mental disorders and apposite treatment of such should be important elements of palliative care. However, it is a legal right in most developed nations for persons of sound mind to refuse unwanted life-sustaining medical treatments. In the United States, the Supreme Court has consistently distinguished such arrangements from controversial measures to actively hasten death, including physician-assisted suicide (PAS; in which case, medical help is provided to enable a patient to end his or her life) and euthanasia (an act in which the physician takes measures specifically intended to end the patient's life) (Snyder & Sulmasy, 2001). At the time of writing (2009), assisted suicide for terminal patients is conditionally approved in the American states of Oregon and Washington, and in certain European nations including the Netherlands, Switzerland, Belgium, and Luxembourg. A 7-year study conducted in the Netherlands revealed that one in five patients with ALS died as a result of euthanasia or PAS (Veldink, Wokke, van der Wal, Vianney de Jong, & van den Berg, 2002). In Sweden, where euthanasia or assisted suicide are outlawed, a population study over a 40-year period revealed that ALS patients had a sixfold increased risk for suicide, and that the risk was particularly high after the patient's first period of hospitalization (Fang et al., 2008). A debate on the legitimacy of the notion and practice of "rational" suicide (Werth, 1996) is beyond the scope of this chapter; however, interested readers might examine the arguments of its proponents (e.g. Leeman, 2009) and opponents, including the American College of Physicians and American Society of Internal Medicine (Snyder & Sulmasy, 2001).

Amidst this controversy about whether rationality and autonomy are sufficient to justify rational suicide, it is a regrettable fact that there is only limited scientific understanding of the prevalence of depression and other major mental illnesses and their respective treatment responsiveness among persons who opt for physician-assisted deaths in places where this is legally permitted (Groenewoud et al., 2004; van der Lee et al., 2005; Hicks, 2009; Steinberg, 2009), in part because referral to a psychiatrist for an independent assessment of capacity is not mandatory. Furthermore, various PA studies on older people who have died from completed suicide consistently demonstrate that a segment of the subjects (which ranges from 5% to 30%) have no clear evidence of psychiatric disorders before their death (Harwood, Hawton, Hope, & Jacoby, 2006). There is a deficit in the understanding of the characteristics of this group of people and the circumstances that have led to their self-destructive acts. Harwood et al. found that among 23 older suicide decedents, about half had significantly abnormal personality traits (most notably the anakastic or obsessive-compulsive subtype), which might have influenced their perception and decision making at a stressful time.

One quarter died within a month of a distressful life event such as major bereavement. Another quarter died within the context of a severe, disabling physical illness.

We have looked at management issues concerning older patients with depression and suicidal behavior who are suffering from major medical disorders with acute symptoms. However, a major difference in this case is that although the patient was suicidal, his wish to kill himself did not appear to be driven by overt depressive illness but rather by existential despair about the destruction of his self-hood by an incurable and crippling disease.

It is often difficult to engage these patients (and their caregivers), who usually consider themselves to be rational. We see that a key role of mental health professionals in palliative care is to help clients to mentally adapt to their physical predicament. The management of suicidal patients with terminal illness but no clear-cut mental disorder is often fraught with anxiety and counter-transference issues on the side of the therapist (Bascom & Tolle, 2002; Boston & Mount, 2006). Psychiatrists ought not to reduce the evaluation and assessment of patients who wish to die to a screening for the presence of an active axis I disorder (Brendel, 2009). We recommend that the patient be evaluated as a whole person: personality type and psychosocial factors that contribute to the wish to die early should be evaluated. The therapist should also gain an understanding of the patient's fears, concerns, life goals and values, coping style, interpersonal issues, and how these and other factors may collectively influence the patient's wish to die (Hicks, 2009; Brendel, 2009). We can then seek to help the patient to find alternative solutions to a hastened death, a process which requires the involvement of family members and other close associates, and transdisciplinary efforts.

In the case of Mr. H, engagement in structured day activities in a rehabilitative unit resulted in behavioral activation, a reduction in the amount of time spent ruminating on the physical disability together with his wife, and the establishment of new roles and networks. The building of rapport allows further professional intervention, which includes psychotherapy augmented with elements of existential therapy (Imes, Clance, Gailis, & Atkeson, 2002), to address empathetically a person's subjective mind/body experience, the impact of the illness on his or her life, the person's existential distress, pain, bodily experiences, thoughts and feelings, as well as his or her efforts to cope or find meaning in the illness. Moreover, in this case, therapy with the patient and his daughter might have helped to build an additional source of emotional support and address his concern about role erosion. His drawing up an advance directive concerning his medical care in the latter stage of his illness and the care plans for his wife might have added to his sense of control, especially given his high degree of conscientiousness. Finally, timely amelioration of the patient's physical discomfort was also possible in the rehabilitation unit.

A review conducted by Bascom and Tolle (2002) provides an excellent framework to systematically explore the areas relevant to suicidal patients with terminal illnesses, which include the patient's own expectation and fears, options for end-of-life care, identification of value systems and sources of meaning for the patient, family/caregiver attitudes toward the hastened death of the patient, adequacy of relief of physical symptoms, the patient's perspective on the experience of suffering, perceived quality of life, and evidence of depression or other mental disorders. The suicidal patient might not be aware of the breadth of alternative options and responses available in modern palliative care.

The rapid growth in the aging population worldwide together with the rising incidence of aging-related medical diseases and medical advances to prolong life might render such clinical scenarios less uncommon. Therapeutic interventions for psychiatric conditions have primarily been studied in the medical domain; however, palliative psychiatry is limited by a paucity of solid evidence derived from patients and families who are living with advanced illnesses, going through the dying process and coping with bereavement (Irwin & Ferris, 2008). Characteristics in the psychiatric, interpersonal, and existential domains among suicidal older adults with terminal illnesses and the degree to which these characteristics are amenable to intervention are also poorly understood (Groenewoud et al., 2004; van der Lee et al., 2005; Hicks, 2009; Steinberg, 2009). The expansion of psychiatric research efforts into these areas has the potential to generate evidence-based initiatives to reduce suicide rates through better recognition and management of psychiatric issues in this patient population. In addition, research evidence would inform the intense and growing ethical debate on the principles of benevolence, non-abandonment, non-malevolence, autonomy, and societal interests that underlie the decision of how society should respond to requests from terminal patients to hasten their deaths.

Conclusions and points for reflection

Suicide in later life is a multidetermined end-point of numerous intermingling age-related physical, psychological, and social problems that additively increase suicide risk in older persons. Very often the presence of other triggering physical problems and stressful social situations mask the core prevailing risk factors such as depression. The at-risk situations and mental states might be elusive even to the experienced practitioners who care for at-risk older adults at different time-points. This is especially the case when many treatment settings for older people overemphasize physical illness. Despite the barriers to risk detection and accurate assessment of multifaceted needs, practitioners are informed by the latest research findings that most risk factors are treatable or largely modifiable.

Let us reflect on the challenges set out below:

♦ How to enhance suicide risk detections by practitioners in different service sectors?

♦ How to integrate care for the multiple needs of at-risk adults in a timely way?

♦ How to meet the specific psychological needs of older adults faced with common late-life challenges such as common physical problems, age-associated degenerative changes including cognitive impairment, terminal illness, as well as changes in life circumstances (e.g. interpersonal losses or change of daily care arrangement)?

Perhaps these three questions should be analyzed together as they represent different facets of a core problem—how should a health care system respond sensibly to the challenges of an individual's body, mind, and social network in the course of aging. These challenges range from normal psychological, social, or physiological changes to pathological processes or social crisis. The thresholds of detecting the various kinds of warning signs are different. As we have seen in the case studies, a failed single step along the pathway to care may result in tragic suicide deaths. Specific training in mental health and suicide risk assessment seems to be the key to enhance risk detection and management by frontline practitioners in different service sectors. In the absence of coordinated care at multilevels, it is unclear whether enhanced professional capacity at the individual practitioner's level will effectively reduce suicidal behaviors. Service delivery should be accessible and assertive enough (e.g. outreaching/community-based services) to reach at-risk elders who might otherwise be poorly engaged with generic services. The NIMH-sponsored multisite PROSPECT study in the United States highlights the importance of early intervention of late-life psychological problems, enhanced access to indicated clinical care predominantly at primary care level, integrated service coordinated by case managers as well as psychotherapeutic interventions tailor-made for the specific challenges in later life (Alexopoulos et al., 2009). Any service model, however, needs adaptations to meet the specific needs of different communities and cultures. Rigorous service evaluation should accompany any program implementation. A well-informed mental health and social welfare policy or strategic planning at a governmental level may be essential for sustaining an effective service model.

References

Abrams, R.C., Marzuk, P.M., Tardiff, K., & Leon, A.C. (2005). Preference for fall from height as a method of suicide by elderly residents of New York City. *American Journal of Public Health, 95,* 1000–1002.

Ahearn, E.P., Jamison, K.R., Steffans, D.C., Cassidy, F., Provenzale, J.M., Lehman, A., et al. (2001). MRI correlates of suicide attempt history in unipolar depression. *Biological Psychiatry, 50,* 266–270.

Alexopoulos, G.S., Meyers, B.S., Young, R.C., Campbell, S., Silbersweig, D., & Charlson, M. (1997). Vascular depression hypothesis. *Archives of General Psychiatry, 54,* 915–922.

Alexopoulos, G.S., Reynolds, C.F., III, Bruce, M.L., Katz, I.R., Raue, P.J., Mulsant, B.H., et al. (2009). Reducing suicidal ideation and depression in older primary care patients: 24-month outcomes of the PROSPECT study. *American Journal of Psychiatry, 166,* 882–890.

Allard, R., Marshall, M., & Plante, M.C. (1992). Intensive follow-up does not decrease the risk of repeat suicide attempts. *Suicide and Life Threatening Behavior, 22,* 303–314.

Barraclough, B.M. (1971). Suicide in the elderly: Recent developments in psychogeriatrics. *British Journal of Psychiatry,* (Suppl 6), 87–97.

Bascom, P.B., & Tolle, S.W. (2002). Responding to requests for physician-assisted suicide: These are uncharted waters for both of us. . . . *JAMA, 288,* 91–98.

Beautrais, A.L. (2002). A case control study of suicide and attempted suicide in older adults. *Suicide and Life Threatening Behavior, 32,* 1–9.

Beck, A.T., Steer, R.A., Kavocs, M., & Garrison, B. (1985). Hopelessness and eventual suicide: A 10-year prospective study of patients hospitalized with suicidal ideation. *American Journal of Psychiatry, 142,* 559–563.

Berger, A.K., Fratiglioni, L., Forsell, Y., Winblad, B., & Backman, L. (1999). The occurrence of depressive symptoms in the preclinical phase of AD: A population-based study. *Neurology, 53,* 1998–2002.

Borson, S., Scanlan, J., Friedman, S., Zuhr, E., Fields, J., Aylward, E., et al. (2008). Modeling the impact of COPD on the brain. *International Journal of COPD, 3,* 429–434.

Boston, P.H., & Mount, B.M. (2006). The caregiver's perspective on existential and spiritual distress in palliative care. *Journal of Pain and Symptom Management, 32,* 13–26.

Bramness, J.G., Walby, F.A., & Tverdal, A. (2007). The sales of antidepressants and suicide rates in Norway and its counties 1980-2004. *Journal of Affective Disorders, 102,* 1–9.

Brendel, R. (2009). On 'Distinguishing among irrational suicide, rational suicide, and other forms of hastened death: Implications for clinical practice' by Calvin P. Leeman, M.D. *Psychosomatics, 50,* 193–194.

Brent, D.A., Perper, J.A., Moritz, G., Baugher, M., Schweers, J., & Roth, C. (1993). Firearms and adolescent suicide: A community case-control study. *American Journal of Diseases of Children, 147,* 1066–1071.

Brommelhoff, J.A. (2009). Depression as a risk factor or prodomal feature for dementia? Findings in a population-based sample of Swedish twins. *Psychology and Aging, 24,* 373–384.

Burkhard, P.R., Vingerhoets, F.J.G., Berney, A., Bogousslavsky, J., Villemure, J.G., & Ghika, J. (2004). Suicide after successful deep brain stimulation for movement disorders. *Neurology, 63,* 2170–2172.

Carney, S.S., Rich, C.L., Burke, B.A., & Fowler, R.C. (1994). Suicide over 60: The San Diego study. *Journal of American Geriatrics Society, 42,* 174–180.

Carter, G.L., Clover, K., Whyte, I.M., Dawson, A.H., & D'Este, C. (2005). Postcards from the EDGE project: Randomised controlled trial of an intervention using postcards to reduce repetition of hospital treated deliberate self poisoning. *British Medical Journal, 331,* 966.

Cedereke, M., Monti, K., & Ojehagen, A. (2002). Telephone contact with patients in the year after a suicide attempt: Does it affect treatment attendance and outcome? A randomized controlled study. *European Psychiatry, 17,* 82–91.

Chan, S.S., Lyness, J.M., & Conwell, Y. (2007). Do cerebrovascular risk factors confer risk for suicide in later life? A case-control study. *American Journal of Geriatric Psychiatry, 15,* 541–544.

Chen, P., Ganguli, M., Mulsant, B.H., & DeKosky, S.T. (1999). The temporal relationship between depressive symptoms and dementia: A community-based prospective study. *Archives of General Psychiatry, 56,* 261–266.

Chiu, H.F., Chan, S., & Lam, L.C. (2001). Suicide in the elderly. *Current Opinion in Psychiatry, 14*, 395–399.

Chiu, H.F., Yip, P.S., Chi, I., Chan, S., Tsoh, J., Kwan, C.W., et al. (2004). Elderly suicide in Hong Kong—a case-controlled psychological autopsy study. *Acta Psychiatrica Scandinavica, 109*, 299–305.

Chochinov, H.M., & Wilson, K.G. (1995). The euthanasia debate: Attitudes, practices and psychiatric considerations. *Canadian Journal of Psychiatry. Revue Canadienne de Psychiatrie, 40*, 593–602.

Clarke, D.M. (1999). Autonomy, rationality and the wish to die. *Journal of Medical Ethics, 25*, 457–462.

Conwell, Y. (2001). Suicide in later life: A review and recommendations for prevention. *Suicide and Life Threatening Behavior, 31*(Suppl), 32–47.

Conwell, Y., Duberstein, P.R., Cox, C., Herrmann, J.H., Forbes, N.T., & Caine, E.D. (1996). Relationships of age and axis I diagnoses in victims of completed suicide: A psychological autopsy study. *American Journal of Psychiatry, 153*, 1001–1008.

Conwell, Y., Duberstein, P.R., Cox, C., Herrmann, J., Forbes, N., & Caine, E.D. (1998). Age differences in behaviors leading to completed suicide. *American Journal of Geriatric Psychiatry, 6*, 122–126.

Conwell, Y., Lyness, J.M., Duberstein, P., Cox, C., Seidlitz, L., DiGiorgio, A., et al. (2000). Completed suicide among older patients in primary care practices: A controlled study. *Journal of the American Geriatrics Society, 48*, 23–29.

Conwell, Y., Duberstein, P.R., & Caine, E.D. (2002). Risk factors for suicide in later life. *Biological Psychiatry, 52*, 193–204.

Conwell, Y., Duberstein, P.R., Conner, K., Eberly, S., Cox, C., & Caine, E.D. (2002). Access to firearms and risk for suicide in middle-aged and older adults. *American Journal of Geriatric Psychiatry, 10*, 407–416.

Cummings, J.L. (1989). Dementia and depression: An evolving enigma. *Journal of Neuropsychiatry and Clinical Neurosciences, 1*, 236–242.

Cummings, J.L. (1992). Depression and Parkinson's disease: A review. *American Journal of Psychiatry, 149*, 443–454.

De Leo, D., & Scocco, P. (2000). Treatment and prevention of suicidal behaviour in the elderly. In K. Hawton & C. van Heeringen (Eds.), *The international handbook of suicide and attempted suicide* (pp. 556–570). New York, NY: John Wiley & Sons.

De Leo, D., Dello Buono, M., & Dwyer, J. (2002). Suicide among the elderly: The long-term impact of a telephone support and assessment intervention in northern Italy. *British Journal of Psychiatry, 181*, 226–229.

Dombrovski, A.Y., Butters, M.A., Reynolds, C.F., III, Houck, P.R., Clark, L., Mazumdar, S., et al. (2008). Cognitive performance in suicidal depressed elderly: Preliminary report. *American Journal of Geriatric Psychiatry, 16*, 109–115.

Draper, B. (1994). Suicidal behaviour in the elderly. *International Journal of Geriatric Psychiatry, 9*, 655–661.

Draper, B., MacCuspie-Moore, C., & Brodaty, H. (1998). Suicidal ideation and the 'wish to die' in dementia patients: The role of depression. *Age and Ageing, 27*, 503–507.

Duberstein, P.R., Conwell, Y., & Caine, E.D. (1994). Age differences in the personality characteristics of suicide completers: Preliminary findings from a psychological autopsy study. *Psychiatry, 57*, 213–224.

Duberstein, P.R., Conwell, Y., Seidlitz, L., Lyness, J.M., Cox, C., & Caine, E.D. (1999). Age and suicidal ideation in older depressed inpatients. *American Journal of Geriatric Psychiatry, 7*, 289–296.

Duberstein, P.R., Conwell, Y., Conner, K.R., Eberly, S., & Caine, E.D. (2004). Suicide at 50 years of age and older: Perceived physical illness, family discord, and financial strain. *Psychological Medicine, 34*, 137–146.

Erlangsen, A., Zarit, S.H., & Conwell, Y. (2008). Hospital-diagnosed dementia and suicide: A longitudinal study using prospective, nationwide register data. *American Journal of Geriatric Psychiatry, 16*, 220–228.

Fang, F., Valdimarsdottir, U., Furst, C.J., Hultman, C., Fall, K., Sparen, P., et al. (2008). Suicide among patients with amyotrophic lateral sclerosis. *Brain, 131*, 2729–2733.

Fountoulakis, K., O'Hara, R., Iacovides, A., Camilleri, C., Kaprinis, S., Kaprinis, G., et al. (2003). Unipolar late-onset depression: A comprehensive review. *Annals of General Hospital Psychiatry, 2*, 11.

Frierson, R.L. (1991). Suicide attempts by the old and the very old. *Archives of Internal Medicine, 151*, 141–144.

Gallo, J.J., Anthony, J.C., & Muthen, B.O. (1994). Age differences in the symptoms of depression: A latent trait analysis. *Journal of Gerontology, 49*, 251–264.

Ganzini, L., Goy, E.R., & Dobscha, S.K. (2008). Prevalence of depression and anxiety in patients requesting physicians' aid in dying: Cross sectional survey. *British Medical Journal, 337*, a1682.

Groenewoud, J.H., van der Heide, A., Tholen, A.J., Schudel, W.J., Hengeveld, M.W., Onwuteaka-Philipsen, B.D., et al. (2004). Psychiatric consultation with regard to requests for euthanasia or physician-assisted suicide. *General Hospital Psychiatry, 26*, 323–330.

Hall, W.D., Mant, A., Mitchell, P.B., Rendle, V.A., Hickie, I.B., & McManus, P. (2003). Association between antidepressant prescribing and suicide in Australia, 1991-2000: Trend analysis. *British Medical Journal, 26*, 323–330.

Harris, E.C., & Barraclough, B.M. (1994). Suicide as an outcome for medical disorders. *Medicine, 73*, 281–296.

Harris, E.C., & Barraclough, B. (1997). Suicide as an outcome for mental disorders. A meta-analysis. *British Journal of Psychiatry, 170*, 205–228.

Harwood, D., Hawton, K., Hope, T., & Jacoby, R. (2001). Psychiatric disorder and personality factors associated with suicide in older people: A descriptive and case-control study. *International Journal of Geriatric Psychiatry, 16*, 155–165.

Harwood, D., Hawton, K., Hope, T., & Jacoby, R. (2006). Suicide in older people without psychiatric disorder. *International Journal of Geriatric Psychiatry, 21*, 363–367.

Hawton, K., & Fagg, J. (1990). Deliberate self-poisoning and self-injury in older people. *International Journal of Geriatric Psychiatry, 5*, 367–373.

Hawton, K., Appleby, L., Platt, S., Foster, T., Cooper, J., Mamberg, A., et al. (1998). The psychological autopsy approach to studying suicide: A review of methodological issues. *Journal of Affective Disorders, 50*, 269–276.

Heikkinen, M.E., & Lonnqvist, J.K. (1995). Recent life events in elderly suicide: A nationwide study in Finland. *International Psychogeriatrics, 7*, 287–300.

Henriksson, S., & Isacsson, G. (2006). Increased antidepressant use and fewer suicides in Jämtland county, Sweden, after a primary care educational programme on the treatment of depression. *Acta Psychiatrica Scandinavica, 114*, 159–167.

Hicks, D.W. (2009). On 'Distinguishing among irrational suicide, rational suicide, and other forms of hastened death: Implications for clinical practice' by Calvin P. Leeman, M.D. *Psychosomatics, 50*, 194–195.

Hynninen, K.M., Breitve, M.H., Wiborg, A.B., Pallesen, S., & Nordhus, I.H. (2005). Psychological characteristics of patients with chronic obstructive pulmonary disease: A review. *Journal of Psychosomatic Research, 59*, 429–443.

Imes, S.A., Clance, P.R., Gailis, A.T., & Atkeson, E. (2002). Mind's response to the body's betrayal: Gestalt/existential therapy for clients with chronic or life-threatening illnesses. *Journal of Clinical Psychology, 58*, 1361–1373.

Irwin, S.A., & Ferris, F.D. (2008). The opportunity for psychiatry in palliative care. *Canadian Journal of Psychiatry, 53*, 713–724.

Isaac, M., Elias, B., Katz, L.Y., Belik, S.L., Deane, F.P., Enns, M.W., et al. (2009). Gatekeeper training as a preventative intervention for suicide: A systematic review. *Canadian Journal of Psychiatry, 54*, 260–268.

Ji, J., Kleinman, A., & Becker, A.E. (2001). Suicide in contemporary China: A review of China's distinctive suicide demographics in their sociocultural context. *Harvard Review of Psychiatry, 9*, 1–12.

Jones, J.S., Stanley, B., Mann, J.J., Frances, A.J., Guido, J.R., Traskman-Bendz, L., et al. (1990). CSF 5-HIAA and HVA concentrations in elderly depressed patients who attempted suicide. *American Journal of Psychiatry, 147*, 1225–1227.

Juurlink, D.N., Herrmann, N., Szalai, J.P., Kopp, A., & Redelmeier, D.A. (2004). Medical illness and the risk of suicide in the elderly. *Archives of Internal Medicine, 164*, 1179–1184.

Keilp, J.G., Sackeim, H.A., Brodsky, B.S., Oquendo, M.A., Malone, K.M., & Mann, J.J. (2001). Neuropsychological dysfunction in depressed suicide attempters. *American Journal of Psychiatry*, *158*, 735–741.

King, D.A., Conwell, Y., Cox, C., Henderson, R.E., Denning, D.G., & Caine, E.D. (2000). A neuropsychological comparison of depressed suicide attempters and nonattempters. *Journal of Neuropsychiatry and Clinical Neurosciences*, *12*, 64–70.

Kleinman, A. (2004). Culture and depression. *New England Journal of Medicine*, *351*, 951–953.

Knox, K.L., Litts, D.A., Talcott, G.W., Feig, J.C., & Caine, E.D. (2003). Risk of suicide and related adverse outcomes after exposure to a suicide prevention programme in the US Air Force: Cohort study. *British Medical Journal*, *327*, 1376–1378.

Langley, G.E., & Bayatti, N.N. (1984). Suicides in Exe Vale Hospital 1972-1981. *British Journal of Psychiatry*, *145*, 463–467.

Lawrence, D., Almeida, O.P., Hulse, G.K., Jablensky, A.V., & Holman, C.D. (2000). Suicide and attempted suicide among older adults in Western Australia. *Psychological Medicine*, *30*, 813–821.

Leeman, C.P. (2009). Distinguishing among irrational suicide, rational suicide, and other forms of hastened death: Implications for clinical practice. *Psychosomatics*, *50*, 185–191.

Lichtenberg, P.A., Ross, T., Millis, S.R., & Manning, C.A. (1995). The relationship between depression and cognition in older adults: A cross-validation study. *Journals of Gerontology Series B: Psychological Sciences and Social Sciences*, *50*, 25–32.

Linehan, M.M. (1993). *Skills training manual for treating borderline personality disorder*. New York, NY: Guilford Press.

Lyness, J.M., Cox, C., Curry, J., Conwell, Y., King, D.A., & Caine, E.D. (1995). Older age and the underreporting of depressive symptoms. *Journal of the American Geriatrics Society*, *43*, 216–221.

Mann, J.J. (1998). The neurobiology of suicide. *Nature Medicine*, *4*, 25–30.

Mann, J.J., & Stoff, D.M. (1997). A synthesis of current findings regarding neurobiological correlates and treatment of suicidal behavior. *Annals of the New York Academy of Sciences*, *836*, 352–363.

Mann, J.J., Waternaux, C., Hass, G.L., & Malone, K.M. (1999). Toward a clinical model of suicidal behavior in psychiatric patients. *American Journal of Psychiatry*, *156*, 181–189.

Mann, J.J., Apter, A., Bertolote, J., Beautrais, A., Currier, D., Haas, A., et al. (2005). Suicide prevention strategies: A systematic review. *JAMA*, *294*, 2064–2074.

Miller, M. (1978). Geriatric suicide: The Arizona study. *Gerontologist*, *18*, 488–495.

Moscicki, E.K. (1997). Identification of suicide risk factors using epidemiologic studies. *Psychiatric Clinics of North America*, *3*, 499–517.

Morgan, H.G., Jones, E.M., & Owen, J.H. (1993). Secondary prevention of non-fatal deliberate self-harm. *The green card study. British Journal of Psychiatry*, *163*, 111–112.

Motto, J.A., & Bostrom, A.G. (2001). A randomized controlled trial of postcrisis suicide prevention. *Psychiatric Services*, *5*, 828–833.

Niederehe, G.T. (1994). Psychosocial therapies with depressed older adults. In L.S. Schneider, C.F. Reynolds, B.D. Lebowitz, & A.J. Friedhoff (Eds.), *Diagnosis and treatment of depression in late life* (pp. 293–315). Washington, DC: American Psychiatric Press.

Nowers, M. (1993). Deliberate self-harm in the elderly: A survey of one London borough. *International Journal of Geriatric Psychiatry*, *8*, 609–614.

Oyama, H., Watanabe, N., Ono, Y., Sakashita, T., Takenoshita, Y., Taguchi, M., et al. (2005). Community-based suicide prevention through group activity for the elderly successfully reduced the high suicide rate for females. *Psychiatry and Clinical Neurosciences*, *59*, 337–344.

Oyama, H., Fujita, M., Goto, M., Shibuya, H., & Sakashita, T. (2006). Outcomes of community-based screening for depression and suicide prevention among Japanese elders. *Gerontologist*, *246*, 821–826.

Parkin, D., & Stengel, E. (1965). Incidence of suicidal attempts in an urban community. *British Medical Journal*, *2*, 133–138.

Paykel, E.S., Myers, J.K., Lindenthal, J.J., & Tanner, J. (1974). Suicidal feelings in the general population: A prevalence study. *British Journal of Psychiatry, 124*, 460–469.

Pearson, J.L., & Conwell, Y. (1995). Suicide in later-life: Challenges and opportunities for research. *International Psychogeriatrics, 7*, 131–136.

Phillips, M.R., Yang, G., Zhang, Y., Wang, L., Ji, H., & Zhou, M. (2002). Risk factors for suicide in China: A national case-control psychological autopsy study. *Lancet, 360*, 1728–1736.

Pierce, D.W. (1987). Deliberate self-harm in the elderly. *International Journal of Geriatric Psychiatry, 2*, 105–110.

Roy, A., Rylander, G., & Sarchiapone, M. (1997). Genetics of suicide: Family studies and molecular genetics. *Annals of the New York Academy of Sciences, 836*, 135–157.

Rubenowitz, E., Waern, M., Wilhelmson, K., & Allebeck, P. (2001). Life events and psychosocial factors in elderly suicides: A case-control study. *Psychological Medicine, 31*, 1193–1202.

Rubio, A., Vestner, A.L., Stewart, J.M., Forbes, N.T., Conwell, Y., & Cox, C. (2001). Suicide and Alzheimer's pathology in the elderly: A case-control study. *Biological Psychiatry, 49*, 137–145.

Rutz, W., von Knorring, L., & Wálinder, J. (1989). Frequency of suicide on Gotland after systematic postgraduate education of general practitioners. *Acta Psychiatrica Scandinavica, 80*, 151–154.

Rutz, W., von Knorring, L., Pihlgren, H., Rihmer, Z., & Wálinder, J. (1995). Prevention of male suicides: Lessons from Gotland study. *Lancet, 345*, 524.

Schneidman, E.S. (2004). *Autopsy of a suicidal mind*. New York, NY: Oxford University Press.

Schweitzer, I., Tuckwell, V., O'Brien, J., & Ames, D. (2002). Is late onset depression a prodrome to dementia? *International Journal of Geriatric Psychiatry, 17*, 997–1005.

Shah, A., Bhat, R., McKenzie, S., & Koen, C. (2007). Elderly suicide rates: Cross-national comparisons and association with sex and elderly age-bands. *Medicine, Science and the Law, 47*, 244–252.

Shulsinger, R., Kety, S., Rosenthal, D., & Wender, P. (1979). A family study of suicide. In M. Schou & E. Stromgren (Eds.), *Origins, prevention and treatment of affective disorders* (pp. 277–287). New York, NY: Academic Press.

Snyder, L., & Sulmasy, D.P. (2001). Physician-assisted suicide. *Annals of Internal Medicine, 135*, 209–216.

Soulas, T., Gurruchaga, J.M., Palfi, S., Cesaro, P., Nguyen, J.P., & Fenelon, G. (2008). Attempted and completed suicides after subthalamic nucleus stimulation for Parkinson's disease. *Journal of Neurology, Neurosurgery & Psychiatry, 79*, 952–954.

Steinberg, M.D. (2009). On 'Distinguishing among irrational suicide, rational suicide, and other forms of hastened death: Implications for clinical practice' by Calvin P. Leeman, M.D. *Psychosomatics, 50*, 195–197.

Stevens, J.A., Hasbrouck, L.M., Durant, T.M., Dellinger, A.M., Batabyal, P.K., Crosby, A.E., et al. (1999). Surveillance for injuries and violence among older adults. *MMWR CDC Surveillance Summary, 48*, 27–50.

Takahashi, Y., Hirasawa, H., Koyama, K., Asakawa, O., Kido, M., Onose, H., et al. (1995). Suicide and aging in Japan: An examination of treated elderly suicide attempters. *International Psychogeriatics, 7*, 239–251.

Tsoh, J., Chiu, H.F., Duberstein, P.R., Chan, S.S., Chi, I., Yip, P.S., et al. (2005). Attempted suicide in elderly Chinese persons: A multi-group, controlled study. *American Journal of Geriatric Psychiatry, 13*, 562–571.

Turvey, C.L., Conwell, Y., Jones, M.P., Phillips, C., Simonsick, E., Pearson, J.L., et al. (2002). Risk factors for late-life suicide: A prospective, community-based study. *American Journal of Geriatric Psychiatry, 10*, 398–406.

United Nations Population Division/DESA (2009). World population to exceed 9 billion by 2050: Developing countries to add 2.3 billion inhabitants with 1.1 billion aged over 60 and 1.2 billion of working age. Press release March 11.

Uncapher, H., & Arean, P.A. (2000). Physicians are less wiling to treat suicidal ideation in older patients. *Journal of the American Geriatrics Society, 48*, 188–192.

van der Lee, M.L., van der Bom, J.G., Swarte, N.B., Heintz, A.P., de Graeff, A., & van den Bout, J. (2005). Euthanasia and depression: A prospective cohort study among terminally ill cancer patients. *Journal of Clinical Oncology, 23*, 6607–6612.

van Manen, J.G., Bindels, P.J., Dekker, F.W., Ijzermans, C.J., van der Zee, J.S., & Schade, E. (2002). Risk of depression in patients with chronic obstructive pulmonary disease and its determinants. *Thorax, 57*, 412–416.

Veldink, J.H., Wokke, J.H., van der Wal, G., Vianney de Jong, J.M., & van den Berg, L.H. (2002). Euthanasia and physician-assisted suicide among patients with amyotrophic lateral sclerosis in the Netherlands. *New England Journal of Medicine, 346*, 1638–1644.

Voon, V., Krack, P., Lang, A.E., Lozano, A.M., Dujardin, K., Schupbach, M., et al. (2008). A multicentre study on suicide outcomes following subthalamic stimulation for Parkinson's disease. *Brain, 131*, 2720–2728.

Waern, M., Rubenowitz, E., Runeson, B., Skoog, I., Wilhelmson, K., & Allebeck, P. (2002). Burden of illness and suicide in elderly people: Case-control study. *British Medical Journal, 324*, 1355–1357.

Werth, J.L. (1996). Criteria for rational suicide. In J.L. Werth (Ed.), *Rational suicide? Implications for mental health professionals* (pp. 55–80). Washington, DC: Taylor & Francis.

World Health Organization (2003). *World health report 2003: Shaping the future.* Geneva, Switzerland: World Health Organization.

World Health Organization (1999). *Figures and facts about suicide.* Geneva, Switzerland: Department of Mental Health, World Health Organization.

Author Index

Subject Index